HIGH PRAISE FOR
KAREN STABINER'S
TO DANCE WITH THE DEVIL

"*To Dance with the Devil* will inevitably be compared to *And the Band Played On*, Randy Shilts's best-selling book on AIDS . . . there is the structure, the interweaving of policy and biography, of cold science and heartbreaking reality. . . . Ms. Stabiner has taken full advantage of a situation that might have intimidated a lesser journalist. *To Dance with the Devil* is compelling, moving and very, very scary, a contrapuntal examination of the disease and of the women whose lives—whose identities—have been forever altered by it." —*The New York Times Book Review*

"BEAUTIFULLY RESEARCHED AND WRITTEN . . . EVERY WOMAN SHOULD READ IT . . . [Stabiner's] contribution to the understanding of breast cancer, of women's health care in general, is invaluable."
—Delia Ephron

"[AN] EXHAUSTIVELY RESEARCHED, DOGGED EPIC OF A WAR ZONE—THE UCLA BREAST CENTER."
—*Los Angeles Times*

"GRIPPING . . . thrusts the reader into a remarkably intimate behind-the-scenes exploration of breast cancer—and the people suffering from it. Stabiner presents a memorable cast of characters in a book that, in many ways, reads like a novel—but whose compelling subject material is all too real."
—*Town & Country*

"Stabiner weaves the stories of doctors, patients, researchers, advocates and lobbyists into a novel-like structure that puts a human face on breast cancer and the war being waged against it." —*The Philadelphia Inquirer*

"COMPELLING AND INFORMATIVE . . . This book is for everyone who wants to make sense of the mystery, learn from what is being done, find out how to get involved or see that she is not alone." —*New York Newsday*

Please turn the page for more extraordinary acclaim. . . .

TO DANCE WITH THE DEVIL

THE NEW WAR ON BREAST CANCER

KAREN STABINER

Delta
Trade Paperbacks

This book contains discussions of cancer treatments and other medical matters. It is not intended as a substitute for the medical advice of physicians.

Manufactured in the United States of America
Published simultaneously in Canada

April 1998

10 9 8 7 6 5 4 3 2 1

BVG

To my teachers,
Barbara Pannwitt
and
John Reque

CONTENTS

HOPE

TO DANCE WITH THE DEVIL

AUTHOR'S NOTE

THERE IS NO SURE WAY TO DODGE BREAST CANCER—NO PROVEN PRE-
ventive, no dependable treatment, no cure. The only certainty is that over 183,000 women will get breast cancer
this year, and about 44,000 will die of it. The mortality rate has
dipped, slightly, since 1989, but that fact is offset by the guarantee
of higher numbers of patients in the years to come, as the baby
boomers age.

It is an unrelenting threat, and a crafty foe. The breast cancer
patients whose stories are part of this book were probably starting
to get sick eight to ten years before I met them. They did not know
it—could not, since neither a mammogram nor a physical examination can detect breast cancer when the first malignant cell divides. It
takes an average of one hundred days for that cell to turn into two,
another hundred for those two to turn into four, and on and on,
until one billion cancer cells reside in a woman's body. Only then
does the cancer elicit a response: the lump or mass that shows up as
a shadow on a mammogram, or under probing fingers, is in fact not
the cancer itself, but a reaction to it, an irritation.

That is what usually happens. But breast cancer is not a predictable disease, and there are always exceptions. It can come roaring
up like a train without brakes and kill a woman almost before she
can grasp what has happened to her. It can loll around in the breast

and never pose a threat to her life. Breast cancer takes a particular delight in fooling people—and if it spreads from the breast to distant organs, there is no way to keep it from killing.

Until 1990, there had been no concerted effort to stop it. Now there is. In that year, geneticist Mary-Claire King narrowed the search for a gene for heritable breast cancer to a stretch of a single chromosome, fairly guaranteeing that someone would locate it in the next few years. In 1991 Dr. Susan Love, a frustrated surgeon; Susan Hester, whose companion had died of the disease; and Amy Langer, Executive Director of the National Alliance of Breast Cancer Organizations, cofounded the National Breast Cancer Coalition, a lobbying group bent on getting increased funds for breast cancer research. Fran Visco, an angry lawyer and a breast cancer survivor, was its first president. In 1992 Congress appropriated an unprecedented $210 million for a new research program, to be administered by the army. And in 1993 the Clinton Administration embarked on a National Action Plan on Breast Cancer, to define for the first time a national strategy for research and health care. In 1994, BRCA-1, the gene for heritable breast cancer that King had spent her life looking for, was found.

New science, a new advocacy movement, a new political commitment, and new money—great promise, just as the advent of managed care and the government's budget crisis demanded greater restraint.

At the same time, the baby boomers inched toward fifty—and a generation spoiled by easy medical answers came face-to-face with a foe that had so far defied the doctors. In a culture obsessed with a woman's beauty and youthfulness, they faced the specter of treatments that would dismantle their physical and sexual identity, bit by bit: the removal of a breast; the possibility of premature menopause from chemotherapeutic drugs. The media told us we could be vibrant well into middle age, even beyond, while breast cancer snickered and plucked women off that path at random.

Most of the women I knew were frightened all out of proportion to statistical reality. Although heart disease was far likelier to kill them, they worried more about breast cancer.

They were more diligent about having mammograms than

about getting their teeth cleaned; they superstitiously made lunch dates after that mammogram to make sure there was no time in the day to entertain bad news. Whenever a headline announced a new risk factor, they tallied their chances again. And because there were so many of them, because this outsize generation defines what is news, there were ever more headlines.

Older women may have escaped the media frenzy, but each birthday put them in more danger. The primary risk factors for breast cancer are being female and growing old.

When Susan Love arrived at UCLA to run its breast program, I approached her about writing a book about that program and the larger effort against breast cancer. The only way to make sense of what was going on was to immerse myself in the subject—to live in that community of doctors, patients, researchers, advocates, and politicians. Love granted me complete access, as did a number of her patients, and in January 1994 I began my research.

The women whose stories I decided to include here represent a range of experience in terms of their age, the severity of their disease, their family background and home life, and the treatment regimen they endured. The one thing they have in common stands in ironic testimony to our lack of understanding: five originally were misdiagnosed, and the other two had more widespread disease than initial tests had shown.

Any university medical center tends to attract patients who are more aggressive about their health than most people—they ask more questions, they demand the best and have the insurance to pay for it. The women in this book belong to a fortunate subgroup—they are not poor women struggling for access to basic care, but lucky, middle- and upper-class women who are receiving some of the best care this country has to offer. And yet no one can promise them a cure. No one can even promise them a consensus, since treatment is an exasperatingly imprecise art. All their doctors can do is make sure they get what those doctors define as comprehensive treatment. This is how bad it is: Every breast cancer patient, even women who could buy a solution if there was one, faces a lifetime of apprehension.

* * *

I was at UCLA on a daily basis between January and September 1994—watching as Dr. Love saw patients, ran clinical programs, attended administrative meetings, and performed surgeries. I regularly met with the patients I was writing about and accompanied them to various medical appointments.

In addition to following the patients, I conducted numerous taped interviews with them, their doctors, and members of their families. Given the nature of the disease, we spent a great deal of time talking about the emotional toll it takes—both on the patients and on the professionals who treat them. When I attribute a private thought or feeling to an individual, it is because that person told me what he or she was thinking or feeling at the time.

Four of the women allowed me to use their names. Three did not, and in the interest of protecting their privacy I changed their names and certain details of their physical appearance. I changed none of the details of their condition or treatment.

I did make one other change—in the journalistic tradition of using people's last names. I do so at first mention, or when someone is referred to by other participants in the story. Otherwise I tend to use first names, for doctors and researchers as well as for patients. This is an intimate community; the detachment of referring to everyone at a formal distance seemed inappropriate.

Between December 1993 and November 1996, I interviewed government health officials at the National Institutes of Health, the National Cancer Institute, and the Department of Health and Human Services; I also interviewed political figures and lobbyists, the army officers who administer the new Defense Department program, the advocates who fought for increased funding and better health care services, other doctors and medical staff around the country, and the hospital personnel who must make sense of managed care.

I interviewed medical researchers around the country who are involved in breast cancer research, and attended regional oncology conferences where new breast cancer studies were presented.

I am not a medical writer by specialty—but women who worry about breast cancer are not specialists either, and it was my job, writing from a reporter's perspective, to translate confusing information into a form they could comprehend.

I am not a breast cancer survivor, either, but I learned in the course of researching and writing this book that that is a fragile distinction. Those of us outside this world tend to divide the population into us, the healthy ones, and them, the breast cancer patients. There is no such line. Yesterday they were on our side; tomorrow any one of us could cross over.

In 1993 the National Breast Cancer Coalition presented President Clinton with petitions containing 2.6 million signatures, representing the 1.6 million women who knew they had breast cancer at the time, and the 1 million who had it but had not yet been diagnosed. One of those women—or her mother or father, sister or brother, husband, child, or best friend—has just finished reading this sentence. This is not the story of other people's problems.

CAST OF CHARACTERS

The Patients

Shirley Barber, a forty-three-year-old career flight attendant whose precancerous condition was diagnosed because of improved mammography technology.

Ann Donaldson,* a forty-six-year-old businesswoman who was diagnosed when she was twenty-seven weeks pregnant with her first child.

Jerilyn Goodman, a forty-three-year-old freelance television producer whose breast cancer was diagnosed five years after the first of several doctors told her that she had nothing to worry about.

Dottie Mosk,* a sixty-four-year-old wife, mother, and grandmother whose breast cancer showed up in a swollen lymph node despite the fact that her doctors could not feel a breast lump or find evidence of it on a mammogram.

Barbara Rubin, a fifty-three-year-old psychologist who rejected her doctor's treatment suggestions and embarked on a self-prescribed regimen of alternative therapies.

Dee Wieman, a forty-five-year-old housewife whose virulent

* Names marked with an asterisk are pseudonyms.

cancer required her to have an experimental bone marrow transplant.

Laura Wilcox,* a thirty-eight-year-old film development executive who had a mastectomy with simultaneous reconstruction, using her own tissue.

The Clinicians

At UCLA:

Dr. Susan Love, Director, UCLA Breast Center

Dr. Larry Bassett, Iris Cantor Professor of Breast Imaging, Department of Radiological Sciences

Dr. Linnea Chap, medical oncologist; Director, UCLA, Research Program

Dr. Ann Coscarelli, Director, Rhonda Fleming Mann Resource Center for Women with Cancer

Dr. John Glaspy, Medical Director, UCLA Joint Medical-Surgical Oncology Center

Dr. David Heber, Chief, Division of Clinical Nutrition; Director, UCLA Clinical Nutrition Research Unit

Dr. David McFadden, Chief of General Surgery, Veterans' Administration Hospital

Dr. Michael Racenstein, Fellow, Department of Radiological Sciences

Dr. William Shaw, Chief, UCLA Division of Plastic Surgery

Dr. Dennis Slamon, Vice-chair, Research, UCLA Department of Medicine; Chief, UCLA Division of Hematology-Oncology; Director of Clinical Research, Jonsson Comprehensive Cancer Center

Dr. David Wellisch, Professor of Medical Psychology; Chief Psychologist, Adult Division

Dr. Michael Zinner, Executive Chairman, UCLA Department of Surgery; Chief, Division of General Surgery

Linda Norton and Stephanie Chang, Clinical Research Unit, UCLA Joint Medical-Surgical Oncology Center

Staff of The UCLA Breast Center: Nurse-practitioner Sherry

* Names marked with an asterisk are pseudonyms.

Goldman, administrator Leslie Laudeman, assistant Connie Long, facilitators Shannon Tucker, Christi Dearborn, Lisa Gotori

At Memorial Sloan-Kettering, New York City
Dr. Larry Norton, Chief, Breast and Gynecological Cancer Medicine Service
Dr. Jeanne Petrek, breast surgeon

At Columbia-Presbyterian, New York City
Dr. Alison Estabrook, breast surgeon

At Stanford University, Palo Alto, California
Dr. David Spiegel, Department of Psychiatry

At the University of California, San Francisco
Dr. I. Craig Henderson, Chief, Medical Oncology, and Director, Clinical Oncology Program

At the Joint Center for Radiation Therapy, Boston
Dr. Jay Harris, Clinical and Education Director

At Massachusetts General Hospital, Boston
Dr. Daniel Kopans, Director, Breast Imaging

The Researchers

Dr. Samuel Broder, Director, National Cancer Institute (1988—April 1995)
Dr. Francis Collins, geneticist, Director, National Center for Human Genome Research
Dr. Bernard Fisher, Director, National Surgical Adjuvant Breast and Bowel Project, University of Pittsburgh; Distinguished Service Professor of Surgery, University of Pittsburgh
Dr. Ronald Herberman, Interim Director, NSABP
Dr. Mary-Claire King, geneticist, University of California, Berkeley
Dr. Malcolm Pike, epidemiologist, University of Southern California

Dr. Mark Skolnick, geneticist and co-founder, Myriad Genetics, Inc., Salt Lake City, Utah

Dr. Harold Varmus, Director, National Institutes of Health

Government Officials

Dr. Susan Blumenthal, Co-chair, National Action Plan on Breast Cancer

Senator Tom Harkin (D-Iowa)

Ed Long, legislative aide to Senator Harkin

Colonel Irene Rich, Director, Research Area Directorate VI U.S. Army Medical Research and Materiel Command

Donna Shalala, Secretary, Department of Health and Human Services

Advocates and Lobbyists

Joanne Bass, partner, Bass and Howes, Inc.

Amy Langer, Executive Director, National Alliance of Breast Cancer Organizations

Fran Visco, President, the National Breast Cancer Coalition; Co-chair, National Action Plan on Breast Cancer

The Private Sector

Giorgio Armani, fashion designer and honorary chair, 1994 Revlon Fire & Ice Ball

Evelyn Lauder, cosmetics executive and benefactor, the Evelyn H. Lauder Breast Center at Memorial Sloan-Kettering

Harmon Eyre, Deputy Executive Vice President for Medical Affairs and Research, American Cancer Society

Ralph Lauren, fashion designer and fund-raiser for the Nina Hyde Breast Center at Georgetown University, Washington, D.C.

Ronald Perelman, Chairman, The Revlon Group, contributor to UCLA breast cancer research and treatment programs

Lilly Tartikoff, fund-raiser for UCLA breast cancer research since 1989

"There are two kinds of people in this country—those who know someone with breast cancer, and those who will."

—Dr. John Glaspy, Medical Director,
UCLA Joint Medical-Surgical Oncology Center

PROLOGUE

ONE IN EIGHT

S LEEP HAD NEVER BEEN A PROBLEM BEFORE.
Shirley Barber was a veteran flight attendant for United
Airlines, and she was proud of her ability to master time.
When she was home, she could go to bed at two and be up making
coffee at seven. When she was flying, all she needed was a four-
hour nap at what passed for night in the time zone she was headed
for.

If she could not sleep—and periodically Shirley caved in after a
late-night flight and lost her rhythm—she could still get by for five
or six days. Then she collapsed, slept for ten hours straight, and
started over again.

No longer. Three months earlier Shirley Barber had been diagnosed with breast cancer, and every night since she had awakened
in the middle of the night and been unable to go back to sleep. Her
professional discipline deserted her. Once awake she tossed and
turned for two hours, maybe three.

She would not dignify the insomnia by turning on a light to
read, and she refused to follow the standard advice about getting
out of bed until she felt sleepy. It made no sense. When sleep was
finally ready to reclaim her she did not want to waste precious time
getting back to bed.

So she lay there and waited to see if the widow down the hill was going to watch television. The woman usually turned it on at about three in the morning—not to watch anything in particular, it seemed, but to fill the empty space where another person so recently had been.

The widow channel-surfed. She rolled around the dial with her remote control, and if she did not find anything she liked she started over. The staccato images bounced out of her bedroom and onto the window next to Shirley's side of the bed, just bright enough for Shirley to watch too. Infomercials, old movies, newscasters reporting from parts of the world where people were supposed to be awake—fuzzy, mute images set to the beat of a stranger's lonesome sorrow.

Shirley watched them mindlessly, eager for distraction. Otherwise the incomprehensible facts of the recent past nagged at her: she was forty-three years old, she had breast cancer, she was getting some of the best medical care in the country, and still no one could say anything definitive about her condition. There was an array of likelihoods and percentages, and that was all. She could live to a ripe old age or be dead before she was fifty. The more she learned, the more she realized how frightfully little anyone knew.

Her surgeon, UCLA's Dr. Susan Love, liked to reassure her patients by telling them, "When you die at ninety of a stroke, we'll know you beat breast cancer." There was a darker message lurking in that reassuring quip—a woman did not know she was cured until she succumbed to something else. So every night Shirley sat up alone, listened to her body, watched the widow's television, and wondered what was happening. She finally slipped back to sleep near dawn, just before the kids got up for school.

Her family took note of the changes from a wary distance. Shirley started going to bed at ten o'clock to compensate for the hours of sleep she expected to lose, and still she woke up groggy. Her husband, Tracy, joked nervously that he had to pour a pot of black coffee down his wife's throat to get her out of bed—and yearned for the days when she had slept like a stone sunk underwater, a sleep so deep and peaceful that he felt comforted by it.

Over the twenty-two years Shirley had been with the airline she had built up a lot of sick leave. She took it and stayed home. She was there when seventeen-year-old Mitch and thirteen-year-old Kimberly got home from school, there to sit down with her family for dinner, there to watch sitcoms after the table was cleared. Shirley was suddenly predictable and dependable, like anyone else's wife or mother.

It frightened them all. Tracy and the kids were used to not knowing if she was coming or going. For her part, Shirley wished for the slightest reprieve—just one day without anxiety, a clear twenty-four hours when she did not think about her health. She had no idea how to stop worrying about the cancer. She felt alone all the time, not just in the middle of the night. For the first time in her life, she felt vulnerable.

MOMENTUM

1

OLD ENEMIES,
NEW ALLIES

OCTOBER 1993: WASHINGTON, D.C.

I T TOOK FRAN VISCO TWO YEARS TO GET INTO THE WHITE HOUSE. THE first time she tried, in 1991, she got only as far as a guarded, locked gate where she loaded boxes containing 140,000 letters onto a conveyor belt. As the boxes were carried away she joked to her friends that they would probably ride straight through, out the back door and into an incinerator. President Bush would never see them.

In fact, no one ever acknowledged that the letters had arrived. She went home to Philadelphia to start over.

On October 18, 1993, she stood in a small room just off the East Room, talking with Health and Human Services Secretary Donna Shalala and Dr. Susan Love, director of the UCLA Breast Center and cofounder of the National Breast Cancer Coalition (NBCC), the two-and-a-half-year-old advocacy group that had twice waged a campaign for a national strategy against breast cancer. They were waiting for President Clinton and the First Lady to arrive, to accept Visco's latest offering. The boxes were piled in a lopsided pyramid at the back of a small stage in the East Room: Petitions that contained 2.6 million signatures, representing the 1.6 million women in the United States who knew they had breast cancer, and the one million who already had the disease but had not yet been diagnosed.

Visco, a forty-five-year-old corporate lawyer, was the president of the National Breast Cancer Coalition. Since May 1991 the Coalition had been fighting for research dollars and a strategy on how best to spend them. In fifteen minutes she would be seated onstage in front of all those boxes, listening to President Clinton outline a plan that was as much Fran's as anyone's.

She and Love had set out to dismantle the civilized conspiracy that had hobbled medicine's progress against breast cancer since the mid-1800s, when American and British surgeons began to define a therapeutic approach. Before that, much of what passed for treatment was based on anecdote and superstition; afterward, on often misguided heroics, as though to compensate for the clumsiness of the past.

It was not a conscious plot; not even willful disregard. It was somehow worse: layer upon layer of silence and neglect, of therapies whose use far outlasted their efficacy, and research budgets that focused almost exclusively on men's diseases. The three most potent threats to a woman's health—heart disease, breast cancer, and osteoporosis—went virtually ignored. There was not enough money to keep women from getting sick, only a desperate scramble to save them once they did.

It did not work. One third of all women who developed breast cancer eventually died of it. That had been true for fifty years—but the Coalition was determined to buy a better future. The National Institutes of Health (NIH), which conducted most of the government's health care research, had to Visco's mind embarrassed itself with paltry breast cancer budgets—$90 million in fiscal 1990, $100 million the next year, and $155 million in fiscal 1992. The Coalition had lobbied until Congress found an additional $210 million for the fiscal 1993 budget, a windfall from the peacetime Department of Defense, which had been led into the fray, kicking and screaming, by Visco and a handful of sympathetic politicians who insisted that breast cancer was a perfectly reasonable topic for army research.

Between the army's two-year program and the NIH, which had managed an $80 million increase in its own breast cancer budget for fiscal 1993, the government had allocated over $400 million in research dollars, almost triple the 1992 budget—enough to jump-start a stalled research effort, the result of too little money and too little imagination. Better still, Visco's proprietary role in the army program had won her the chance to change the way that money was spent. The government's delicate label for patients was "consumers." Fran Visco would be the first consumer to actively participate in the grant review process, which meant that she could help to steer the money away from endless treatment regimens and into more promising work on prevention or cure. The Coalition had won not just money, but authority. Patients had their foot firmly inside a door that had always been closed to them.

The East Room reception was the crowning event of National Breast Cancer Awareness Month, and Visco had organized it down to the last detail. Ronald Perelman, the billionaire owner of the Revlon Group and one of the Coalition's financial angels, had underwritten part of the petition drive, but as usual the effort had depended on volunteer labor and donated supplies, and Visco was determined to acknowledge that contribution. She did not want celebrities like Revlon models Lauren Hutton and Veronica Webb onstage, or even in the front row of the audience, because they would distract the media. She insisted that many of the seats in the East Room be awarded to "just folks" who had collected signatures. If the Coalition was to grow and sustain its effort, she needed people, lots of them, all around the country. Rewarding the volunteers was the best way to ensure that they went home and got back to work.

She knew what she wanted President Clinton to say to them. More than anything, Visco wanted him to refer to breast cancer as an epidemic. An epidemic required a solution, however long that took. If he started using the word it would be easier to get funding next year.

She knew what the resistance was. Visco had debated the linguistic point on countless radio talk shows with scientists who preferred the formal definition of the term. Breast cancer was not a true epidemic like AIDS. It had not exploded out of nowhere, nor did it spread from one person to another, nor was there as dramatic a rise in incidence. *Epidemic* was a literal distinction, they reminded her, not an emotional state.

Visco was always quick to reply that there was a second defini-

tion of epidemic—an ongoing, inexplicable increase in incidence—
that certainly applied to breast cancer.

The more she had to explain it the angrier she got. Surely the
numbers were convincing without her help: 182,000 women got
breast cancer every year and 46,000 died. Between 1990 and 2000
nearly a half million women would die of the disease, the most
commonly diagnosed cancer in women and the second most fatal
after lung cancer. Among African-American women it was the most
lethal cancer because it often was detected at a later stage. A
woman's lifetime risk of developing breast cancer—the chance that
she would develop the disease if she lived to be eighty-five—was
one in eight, up from one in twenty when Visco was born.

Worse yet, there seemed to be nothing a woman could do to
improve her odds. Cigarettes caused lung disease, and that simple
causal link gave a woman an obvious tool: the best way to avoid
lung cancer was to stop smoking or not start. Breast cancer had so
far resisted medicine's best hunches about prevention. It claimed
vegetarians, women on low-fat diets, women who were fat, women
who were thin and fit—anyone.

Other ailments presented a greater statistical danger. A
woman's lifetime risk of developing heart disease was one in two;
adult-onset diabetes or alcoholism, one in three; a stroke, one in
five; a hip fracture, one in seven. But rational fact was no consolation. Women reported that they were more frightened of breast
cancer than of heart disease, the most serious health threat they
faced, in great part because there was nothing they could do to
protect themselves. Life was roulette when it came to breast cancer.
As far as Visco was concerned, the government had to make up for
lost time and find some answers—if not a cure, which was what she
dreamed of, then at least a prevention strategy women could depend on.

Medicine could not even fight breast cancer to a draw. If one in
eight did not qualify as an inexplicable increase, what did?

Visco tried to convince the White House speechwriters of her
position, but a few days before the reception she got an apologetic
call from one of them. Despite her arduous lobbying, the President

probably would not refer to breast cancer as an epidemic. There were, the speechwriter said, "political implications" to consider.

It was Visco's one tactical defeat, but she decided to yield rather than alienate the scientific community even further. The people at the NIH were already irritated because the Defense Department controlled $210 million in research money that they believed properly should have gone to the NIH, and cranky about the upstart lawyer who fancied herself a breast cancer expert. Researchers were not used to intruders from the outside world, whether they were army officers or advocates. The NIH had functioned since 1887 in collegial isolation, set apart both by geography—a sprawling 300-acre campus in Bethesda, Maryland—and by the impenetrable nature of its research, which attempted to understand the fundamental rules of the human body, how it stayed healthy and why it fell ill. The National Cancer Institute (NCI), created by a special act of Congress in 1937 and the largest division of the NIH, enjoyed even greater autonomy thanks to a "bypass budget" that circumvented Congress and was signed directly by the President.

These were the bastions of basic research. The native dialect was intimidating, spoken only by an elite corps who believed that answers about specific diseases came not from studying those diseases but by amassing a body of general knowledge. They considered earmarked research, in which scientists spent targeted money on a particular disease, to be a lesser challenge and a potentially dangerous distraction.

Basic researchers insisted that the key to a particular disease could come from anywhere—from the study of how yeast cells behaved, from research into a virus implicated in other ailments. Limiting the scope of a scientist's work was like putting blinders on him, and critics of the Defense Department's earmarked program worried that it might by definition exclude research that would lead to an answer.

As far as Visco was concerned, basic research was nothing more than a polite euphemism for benign neglect. The scientists feared that special interests would dismantle the nation's research effort, steal money from basic research to fund their own agenda. Visco felt the NIH was out of touch with reality, engaged in a grand intellectual exercise while people who needed practical answers suffered and died. The NIH was part of the government, supported by taxpayers' dollars. It was time for scientists to better serve the people who paid them.

She fully intended to live up to their nightmare scenario, to demand even more money and insist on a voice on how it was spent. The NIH had every reason to be upset by the Defense Department program. It was Visco's pet project, a model for an eventual invasion of the inaccessible NIH. The days when researchers and politicians made decisions about women's health—or simply opted to ignore it—were over.

Money and attention. She had been after them ever since September 17, 1987, the day she dutifully went in for a baseline mammogram on her way to work at the law firm of Cohen, Shapiro, Polisher, Sheikman and Cohen in Philadelphia. She was thirty-nine, almost forty, and her doctor liked women to have their first mammogram at that age.

On her lunch hour she and one of the partners went downstairs to watch a parade celebrating the two hundredth birthday of the Constitution. When she got back to her office there was a message from her gynecologist, asking her to call him right away.

He told her that the radiologist had already phoned to say he saw something on the film.

"They're fairly certain it's malignant," the gynecologist said. He had the name of a surgeon, and he wanted Fran to schedule an appointment immediately.

Obediently she picked up the phone and called the surgeon, only to be told she would have to wait two weeks to see him, at which point they could talk about scheduling the surgery. She did not want to wait that long, so she called her husband, who knew another surgeon who agreed to see Fran right away. Within two weeks Visco had a lumpectomy and was ready to begin a regimen of radiation and chemotherapy. Still, she could not help but think: "What do women do who *don't* have connections?"

The oldest of four children in an Italian Catholic family in Philadelphia, Visco had spent her life railing at injustice, both personal and political. She had always dreamed of being a lawyer—and if her parents did not have the money to send her to law school, if most girls in the mid-sixties had more traditional goals, she refused to surrender to circumstance. She simply worked her way through. She marched against the Vietnam War, stuffed envelopes for mailings, and wrote letters to politicians—and once she became a lawyer she worked for women's rights.

She married twice before she found the right guy, and at thirty-nine had a son and embarked on a new life as a working mother. She had become someone quite different from what her family and society had expected her to be, but Fran Visco had always behaved as though the world order had a question mark at the end. Reality was there to be challenged.

Breast cancer became her new cause. As an activist, Visco had faith that change could be enforced, that the collective will could alter medicine's path. That was the point of the petition drive, the DOD program, and this presidential reception: to consolidate the effort against a foe that for too many years had had its headstrong way. She did not allow herself to contemplate the alternative—that breast cancer was devious enough to evade even the most dedicated scientific assault.

This was the day change began. Visco bought a new black suit to commemorate the day and traveled from Philadelphia with her mother, her husband, and her seven-year-old son. She wanted them all to witness the historic events of October 18.

Dr. Susan Love had not thought to buy a new suit or bring her family with her. She was in the same coral jacket and skirt that she often wore to testify before Congress or speak to women's groups. She wore flesh-toned support hose, the reflexive choice of a woman who got dressed in the predawn dark and spent long hours on her feet in the operating room, and a pair of generic low-heeled pumps.

Love was always zipping in and out of a city in a single day, one suit in a carry-on garment bag, hurried good-byes to Helen Cooksey—the surgeon who for eleven years had been Love's companion—and their five-year-old daughter, Kate, and a mad dash to Los Angeles International Airport. Helen and Kate never came with her when she was working. What fun was there in watching her departing back?

It was hardly her first public appearance, and she had met the President and Hillary Clinton several times before. When they arrived she moved to the doorway of the East Room and waited to be announced, the same as always. By dinnertime she would be on a plane back home.

She stepped over the threshhold—and in that single moment everything changed. Love suddenly had a visceral sense that this was emphatically not business as usual. She had long since learned the surgeon's disciplined detachment, which enabled her to tell the last patient on a Friday afternoon that she had breast cancer, and then go fly-fishing on Saturday without a care in the world. This was different. The air was charged with feeling.

The women and men in the room, most of them NBCC members, rose to their feet in a raucous standing ovation. The lights from the television cameras bleached the room. Love glanced over at the boxes full of petitions and thought, These are our people. We did this. She knew there was a chair on the stage behind her, and she knew she was supposed to sit down, but as she and Visco did so, Donna Shalala gestured to them to get back up and acknowledge the continued applause.

They made a funny pair: Love, a large, broad-shouldered woman prone to big gestures and explosive laughter; Visco, a short, compact woman with wistful eyes and an apple-cheeked grin. Two and a half years ago they had been strangers. Now they were a formidable partnership, a symbol of potential and hope to thousands of women across the country.

They had managed along the way to make their share of enemies, people who found Visco abrasive and Love outrageous. None of those people were in the East Room of the White House.

Neither of them seemed to know what to do in the face of all the clapping and yelling. Visco raised a clenched fist above her head and Love slung a companionable arm around her friend's shoulder. Donna Shalala embraced Visco from the other side, and just for a moment it looked as though Visco might start to cry. Her fist fell to her side and her grin began to wobble at the corners.

Love had spent her career steadying patients who stared over the edge of the abyss and started to crumble. She tightened her grasp on Visco's arm and leaned toward her. "Congratulations," she whispered fiercely. Visco took a breath, straightened her shoulders, and found her smile, just in time to shake hands with the President and Mrs. Clinton as they made their way onstage.

The applause swelled again. It was too much even for the stalwart Dr. Love. She stared out at the crowd and thought to herself, Shit. I should have brought Helen and Kate.

And perhaps bought a new suit—not because she cared about such things, but because it would help to mark this remarkable day.

It was almost too easy to draw up a roster of enemies—anyone who had voted against the $210 million Department of Defense appropriation for breast cancer research; the Pentagon officials who loudly proclaimed that they would gladly place the program up for adoption; the National Institutes of Health, with its sorry history on women's health problems; and the National Cancer Institute, which had already tried to wrest control of the money away from the army.

That was just the surface, though, the immediate squabble. The true foe was tradition. Doctors continued to depend on combinations of surgery, chemotherapy, and radiation, despite their hit-and-miss success rate, because these were the only tools they had. Medicine embraced action and discouraged inquiry. Skeptics within the medical community suggested new remedies and watched their work go ignored for years.

And in a culture that revered the female breast, patients were loath to demand attention. Breast cancer was a secret shame, to be endured without complaint. When the first few activists stepped forward in the late 1970s and early 1980s—Rose Kushner, pioneer patient advocate, and Nancy Brinker, founder of the Susan G. Komen Foundation and a survivor as well—they were after specific revisions in the status quo. Progress meant better early detection or the end of the standard one-step surgical procedure, in which a woman who was having a surgical biopsy would not know until she woke from the anesthesia whether she still had a breast. They had not yet found a voice loud enough to demand wholesale change.

With few exceptions, women accepted silent isolation as a side effect of their disease. The good doctor and the good patient were extremely well-behaved.

Then technology and the population curve collided, and a whole new generation of women faced the disease. Improved mammography equipment enabled doctors to detect more cancers, even some early forms of the disease that did not produce a palpable tumor. The baby boomers headed toward middle age, and as they did their risk of breast cancer increased. When they got sick, the media took notice. Suddenly breast cancer was a public issue.

Like Visco, many of these women were used to making noise to get results. They were not satisfied with incremental tinkering—a different chemotherapy dosage schedule, a faster-acting anesthetic. They demanded attention, participation, and an attitude shift; that is, they wanted more money spent, they wanted a voice in how it was spent, and they wanted prevention, as well as improved treatment, to become a research priority.

They wanted to be compensated for all the years lost.

Hillary Rodham Clinton was the first to speak. "We are here to reiterate this President's and this Administration's commitment to working with you in this room, and advocates and scientists and doctors and nurses and citizens all over this country, to work tirelessly, persistently, and relentlessly against the enemy known as breast cancer," she said, "and to do all that we can do to end this epidemic."

Visco smiled when she heard the word *epidemic*. Mrs. Clinton did not have to worry quite as much about diplomacy and balance as her husband did. Maybe someone would quote the First Lady.

"Now it is my great, great pleasure," Mrs. Clinton continued, "to recognize someone who many of you know as the founder of the Coalition, others of you know as the director of the UCLA Breast Center, but many of us know as"—she paused—"*the* Dr. Susan Love, who is going to make a *difference* in breast cancer. . . ." She was cut off by another noisy round of applause. Love was not scheduled to speak, but the First Lady motioned her over to the podium. The crowd was not going to settle for her mute presence.

Love shoved her oversize red glasses up to the bridge of her nose and made her way to the microphone.

"Thank you," she said. "It's very exciting for all of us to be here, and it's a tribute to all of your work and all of your effort."

She hesitated. Susan Love was an Irish Catholic who had considered becoming a nun as seriously as she had thought about being a doctor. She had left formal Catholicism behind twenty-five years ago, but the notion of being called by God, of being tapped on the shoulder to do a particular job, stayed with her still. She had not planned to become a breast surgeon and an activist. Susan Love had wanted to be one of the boys, performing big, lifesaving surgeries with the best of them. But fate had handed her a different life, one molded by her desire for a "relevant" existence, and by the demands of patients who had suddenly found their voice.

This was her calling, as surely as if she had taken vows. Her critics accused her of grandstanding, of allowing herself to become a media celebrity, hardly a dignified role for a serious physician to assume. They did not understand the nature of her desire. For all her bushwacking irreverence, Susan Love wanted to please God— and she believed that her mission, her religious crusade, was to eradicate breast cancer.

It was the center of her life; everything else was merely a matter of style and tactics. She held on to the podium and looked at the expectant faces in the audience. By now Love had a polished public voice, for not a week went by without a speech or a sound bite. It deserted her. She could not make this simple declaration of intent without a break in her voice.

"We're going to eliminate breast cancer," she said. She thought of her daughter, Kate, who liked to tease that Mommy had better get rid of breast cancer because she, Kate, was going to be too busy being a ballerina to bother. "And we're not going to let it go on to another generation. Thank you."

The woman who should have made the next speech was dead. Sherry Kohlenberg had tutored Fran Visco in the art of congressional lobbying in the early days of the NBCC, when by rights she should have been in bed. Visco had painful memories of Kohlenberg waiting outside a senator's office, wig askew, face wan and sweaty. Her cancer had already metastasized, but if she could not beat the disease she was determined to make progress against a federal bureaucracy that had so long ignored it. She had kept on almost until her death the previous July.

Her husband and young son were in the audience, and before Hillary Clinton turned the podium over to Visco she asked them to rise, Larry Goldman wearing a wistful smile, his bewildered son clutching a book, eager to resume his position on his father's lap. They were casualties too. Before she died Kohlenberg had asked the President for one thing: not to forget the ones who were left behind.

Then Visco stepped forward. She offered the people in the room her congratulations, but the last thing she wanted was a room full of complacent activists. She was here to lay out her agenda.

"Money for research is not enough," she said. "Too many women die because they do not have access to quality screening and treatment. Women with breast cancer are tied to jobs because they cannot afford to lose their insurance—or they cannot find jobs because of what their diagnosis will do to an employer's health care costs. And they cannot find insurance on their own because of pre-existing condition restrictions."

She wanted to redefine the problem. Breast cancer was not just a women's health care issue. It was a social malady that ate up families, and anyone who thought he was immune to its effects—any husband or father, any son or daughter or sister, any woman who hid behind age statistics or a clean family history—was fooling himself.

"One of the many compelling messages that accompany these petitions is that of my son, David, who is seven, and who's here today." Visco smiled at the boy, who sat stiffly in a dark gray jacket and dress shirt, his father's arm around his shoulder. David hid his face in his hand when his mother pointed him out, making it impossible to tell if he was overcome by sadness or by the embarrassment of having his mother reveal in public what he had done.

She took a moment to compose herself. "And his note reads: 'Mr. President, please stop this disease. I want my mom to live forever.'"

* * *

At the end of her remarks Visco addressed the President directly. "We know that as the son of a breast cancer survivor you know firsthand the devastation of this disease," she said. "I want to thank you and Mrs. Clinton for today, and the beginning of our new partnership, a partnership to obliterate this disease. Thank you."

As she spoke the President closed his eyes for a moment and turned his face heavenward, as though trying to keep his feelings under control. A year and a half ago the President's mother, Virginia Kelley, had suffered a recurrence of the breast cancer that had been first diagnosed in 1990. Within months he would become one of the ones left behind.

The next speaker was Health and Human Services Secretary Donna Shalala, whose job it was to introduce Clinton, her "friend and boss." A tiny, stocky woman who favored impeccably tailored designer suits and let intimates call her "Boom-Boom," Shalala was like some sophisticated descendant of the Wizard of Oz. She promised to do only the magic tricks she knew she could perform, and as a result those who felt beholden to her, like the breast cancer advocates, came to believe she could do almost anything.

She administered what looked like a rosy future. The HHS umbrella extended over the NIH's increased breast cancer budget as well as the Women's Health Initiative, a $625 million, fifteen-year research effort announced in 1991 by then-NIH director Dr. Bernadine Healy in an attempt to bring women's health research into parity with men's. Shalala was a vocal supporter of the Defense Department's allocation for breast cancer research, and Clinton was about to put her in charge of devising a national strategy against the disease. The history of breast cancer research was marked not just by inadequate funds, but by a fundamental lack of organization: researchers duplicated each other's efforts while such basic requirements as tissue banks, to store tissue samples for research and study, went begging. Shalala had $10 million to spend on an action plan that would enforce order on chaos—to make sure no one misspent the government's new riches.

In truth, she presided over a troubled kingdom. Five months earlier Healy had abandoned her approved comments before the House of Representatives Appropriations Committee to complain about Clinton's proposed $10.67 billion budget request for the NIH in fiscal 1994. What looked like a 3.2 percent increase, she had charged, was in fact creative accounting and money for new programs. The funding for basic research would actually be one percent lower than in the previous year—slightly over four percent, when biomedical inflation was taken into account. The final budget figure for 1994 was slightly higher—$10.9 billion—but still meager compared to the nearly nine percent annual increase of the 1970s and 1980s. And Shalala was waiting for a report on the Women's Health Initiative, whose design and escalating price tag had been criticized since its inception. Research was not as rich as it seemed to the people in this room.

Still, it was the perfect moment for a push. Shalala could think of no one at the senior level of this Administration whose life had not been touched by breast cancer. Each one had a close friend or family member who suffered from the disease—and it changed people, she could see it. Shalala had lost two aunts on her father's side to the disease, and a third aunt was in remission. Once the issue was no longer a theoretical one, once it came down to the threat of losing someone you loved, it was hard to turn away. Practical considerations like a balanced budget became an obstacle, not an excuse. Defense Department spokesmen liked to tell anyone who would listen that the $210 million appropriation was a one-time expenditure, but Shalala had already advised Visco to keep the pressure on. Shalala thought the program might have a longer life as long as Clinton was in office.

The President stepped to the podium and joked that he had won the lottery to be the one man who got to speak at this event. Then his tone changed. "In the three minutes since the beginning of this talk another American woman has been diagnosed with breast cancer," he said. "If I speak for twelve minutes another woman will die of it, in the course of these remarks. We know that one in every three women does not receive the basic services, like mammography, that help to detect breast cancer. And the cost of not dealing with this amounts to about six billion dollars a year to this country, over and above all the human heartbreak involved."

To him, an assault on breast cancer made economic sense, even if it involved spending more money. There was, Clinton said, "no excuse for why we would spend so much money picking up the pieces of broken lives, when we could spend a little bit of money trying to save them.

"I appreciate the reference to my brave mother," he said, glancing over at Visco, "who struggles on with her breast cancer condition and who has resumed her remarkable life, but who also knows how much more we need to do."

He set forth his plan. In mid-December Secretary Shalala would hold a meeting to initiate a National Action Plan on Breast Cancer, which would establish a national health care strategy, research priorities, and political policy to outlast even the Clinton Administration's commitment to it. He promised a new emphasis on prevention and improved methods of early detection. He explained that doctors around the country would offer discount mammograms the next day, in observance of National Mammography Day. And while his health care reform package included payments for screening mammograms only for women over fifty, he tried to reassure the audience: any women under fifty whose doctor specifically recommended a mammogram would be reimbursed as well.

The intended message was clear. Breast cancer ate away at the integrity of the American family and had done so for far too long. The Clinton Administration had both a personal and a political commitment to change that—and, thanks to a hefty nudge from the advocates, it had the beginnings of a working plan.

Clinton walked over to a small table to sign the proclamation for National Mammography Day, but Visco, a paralyzed smile on her face, had to be herded into place by Shalala. Delight had invaded every cell of Fran's body. She looked as though at any moment she might levitate and float buoyantly around the room.

Now that the speeches were finished, she could relax and enjoy her victory celebration—the payoff for two and a half years of diligence that sometimes left David wondering when he was going to see the mother he wanted to live forever. She blinked as the flashbulbs went off and the President pressed a souvenir signing pen into her hand. She stood by as he gave another pen to Dr. Love and kissed her cheek. Then he called out, "We're adjourned," and walked off the stage to talk to members of the audience.

Visco stood rooted to the spot. It was over. The NBCC had engineered an official federal commitment to fight breast cancer. More to the point, the army money was earmarked for breast cancer research. Science went where the money was; the new research budget fairly guaranteed a stampede. The final deadline for grant proposals for the DOD money was just over a month away, November 30. Once a scientific review of the proposals was completed, a new panel, made up of researchers, doctors, and advocates, would decide which of the qualified applications were relevant to the community—that is, which ones moved in the direction that women like Fran thought was appropriate.

One of the Coalition members who had been in the audience came up to her, and Visco started going on about what a great day it was.

"But Fran," said the woman, mindful of the distinction between getting money and getting results, "where can we go from here?"

It was as though someone had thrown cold water in her face. Triumph faded. Other people came up to congratulate her—newscaster Linda Ellerbee, who was a patient of Susan Love's, Secretary Shalala yet again, the First Lady, Lauren Hutton—but Visco seemed unable to shake off the gloom that had suddenly descended upon her. They flitted around her and moved on. She glanced about in momentary confusion, numb with sudden exhaustion.

Her friend was right. Fran had worked tirelessly for two years just for the chance to make things better, but tomorrow the Coalition had to get back to work, in a suspicious, sometimes openly hostile, environment. They had to figure out how to spend the money and hope that something they funded would yield results. They had to convince Congress that the DOD program should continue. They had to worry three years before the next election about what would happen if Clinton did not hold the White House, since Visco believed that she would not be able to get within ten feet of a congressional office door if the Republicans were in power. She had already started to think about pursuing private money more aggressively in case that distressing day arrived.

It was all so tentative. Even Shalala had issued a warning not to like her too much. "All of my experience in movements," Shalala had said, "is that you've got to have a Left. You have to have people screaming at you, keeping your feet to the fire, or you don't keep the momentum up."

Visco had to badger even the people she perceived as her allies. There were no guarantees.

She was back to earth—a wife, mother of a seven-year-old son, friend to two women who had died of breast cancer before they could see this day. Six years out from her own diagnosis. All the money in the world couldn't change that.

2

ALTERNATIVE MEDICINE

JANUARY 1994: UCLA

THE PEOPLE IN UCLA'S GENERAL SURGERY WAITING ROOM WERE VERY busy not meeting each other's gaze when the side door swung open and Dr. Susan Love strode in, the pockets of her rumpled white lab coat sagging under the weight of a fat leather appointment book and a worn man's wallet crammed with bits of paper, and her signature accessory, a long string of pearls, swinging to and fro. She leaned forward when she walked and took big, rolling steps, like someone making her good-natured way through a stiff wind.

The cream-colored slacks under her lab coat were frayed at the hem in back, and the heels of her sensible black pumps were scuffed raw. She was not a careless woman, but she did have priorities, and clothes were not among them. Love wore suits because they bought her professional acceptance, and chose shoes that still felt comfortable at the end of a long day on her feet. When they wore out she replaced them. Between purchase and discard she ignored them. An immigrant from the East Coast, she nurtured a vestigial loyalty to dark clothes in winter and light clothes in spring. Beyond that, she consigned her appearance to a personal shopper at Nordstrom's department store, who coordinated outfits so that Dr. Love lost not a moment debating which blouse or belt to wear with the peach skirt.

She had pared grooming down to an equally efficient minimum. Dr. Love liked to scandalize patients by telling them she would be perfectly happy with a crew cut, but in the interest of not standing out she settled for a short permanent she could comb with her restless fingers. As soon as the corkscrews began to unwind she got a new permanent. Wet, dry, mussed, covered by a surgical net for six hours, her dark brown hair, only recently stippled with gray, always looked the same. She owned contact lenses but rarely bothered to wear them.

She wore no makeup on her freckled face, and when some network television makeup artist got hold of her before an interview she always looked startled and overdone, like a kid caught at her mother's vanity table. The only adornment she allowed herself was jewelry—the pearls and an ankh, an ancient symbol of life, on a chain around her neck; big gold earrings, and above one of them a small stud in the shape of a labrys, the Amazons' mythical double-bladed ax. She wore several gold rings, including a thick band on the ring finger of her left hand that symbolized her relationship with Helen. The workday wardrobe was a nod to propriety; the plain face and the ring were quiet reminders that she was not one of the gang.

She leaned back against the reception desk and considered her audience. The General Surgery waiting room was just that, a holding tank for patients facing everything from mastectomy to gallbladder surgery. The first thing Love had to do was gather her patients together, a brief game of musical chairs that spelled the end of a woman's privacy. Everyone in the room was about to find out who was suffering from breast cancer.

"I'm Dr. Susan Love, director of the UCLA Breast Center," she said. She had been giving the same introductory speech every Wednesday and Friday afternoon for a year, the same cheery delivery, the same punch lines peppered throughout. She spoke in a loud, insistent voice, as though trying to convince a handful of reluctant campers that the summer really was going to be a lot of fun. "Whoever's here for the multidisciplinary clinic, why don't you all kind of move over here together so you can see me."

One woman who had been sitting out of sight behind a big aquarium moved to a seat toward the rear. A man who had come to

General Surgery with his wife for something else quickly got up and took a seat on the other side of the room. Now there was a little nest of women in the center of the room, some alone, some accompanied by family or friends. Each one of them had already been diagnosed with breast cancer.

They came for the Breast Center's multidisciplinary clinic because it promised to make the immediate consequences of that news somewhat easier to bear. The multi, as everyone called it, was the centerpiece of Love's program at UCLA, designed to right as many wrongs as possible given the fact that she was limited to the same problematic treatments any doctor used.

The traditional model for breast cancer treatment required a woman to follow a chain of referrals until she collected all the specialists she needed—doctors who might not know each other or ever speak face-to-face. After a series of overlapping duets, someone would tell her what she ought to do. In addition to coping with her diagnosis, she had to endure the anxiety of wondering when they would all discuss her case, and whether they would ask the questions she thought of while she waited.

This clinic flipped the process around so it accommodated the patient, not the doctors. Love assigned a lead doctor to each patient, depending on the nature of the case, but a woman who invested one afternoon at UCLA got to see specialists in every relevant discipline—surgery; medical and radiation oncology, in case she needed chemotherapy or radiation treatments for her cancer; radiology, which offered an array of imaging techniques; mental health, either a psychiatrist, psychologist, or social worker to tend to her spirit; and plastic surgery. A pathologist reviewed all her slides and a radiologist studied her existing mammograms and scans. Toward the end of the afternoon Love conducted the multi conference, where all the doctors met to confer on the cases. They did so because Love was weary of the ambiguities of standard treatment, and determined that they hash out their answers together.

Afterward the lead doctor returned to provide his patient with a recommendation for treatment. She would get as much of a consensus as medical science allowed.

*   *   *

It was twelve thirty. By five o'clock the patients would all be on their way home with a plan, but right now all they had was a kernel of trouble and lots of questions. The women glanced at each other, instinctively trying to gauge where they ranked on the continuum of bad news. The psychologists had a term for this—"downward comparisons." A woman with breast cancer tended to look for someone who was worse off than she was, and took comfort that she wasn't at the bottom of the heap. A middle-aged woman pitied a young woman with a husband and small child, and that patient, in turn, told herself she was better off than the woman who had come to the clinic alone.

They looked up at Dr. Love like so many schoolgirls in a row, ready to do whatever she asked of them.

"The whole idea behind the multidisciplinary clinic is that you get to sit still and we all come to you, instead of the other way around," Dr. Love explained. "Now, I had a thriving practice back in Boston, where we tried to do this, so you all must think I moved out here for the weather. That's part of it—but I also wanted to see if we could do this in a university setting. What good was I doing in private practice, if I wasn't teaching anybody else how to do it?

"Anyhow, you're going to sit in an examining room and we'll all come to see you. Then you get an hour's break, while we sit down and discuss your case. We don't get a break. You can watch videotapes down the hall at the Rhonda Fleming Mann Resource Center for Women with Cancer"—and here she smiled at the counseling center's unwieldy name, took a breath, and waited for a laugh—"or you can go downstairs to the deli for a frozen yogurt, if that's how you like to deal with stress."

Her audience had loosened up slightly, but Love knew from experience that they would not remember most of what she said. As soon as a woman heard the words *breast cancer* her ears stopped working. She forgot her questions unless she had written them down beforehand. She nodded and listened to the doctors, but by the time she got home most of what she had heard was spaghetti, tangled up in a sorry mass that only got more confusing the more she tried to figure it out.

So Love offered them each a tape recorder and cassette and suggested that they record their conversations with the doctors.

Love believed in information, as much as a woman wanted, usually more than she was used to, and could easily spend an hour with a patient, drawing diagrams and writing upside down and backward, so the woman could read as she drew, answering questions and then answering them again. She thought it was demeaning to do anything less. Women were not children, to be shielded from the truth. The only way they could make a reasonable decision was to hear all the facts.

Besides, a tape was a good defense against an hysterical relative. "That way when your aunt Margaret starts bugging you about what the doctors said," she told them, "you can just give her the tape and go to the movies."

Love introduced them to the frizzy-haired blonde who had been standing silently at her side.

"This is Sherry Goldman," Dr. Love said. "She's our nurse-practitioner. She's the one you can go to with any questions. You go home and think, 'Who was supposed to order that mammogram?' Sherry. She's the glue who takes care of all the scheduling. I call her Elmer."

Goldman had her timing down pat. She waited just a beat, smiled at the crowd over her round tortoiseshell spectacles, and said, "El*ma*." The message was clear. Women ran this place, and the women who came to see them would be made to feel comfortable.

Dr. Love gestured at the three white-coated students who stood behind Sherry. "You will be seen by full grown-up doctors, but in addition there's an assortment of medical students and residents," she said. "You have my permission to yell at them and ask them questions. We can't sit around ten years from now bitching that doctors don't know how to talk to patients if we don't train them. So this is your chance to contribute to the future of medicine.

"I always feel like I ought to fire a starter's gun and say, 'Ready, Set, Go,' " she joked. Then she turned and marched out of the room. A General Surgery nurse herded the patients out behind her and guided each one into an examining room.

One quarter of the women in the waiting room would likely never return because their insurance or their managed care group would not stretch to pay UCLA's multidisciplinary fees. Managed care had turned medicine on its head: private practice doctors had always made more by doing more, but managed care doctors, who received a flat per-patient fee or found their fee schedules challenged, increased their profits by doing less.

Just as women began to learn what they ought to ask for, they had to wonder whether they would be able to get it. Many of them paid out-of-pocket for a second opinion from Dr. Love—ammunition if they needed to fight their HMO to authorize a particular treatment. All she could do for those women was tell them what she would do if they were her patients, and encourage them to demand equivalent care.

The rest of the women who attended the multidisciplinary clinic—the wealthy ones who had private indemnity insurance, or the ones whose plan allowed them to pay a higher percentage for the opportunity to choose doctors outside the approved network— were shopping for services. Traditionally a university medical center drew patients who were white, wealthy, well-educated, and slightly younger than the norm—a valuable group whose medical coverage was more elastic than the HMOs. Competing breast centers all over the city aggressively courted these patients. It was Love's job not just to recommend treatment, but to outsell the competition, to anticipate and address any perceived disadvantages of coming to UCLA.

She had to figure out a way to defend the location—or rather, the lack of one. Love had arrived at UCLA in the summer of 1992, at the tail end of a university real estate boom gone sour. Doctor after doctor had rented sumptuous office space in UCLA's new medical center, but managed care cut into profits and made it hard for them to pay the rent. No one was prepared to rent space to the Breast Center for a dedicated center on the promise of big numbers or the hope of finding a wealthy private donor to foot the bill, which was why this group met twice a week in the General Surgery waiting room and shared its examining rooms. The Center's offices were wedged into a suite of oncology offices around a blind corner at the end of the fifth floor hall, identified only by a piece of paper with an arrow on it, taped to the wall.

Over at St. John's Hospital in Santa Monica, just a few miles away, women sat in a tastefully furnished waiting room exclusively for breast cancer patients, or sipped tea while they watched an educational video in a little library. Love had to convince women that what looked like less was in fact more.

She was determined to find a patron, but until then Love pretended that the bare-bones operation was a badge of honor, a matter of priority, not necessity. She learned quickly how to market disadvantage, and often told patients, "Other hospitals have marble on the counters and carpets on the floor. *We* have programs."

She also knew that some women got nervous about UCLA being a teaching hospital, where portions of their care would be delegated to anonymous interns and residents. That was why she instructed the women to give "the baby docs" a hard time. Breast cancer patients felt that they had suddenly lost control of their bodies. The last thing they needed was to feel that they were at the mercy of untrained hordes of students who roamed the halls looking for mistakes to make.

The trickiest issue, though, was that of celebrity. Women came to UCLA to see Dr. Susan Love, the nationally recognized advocate, the woman the President had kissed on national television, the one who had written the bestselling *Dr. Susan Love's Breast Book.* Her name was the one with marquee value, so she had to be careful not to make promises she could not keep. Her travel schedule was booked six months in advance. Love saw patients at the multi, but she could hardly see all of them. The success of the Breast Center depended on her ability to get women to trust other members of the team, even as she promised them, as she had every Wednesday and Friday for a year, that she was personally aware of each case. Love had to bless every patient herself. Otherwise they would go somewhere else.

They were particularly insecure—just diagnosed, uncertain about how to proceed, doubting their ability to make the right move. Two weeks ago they had not yet felt the lump or seen the shadow on what they had responsibly scheduled as a routine mammogram. Now they were reeling.

The multidisciplinary clinic was supposed to help them cope. When Love moved to UCLA from her private practice in Boston, it was with a mandate to establish such a clinic as part of a comprehensive new breast care program, underwritten for the first two years by the Department of Surgery.

The Breast Center offered an array of programs—a diagnostic clinic every Thursday for women whose problems sounded benign, time for follow-up patients on Wednesday and Friday mornings, and a program for high-risk patients on Tuesdays. Love operated every Monday and Tuesday, and saw both diagnostic and follow-up patients. But the program she cared most about was the multi. The rest was a holding pattern; the multi was progress.

It had been harder to set up than she had anticipated. Six months to get the Breast Center staffed—an administrator, a nurse-practitioner, a computer specialist to set up a patient database, three facilitators to field phone calls and manage the surgery schedule, and an assistant for Love. Another six months once the multi was under way to weed out doctors who were uncomfortable with the collective approach and replace them with what she hoped would be a permanent team. It was only in the last few months that the multi had begun to live up to her expectations.

It was not the way doctors were used to practicing medicine. The multi clinic cost a patient between $350 and $800, depending on how many specialists she saw, but the profit from the initial consultations went to the Breast Center itself. An individual doctor made money from a patient only if she came back to him for treatment. A surgeon who worked alongside Dr. Love might see four patients and operate on only one, not a good return on his investment of time.

The standard diagnostic and follow-up appointments were a more dependable source of profit, although Love's travel schedule and her tendency to spend a long time with each patient kept her volume lower than it might have been. The high-risk program, for healthy women whose family history increased the likelihood that they would someday develop breast cancer, gobbled profits like the multi did—a woman got the services of an oncologist, a psychologist, a nutritionist, and a physical trainer for the price of a single appointment.

Love had managed to find a handful of doctors committed to the multi concept, but it required a measure of coddling and wheedling, flattery and cheerleading. It was not good business, though she believed fervently that it was good medicine. She was all too aware of the grumbling among faculty members at UCLA who resented the fact that the Department of Surgery carried the Breast Center and guaranteed Love a $300,000 annual salary, the highest of any doctor at the level of associate professor. Most doctors got along with a smaller staff and took home the income they generated from performing procedures, but Love had been promised $300,000 no matter how much she earned from surgeries. Some of her colleagues hoped, not so secretly, that she would fail.

She didn't care what they thought. The Breast Center still had six months until it was supposed to break even. If it was losing money it was because she needed a marketing plan, advertising, support from UCLA, a donor with deep pockets. It was not because the concept was flawed. If anything, Love felt that medicine was flawed, expecting women to tromp all over town looking for answers.

Still, every week she reviewed the numbers and faced a sorry irony: more patients was good news.

3

THE MAZE

LAURA WILCOX REGARDED THE HOSPITAL SMOCK WITH WEARY RESIGNA-
tion. No matter what a woman looked like in her street
clothes, her shoulders tended to slump once she put on that
faded blueberry-and-cream wrap-top with UCLA MEDICAL CENTER
stamped in a big circle on the back. She was wearing a crinkly, long
floral print in sunny shades of yellow and gold that made her look
lighthearted and young, even though she did not feel that way. The
smock lay in a puddle on the examining table, dull but insistent.
With a shrug she slid her dress over her head.

Laura carefully folded it over the back of a chair, tucked her
ivory silk bra inside, and put on the gown. She sat down, her back
straight, her smile fixed, as though she were waiting for a friend for
lunch. She was not about to get up on that examining table until
she had to.

This was the last place she had expected to end up, and all of
it—the vivid makeup, the neatness, the perfect posture—was an
attempt to preserve the illusion of health. Laura had gone through
life being told she was beautiful. In her twenties, briefly, she had
been a model—not on the runway, which might have betrayed a
certain skittishness, but in magazines, wearing skimpy Italian outfits that showed a lot of leg. She was used to people paying attention to her because of the way she looked—and although she had

not modeled in over fifteen years, she worked hard to protect and refine that look.

She knew just how to present herself for best effect, chin up, head tilted slightly to the side to display a long neck under a cascade of thick black hair. Her full, rosebud mouth was painted a deep, matte red, and her dark brown eyes were rimmed with black mascara. The preparation had taken a brittle effort earlier that day, but she believed in the self-fulfilling prophecy: If she looked well she was well.

Laura was a production executive for a television personality who wanted to break into movies, so she spent most of her working hours trying to woo writers whose books or scripts she might want to option. At thirty-eight she was painfully aware that most development executives were younger, in their late twenties or early thirties. She tended her body diligently—vitamins, daily meditation, no red meat, and three hundred sit-ups a day to maintain the flat stomach she was so proud of. She analyzed herself with a dispassionate eye, and curled her hair, or cropped it, or changed her makeup, to keep the look fresh.

When she decided in 1988 to have silicone breast implants, it was not because she wanted big breasts to impress men. She simply considered her tall, curvy frame and decided that her A-cup breasts were out of proportion. So she fixed them. If she could not position herself as a wunderkind, she could lay claim to being a beautiful woman with brains. That would buy her enough time to become an independent producer, a job where she would have the autonomy to age gracefully.

She took stock as she waited for Dr. Love. Work was not a problem. She had a good job and an ambitious boss, health benefits, and enough vacation time to disappear for a lumpectomy without being missed. The problem was her personal life, or the lack of it. Laura was single despite a couple of promising romances, and more obsessed every day with the desire to settle down and have a family. Time was running out. If her hands fluttered just a bit and a thin vertical line appeared between her brows, it was because her scenario for herself did not include any more downtime for illness.

* * *

Laura had been diagnosed with breast cancer for the first time in 1988, just nine months after her implant surgery. The surgeon said she qualified for a lumpectomy and radiation rather than a mastectomy, but since she had one positive lymph node—an indication of significant risk that the cancer would recur or metastasize, escape through the bloodstream and eventually spread to distant organs—she also had chemotherapy.

She felt a second lump in her right breast in October 1993, and decided to wait to see if it disappeared when she got her period. It didn't. She had a surgical biopsy in late December, and the report showed a malignancy.

Laura rattled off the details to Dr. Love with a false detachment, as though she were reading the weekend grosses on a new movie. Her voice wavered only slightly as she got to the important question. She wanted Love to tell her: Why did she have breast cancer twice? Was this a new cancer, or had the old one come back to kill her?

Love asked her to hop up on the table and began her exam, which more than anything resembled a game of Simon Says. Hands on your waist. Hands above your head. Clench them tight. Lean forward. She was looking for telltale signs of more cancer, a tightening or dimpling of the skin above a tumor, or a new asymmetry that might mean trouble.

She asked Laura to lie on her back and stretch one arm above her head. As Love reached to palpate Laura's right breast she closed her eyes. She always did this part of the exam with her eyes closed, swearing that her fingers worked better when her other senses didn't get in the way. Slowly she felt around the breast and across it, and then had Laura raise her left arm so she could examine that breast. She helped Laura sit up so that she could feel under her arms for swollen lymph nodes. She found none.

When she was done she left the room so that Laura could put her clothes back on. Love had a set of immutable rules about proper examining room behavior, all designed to even out what she saw as an impossibly inequitable relationship. She always had the patient get dressed after an exam and threatened that otherwise she would have to disrobe to even things out. She never stood with her hands folded across her chest, which would make her seem inaccessible. She tried never to stand near the door, which made the patient feel that the doctor was in a hurry. Love had been known to breeze into a room and sit on the floor, legs splayed, her notes in her lap. She often sat on the footstool the patients used to step up onto the table. It was a conscious maneuver. These women felt helpless enough without having to assume a supplicant's posture, staring up at the all-knowing physician.

Love had not yet seen the pathology report, but when she came back into the room she told Laura that this probably was a local recurrence, "leftover" cancer from the 1988 surgery—not an indication that the cancer had spread, but a portion of the tumor that the surgeon simply had failed to get, "which doesn't mean the surgeon's bad, just that they missed some." She hoped she was right. Residual cancer like this was usually a matter of housecleaning: Laura did not have breast cancer again; she had it still. Ten percent of lumpectomy and radiation patients had these recurrences, as did eight percent of women who had mastectomies. Any surgery left some breast cells behind, and any of those cells could be malignant.

Love would have been more concerned if the lump had appeared six months after treatment—or if it were a new, more aggressive primary cancer, unrelated to the 1988 diagnosis, or a distant recurrence in an organ, proof that the original cancer had escaped Laura's breast and posed a systemic threat. This was an indolent cancer. Chemotherapy was designed to decrease the number of cancer cells in the body to a manageable level, so that the immune system could fight the rest off, but it did not necessarily vanquish all the existing malignant cells in the breast. Radiation was supposed to do that, but it worked best on cancers that were dividing rapidly. Laura's cancer had loped along and eluded it.

It seemed nothing more than unfinished business, a fragment of cancer that had taken five years to alert its host to its enduring presence. It had to come out, but Laura did not have to be any more frightened than she had been the day before she found it.

"You'd have to be God, I guess, to get it all," said Laura, relieved. "You know any like that?"

"I know some who *think* they are," said Love. She gestured at the silent resident who had stood all this time in the corner of the room, taking everything in, and asked Laura if she would mind letting him feel the lump as well.

"Oh, I'm used to it," said Laura, lying back down.

Love flashed a wicked grin. "They say the most frequent side effect of breast cancer is that you say, 'Hello,' and immediately start unbuttoning your blouse."

B y three thirty the doctors, residents, and medical students had trailed into a cold, crowded conference room behind the examining rooms, which they borrowed while another room was being remodeled for the Breast Center. This one was too small for the eighteen people who crowded into it, and so by necessity a hierarchy had developed.

As Love put it, "The grown-ups had to come to the conference," though a subordinate, a younger doctor, medical fellow or resident might have seen the patient. The members of the core team took their seats first—Dr. Love and one of the other surgeons, usually Dr. David McFadden, Dr. Robert Bennion, or Dr. Darryl Hiyama; oncologists Dr. John Glaspy, medical director of the UCLA Joint Medical-Surgical Oncology Center, or Dr. Dennis Slamon, chief of the UCLA Medical Center's Division of Hematology-Oncology and director of clinical research at the Jonsson Comprehensive Cancer Center; Dr. Larry Bassett, Iris Cantor Professor of Breast Imaging in the Department of Radiological Sciences; radiation oncologists Dr. Guy Juillard or Dr. Robert Parker; psychologist Dr. David Wellisch or social worker Carol Fred from the Rhonda Fleming Mann Center; and Sherry Goldman, the Breast Center's nurse-practitioner. If a patient required plastic surgery, Dr. William Shaw, chief of the Division of Plastic Surgery, would join the group. The personnel might change from one week to the next, but the idea was always the same, a senior staff member from each discipline. Slamon, who had enthusiastically pursued Love for this job, sometimes dropped in even on days when Glaspy was scheduled to attend—not so much to offer medical advice as to keep tabs on the fledgling effort.

The half dozen young doctors who worked alongside them took the remaining seats, and the residents and medical students edged into chairs shoved snugly against the back wall. When everyone was in place the pathologist took his seat in front of a microscope connected to a Sony color monitor. The two radiologists sashayed sideways from the light box to their pile of mammogram films to make their presentations. The last doctor to enter the room had to sit on top of a small refrigerator in the corner.

They were here to impose what order they could on the information they had collected. Breast cancer was a devious disease—a family of diseases, really, that began at the same site but behaved with frustrating variability. Or rather, with an incorrigible will: while patients talked about being survivors and marked each anniversary of their diagnosis, doctors always kept a wary eye on the horizon and spoke darkly of predestination. Love had come to believe that there were three categories of disease: one third of all breast cancers were so virulent that they would kill a patient regardless of when the cancer was discovered or what treatment she had; one third were so indolent that they might laze around in the breast for years without posing a systemic threat; and one third existed in the middle ground—they required and responded to treatment. It was a neat enough analysis, except that there was no sure way to figure out which category a woman belonged to.

The clinician's only hope was to intrude on the process before the cancer colonized the liver or lungs or bone, and a woman developed demonstrable metastatic disease. If doctors got there first they had a chance of breaking fate, depending on how aggressive the disease was. If they missed that single moment and the cancer invaded the body, they were reduced to palliatives and experiments. Metastatic cancer was incurable. Eventually it had its way.

Doctors had devised a set of staging criteria called the TNM system—tumor, nodes, metastases—to define the severity of a woman's disease. But the longer they tried to shove symptoms into one of four overlapping classifications, the more frustrated they became with those categories. They judged the size of the tumor, the presence and location of swollen lymph nodes, and the existence of obvious metastases in other organs, and then they sorted: Stage 1 was a tumor that was two centimeters or less in diameter with no lymph node involvement. Stage 2 could be several kinds of cancer—a small tumor with positive but mobile axillary lymph nodes; a medium-size tumor, up to five centimeters, with either positive mobile nodes or negative nodes, or a large tumor, over five centimeters, with negative nodes. Stage 3 was a large tumor, over five centimeters, with positive mobile nodes, or a small tumor with fixed nodes. Stage four meant that a woman's cancer had obviously spread.

Staging determined the kind of treatment a patient received. Early-stage localized disease often meant choices—mastectomy or lumpectomy with radiation, the radiation intended to kill any lingering cells elsewhere in the breast. A patient would need a lymph node dissection, in which a surgeon removed a cluster of about ten to fifteen of the thirty to sixty lymph nodes located in a woman's armpit. Lymph nodes were the accepted, if imprecise, indicator of the likelihood of micrometastasis, the as-yet undetectable presence of cancer cells in distant organs, the invisible step before demonstrable disease. Negative nodes and a small tumor meant that a woman could avoid chemotherapy. But once there was evidence of possible systemic disease—a larger tumor, or positive lymph nodes—chemotherapy was added to the arsenal. Late-stage disease meant chemotherapy, and possibly experimental high-dose chemotherapy.

Staging was just the beginning. There were myriad prognostic indicators to consider, and deception everywhere: cancer cells that were markedly abnormal in their appearance were said to be poorly differentiated, and usually were more aggressive than the well-differentiated cells that resembled their benign siblings—but not always. As a rule, in fact, most breast cancer was poorly differentiated.

The pathologist determined the nuclear grade of a breast cancer by evaluating the appearance of the cell nuclei and ranking it on a scale of one to three or one to four, the higher number predicting a more aggressive, more rapidly dividing cancer. It was at best what Love called a piece of "circumstantial evidence": A bizarre-looking cancer could turn out to be slow-growing, and the reverse could also be true.

Another test determined the S-phase, an analysis of cell division. A high S-phase number meant lots of dividing cells. A low S-phase, to be devoutly wished for, identified a more sluggish cancer. The same test also measured the DNA in tumor tissue. If it was the proper amount the tumor was considered diploid, and if it was abnormal the tumor was called aneuploid, and might prove a more aggressive form of the disease.

Estrogen and progesterone receptor tests determined whether a tumor was likely to respond to hormones; the ones that did tended to grow more slowly, and might also respond well to a hormone treatment.

Technology was easier to manipulate than the disease itself. Improvements in mammography enabled doctors to diagnose a new class of breast cancer—not invasive cancer, which had the ability to escape the breast and spread, but DCIS, ductal carcinoma in situ, which literally meant "in place." Love called it precancer, betrayed by tiny specks called microcalcifications that showed up on mammogram film, but even that evidence was unreliable.

Although eighty percent of calcifications were benign, the only way to make sure was to perform a surgical biopsy. Even if there was DCIS, it turned into invasive cancer only thirty percent of the time. Since there was no way to predict if it would, the standard response to extensive DCIS was a mastectomy. The same early detection method that might enable a woman to have a lumpectomy instead of a mastectomy also threatened her with more surgery than anyone was sure she really needed.

What the doctors wanted was a glimpse of the timeline, a sense of whether the patient had arrived in time for treatment to do her any good; the categories were nothing more than an attempt to tame mystery. The problem was that there were biological exceptions to every man-made rule, supposedly compliant cancers that went on a rampage and angrier disease that responded to treatment. The ability to describe the criminal perfectly did not necessarily translate into capture.

Women over fifty accounted for approximately seventy-eight percent of all breast cancer cases—advancing age was the greatest risk factor for the disease—but this multidisciplinary clinic was the harsh exception. Love glanced at the birth dates listed on the scheduling sheet and winced: one woman was fifty-five, one was forty-two, and the other five were younger than that. Breast cancer liked to break its own rules.

The person nearest the door turned off the overhead lights so that everyone could easily see the mammograms on the light board on the wall. The first of the day's seven patients was a thirty-four-year-old who had waited three years to see a doctor about a lump because she had no insurance to pay for treatment if it was malignant. She finally had a mastectomy, but now the cancer had recurred. There were two choices: Treat the recurrence as a local problem, with radiation to the site, or treat it as evidence of systemic disease and bombard her with experimental high-dose chemotherapy and a transplant. The former might not be enough to prevent the disease from spreading. The latter, which could cost over $100,000, was the most aggressive treatment currently available.

What the newspapers called a bone marrow transplant was more formally known as high-dose chemotherapy with autologous stem cell rescue, which was exactly what the stem cells were supposed to do—rescue a breast cancer patient from a chemotherapy regimen so toxic that it would kill her without intervention. The patient received chemotherapy that was about ten times stronger than the standard dose—followed by an infusion of her own stem cells; young, healthy bone marrow cells that had been plumped up with a synthetic growth hormone. The chemotherapy was supposed to kill the cancer. The enhanced stem cells were supposed to keep the chemotherapy from killing her.

It was an expensive, experimental procedure intended for women who had run out of options—at first only those patients with demonstrable metastatic disease were eligible for the experimental treatment, although recently doctors had begun offering the treatment to women with ten or more positive lymph nodes and no evidence of distant metastasis. The theory was that if some chemotherapy was good, more chemotherapy was better, but so far it was only a theory. There was at least a five percent mortality rate from the procedure itself, and no definitive data on whether it improved survival rates.

Duke University's Dr. William Peters first used the bone marrow transplant to treat metastatic breast cancer patients in 1982.

By 1989 only 265 patients with advanced disease had received the regimen of high-dose chemotherapy coupled with the lifesaving transplantation of harvested bone marrow cells. Four years later that number had almost quadrupled; it was the nation's largest transplant program.

After more than eight hundred transplants, Peters had positive results. He found that the procedure improved both disease-free and overall survival: fifteen percent of the women experienced complete remission, and of that group, twenty-three percent were still disease-free at five years, an eternity for a woman under a death sentence. Still the medical establishment was hesitant. The *Journal of the American Medical Association* had published an article in November 1993 that stated, "survival rates after treatment have not shown consistent improvement." Although high-dose chemotherapy showed "promise," according to the *JAMA* article, a great deal more research needed to be done.

It was hard to tell whether the treatment worked or certain patients just got lucky. But this patient was a young woman with children, for whom doing less seemed insufficient. Dr. Glaspy was in charge of the experimental stem cell transplant program, one of only two major research programs in southern California, and he attended the multi conference when Dr. Love found transplant candidates on the roster.

He had several options to offer the patient. UCLA conducted a randomized clinical trial, in which patients were assigned either to receive a transplant or to be part of a control group that got standard treatment. If a patient wanted to be sure she got the most aggressive therapy, she could enroll instead in a study that compared two different high-dose regimens. Or, if she was convinced that one set of drugs held more promise than the other, she could make the choice herself. Given the odds, Glaspy was not about to pressure a woman to take part in the randomized trial. She had to decide if she was willing to risk not receiving the experimental therapy—or even risk letting someone else decide which drugs she would get.

A dour, heavy man who seemed older than his forty-one years, Glaspy listened to the debate, his eyes fixed on the conference table, and then wearily gave his opinion. The woman would choose a transplant but it wouldn't work. She would continue to recur locally in a repeating cycle of anxiety and surgical resolution, until finally the cancer figured out how to escape into her bloodstream and kill, rather than torture, her.

He sighed and considered his clasped hands. In his business it was important to come to terms with the fact that patients died, and he had long since drawn a line. He was sad when older women died, but he accepted it. Young women dying upset him. Young mothers dying made him furious. This woman would likely suffer greatly before she died. It simply was not acceptable—but at the moment the only thing he could do was crack wise about it.

"I told her she's not terminally ill," he said. "She's incurably ill."

The next case for consideration was Laura's. By comparison it was clear-cut. Love firmly believed that the invasive cancer had been left at the site by the surgeon who performed Laura's 1988 lumpectomy. The problem was that the pathologist's slide also showed extensive ductal carcinoma in situ, or DCIS.

The warped cells on Laura's slide ran right up to the edge of the slide. In pathology jargon she had "dirty margins," as opposed to a clean rim of healthy tissue at the edge of the slide. Dirty margins meant there was still DCIS in her breast. There was no way to remove all of it short of what Love called a "salvage mastectomy," a cleanup operation, with immediate reconstruction. According to current data, Laura would have the same survival rate as if she had had a mastectomy in the first place.

The psychology resident who had seen Laura issued a warning. The patient was anxious, wasn't eating, wasn't sleeping, and joked that having low self-esteem and being single must be risk factors. She was terribly worried about whether men would find her appealing—or rather, about what she had to do to make sure they did. She was more fragile than she appeared to be.

The doctors continued down their list. A forty-year-old who had had a lumpectomy and radiation wanted advice on whether to take tamoxifen, a relatively new drug still being studied in clinical trials for its ability to prevent recurrence and possibly prevent malignancy in the first place.

A pregnant twenty-seven-year-old wondered if there was some way to save her breast and keep the baby.

A thirty-nine-year-old who had already had a mastectomy and begun her chemotherapy came to UCLA to ask if she could quit the drugs because they would throw her into premature menopause and she wanted to have a child.

A fifty-five-year-old wanted to go back on estrogen replacement therapy for menopause because it gave her energy. She preferred not to think about whether it also sped tumor growth.

The last patient, forty-two, was mostly sad. After two excisions for an invasive cancer, her pathology slides still showed dirty margins. She was polling doctors to convince herself to have the mastectomy they all said she had to have.

By the end of the conference the doctors looked like they had had the air pumped out of them. Treating young women was hard in a particular way. Chemotherapy often threw them into premature menopause, putting an abrupt end to their fertility and leaving them with harsh symptoms, for which they were advised not to take hormones. The very things that could save them—could, not would—were likely to rob them of the life they hoped to lead.

At five o'clock Love knocked on the door of Laura's examining room, grabbed some paper from a cabinet, slumped on the footstool, and began to draw. Things were not as simple as she had hoped. They might have considered another wide excision for the remnants of Laura's invasive cancer, but the DCIS, the precancer, changed everything.

Love explained the distinction between precancer, which she called "rust on the lining of the duct," and real cancer. There were three stages to precancer—intraductal hyperplasia, where a lot of normal cells were crowded into a duct; intraductal hyperplasia with atypia, "where some of the cells start to look weird," and DCIS, in which the cells officially were weird, by which she meant malignant. All these conditions existed only within the duct, and lacked the ability to escape into the bloodstream. Love likened DCIS to toddlers who had not yet learned to walk.

"It's not more aggressive, not likelier to kill you," explained Dr. Love, "but since it doesn't make lumps, it's hard for the surgeon to find it or radiation to kill it. With hindsight, you're not a good case for a lumpectomy." She paused. "Chemotherapy won't get these cells either."

Laura listened attentively to Love's biology lesson, but as the surgeon started eliminating treatments Laura's smile began to fade.

"The bad news is the best way to deal with this is a mastectomy."

Laura inhaled sharply, and did not let her breath back out again for a long time.

"And you have more concern with having to take the nipple out, since all the ducts lead there."

No breast. There it was, after six years of thinking she had got off with a small scar. Until this moment she had allowed herself to imagine a side exit, maybe another lumpectomy, but no longer. She was going to lose her breast. Not an acceptable option for a woman who carried such a clear picture of the ideal female form in her head, who had asked the implant surgeon to operate a second time to reduce the size just a bit, to bring her closer to that perfect mental image. If she could not tolerate a discrepancy in size, she was hardly ready for a standard mastectomy and a prosthesis. She was not going to stuff a clumsy foam pad in her lacy silk bra.

Laura had the cold strength of someone who had already endured too much—not only her cancer, but her mother's early death the previous spring after years of drinking and drug use. She had come to anticipate trouble, and the more it came her way, the more determined she was to conquer it. In anticipation of bad news she had already gone to see Dr. William Shaw, the UCLA plastic surgeon who specialized in microsurgery and was a pioneer in what he called "free-flap" reconstructive surgery. He had told Laura that he could remove a section of her own skin and tissue from her abdomen or buttocks, place it where her breast had been, and reattach the blood supply. She would have no sensation in the breast, but it would look real. He could even fashion a nipple and match the color of her own nipple with a tattoo.

As though through a fog, Laura heard Dr. Love encouraging her to have the immediate reconstruction. "The first day you'll feel like a truck ran over you, and you'll be right," said Love, "but by the next day you'll start to feel like yourself again." Laura forced herself to focus. She could get rid of the cancer and still look like herself. The plastic surgeon would work on her at the same time that Dr. Love performed the mastectomy, so she would wake up from the anesthesia with something that resembled a breast. She would never have to confront a flat scar. That was pretty good news.

She sighed. "I just want to take care of it and deal with the reconstruction. I saw another plastic surgeon and he said he didn't want to do expanders for six months," she said, referring to a reconstructive process often used for women who have had radiation, which makes breast skin more fragile. An expander was a hollow sack that was inserted behind the muscle and filled, over a period of months, with increasing amounts of saline solution, until it was the size a woman wanted. Then the surgeon replaced it with a permanent implant—but Laura was not prepared to do anything that took so long.

She was emphatic. "I don't want to go around without anything for even three *weeks*."

By six Love was back in her office, organizing her conference notes for her assistant, Connie Long. All the day's recommendations would be faxed or mailed to the women's physicians—in part because some women would go back to those doctors for treatment, in part because UCLA had a reputation for stealing patients. Love could hardly prevent a woman from choosing to have her treatment at the Breast Center, but she could not afford to be cavalier about the doctors they deserted. She needed referrals from those doctors to build a practice.

A year and a half after she moved to UCLA, a year after the multidisciplinary program officially got under way, Love was still the new kid in town. Many UCLA doctors continued to refer their patients to her predecessor, Dr. Armando Giuliano, even though he had left the university for St. John's Hospital. They had all sorts of reasons to distrust her: she was outspoken, she was pushy, she was a woman, she was gay, and she did little to ingratiate herself with her peers. She never visited her office in the main hospital building, where she might have had the chance to socialize with her colleagues—and worse, she loudly proclaimed it a waste of time. Her

clinical responsibilities were far more important than academic camaraderie.

She refused to answer her beeper when she was with a patient
because it rattled people to be interrupted, but that translated into a
reputation for not returning doctors' phone calls. She told affluent
women that the only thing their money guaranteed them was too
much medical care, delivered by doctors who wanted to keep their
profit level high and their risk of malpractice charges low—and in
attacking what she sincerely believed to be overkill she managed to
offend hardworking potential allies as well.

She had just learned, to her fury, that the university's own Physicians' Referral Service did not necessarily direct a woman's call to
the Breast Center. There were general surgeons at UCLA who performed breast surgery and expected referrals, and Love's name was
merely one of the names on the rotation. She got every fourth or
fifth call, and the rest of the patients disappeared into the UCLA
system.

It made no sense to her. How was she supposed to build a
center if her own university did not support the effort with referrals? But the other doctors had seniority. Love would have to settle
for her fraction of the cold calls that came in and figure out another
way to build her practice.

She needed to cultivate relationships. Her dream depended for
its success on the goodwill of strangers, a hard path for a woman
used to being alone.

4

A DOCTOR'S EDUCATION

SUSAN LOVE THOUGHT OF HERSELF AS HER PARENTS' ELDEST SON. THE first of five children, she grew up in strained counterpoint to her mother, Peggy, a pretty woman who seemed to Susan to care far too much about appearances—not just the way she and her husband and children looked, but what other people thought about them. It struck Susan as appropriate that Peggy liked to paint. Life was all about surface impressions.

Susan was her opposite: as methodical as Peggy was instinctive, as defiant as her mother was eager to assimilate. In a funny way she seemed older than her mother. Certainly more responsible. She was the ringleader, the role model to three sisters and a brother growing up in suburban New Jersey. They might enjoy their mother, but Susan felt they looked up to their older sister. Her next sister, Chris, was creative and artistic like Peggy; Debbie was the sweet child, the happy one; Mike and Betsy, eight and twelve years Susan's juniors, were her eager acolytes.

It was easier to get along with her father, James, a kindred spirit, a quiet man who liked to read books. Peggy Love was too mercurial. Her daughter preferred a well-defined path.

Until Susan was thirteen life was predictable enough: she was a bright, personable kid who studied hard and was intent on learning to do the Twist. But when her grandfather died, the import-export business he ran with his son faltered. James Love was suddenly the unemployed father of five, with his family's stable life in jeopardy. A machinery manufacturer provided salvation in the form of a job in Puerto Rico, so in 1961 he picked up his family and moved. Susan Love enrolled at a Catholic school run by the School Sisters of Notre Dame, a teaching order of nuns.

Academics were not a problem. Susan's transplanted social life, however, was a minefield of cultural surprises. At one party she hopped right onto the dance floor to display her prowess at the Twist, only to find the nuns staring at her in horrified silence, her new friends and their parents regarding her with condescending suspicion. Teenagers back in New Jersey might well dance the night away without attracting any attention—but within the Catholic community of Puerto Rico it was considered wanton behavior, the mark of a loose woman. Susan Love had no idea what a loose woman was. All she knew was that she had broken a social rule without knowing it existed, and that people treated her differently from then on.

She learned early in life that there was safety in solitude—that the presence of others fairly guaranteed misunderstanding of even the most innocent behavior—and she retreated into private pursuits, bicycling alone to daily mass at the church, concentrating hard on her schoolwork. Sister Ines was a particular inspiration, a charismatic young nun, just twenty-one, who possessed a grace and enthusiasm that Susan badly wanted to emulate. Sister Ines taught biology and chemistry. Thirteen-year-old Susan decided to walk in her footsteps one way or another. Either she would become a nun or a doctor.

Within a year the company transferred James to Mexico City and the Love family moved again. His wife, Peggy, was thrilled, since she had grown up there. She registered Susan at the American School Foundation, which she had attended—and Susan did her best to fit in at the school everyone called "Gringo High." She was valedictorian of her senior class and received a National Science Foundation Award for excellence, but the dream of being a doctor was still comingled with the notion of being a nun. The convent appealed to her because it promised boundaries—prohibited spontaneity and awarded selflessness. She couldn't get into trouble if there was no dancing allowed.

She enrolled in the College of Notre Dame of Maryland in Baltimore, and two years later decided to enter a convent in Connecticut run by the School Sisters of Notre Dame, the order that had run her school in Puerto Rico. The nuns, impressed with her science background, enrolled their new postulant in Fordham University's premed program.

But the convent was no longer the haven Susan Love had imagined. The Catholic Church was in chaos in the 1960s. The Berrigan brothers, two activist Catholic priests, demonstrated against the Vietnam War, pouring blood on draft records and setting them afire. Priests held folk masses wearing street clothes and playing guitars. Nuns gave up their habits. Even the strictest orders softened the rules and allowed street-length dresses and lighter head coverings.

Love had come to the church expecting the reassurance of structure and discipline. Instead she found turmoil and doubt. She asked for and received permission to wear her habit to classes, to remind herself and her fellow students that she was separate from them, but it was not enough to make her feel secure.

With much of the ritual stripped away, it was all too easy for her to start questioning her choice. At five o'clock in the morning Love understood what she had done, and why: the pale early sun poured into the chapel and lit the rows of women in black habits, anointing their faces as they sang Gregorian chants. Love felt God at dawn. Later in the day, when she was cleaning bathroom tiles with a toothbrush, she found it harder to grasp the meaning of her new life.

She began to wonder if she was simply not up to the task. Over and over she read the New Testament parable of the rich aristocrat, a good man all his life, who approached Jesus Christ and asked to follow him. Christ said that he could as long as he gave up his great wealth—but the man was "overcome with sadness" at the suggestion. His worldly pleasures kept him from taking his place alongside the son of God. Love worried that she was like the rich man, unable to attain goodness. For months she agonized over whether she ought to leave the convent, and how great a disgrace that would be.

Near Christmas, Sister Ines arrived at the convent for a visit to the mother house, and Love sought her out. Perhaps she had a suggestion about how her ex-student might make peace with herself and become a nun. Susan confessed her anguish and asked her what to do.

Sister Ines spoke without any hesitation. "God does not want you to be crazy," she said. If Susan was as miserable as she sounded, surely there was some other way she could find to do good work in the world. The important thing was to do it, not to waste time struggling to fit in.

Love left the convent in January 1969. She continued to attend Fordham University, and during her junior and senior years threw herself into a variety of social projects, including a Police Athletic League summer arts and crafts program in the South Bronx and Harlem. She ran a teen center there as well, but still a sense of failure haunted her. God had shown her an opportunity and she had been unable to take it. She would have to work even harder, in case she was lucky enough ever to receive another chance at grace.

She chose a punishing path for herself. Medical school was hard enough, with its long hours and difficult classes, but in the late 1960s Love also faced a quota system. When she went in for her interview at SUNY's Downstate medical school campus in Brooklyn she was told flatly that if she proceeded with her application she would be killing a young man—taking up a spot in the class that could better be filled by a boy looking for a military deferment to avoid service in Vietnam. The admissions official did his best to discourage her, which had the opposite effect.

By the end of her first two years in medical school she had decided to become a cardiologist. She refused to consider pediatrics because she could not bear the thought of hurting a child without being able to explain that the needle that caused the pain carried valuable medicine. She was not interested in surgery because surgeons were plumbers, admired by their patients but disdained by their colleagues. Internists were the smart ones, and specialists the top of that heap. She liked the cardiologist who taught her—and she found the idea of a cardiologist named Love to be irresistible. She could imagine the slogan: "Send your broken heart to Dr. Love."

She often looked back on that decision as the first of what she called the many "foretellings" in her life. Love was not the sort of person who liked to analyze her psychological motivation—why she made a decision, or why she changed her mind. She preferred to think that the universe had a sense of humor. Every time Love made a definitive pronouncement about her future, fate sent her on a detour.

In her third year of medical school she began six-week rotations on various services, and at the end faced an unexpected truth. Surgery turned out to be the one rotation she enjoyed. Everything else seemed to her like so much "mental masturbation"—lots of talk and no solution. Neurologists could pin down the exact location of a brain lesion but could not help the patient. Surgery was literal: either you helped or you didn't. At least a surgeon had a straightforward chance.

Surgery was supposed to be out of reach for a woman, the one medical discipline known for its conservative, boys' club mentality. She decided to barge in and demand membership.

When she began to interview for a residency she found that the social climate had changed dramatically. The women's movement had begun, and instead of quotas to keep her out medical schools wanted to bring her in. Everyone needed a token woman, and there were few to go around, particularly in surgery. Love was much in demand.

She began her surgical residency in 1974 at Boston's Beth Israel Hospital, determined to prove that she could more than keep pace. Love was a reckless zealot, exhibiting the same disregard for her own well-being that the men did, pushing herself to the physical limit, indulging in all the stress-related behavior of the stereotypical harried man of medicine. She chain-smoked on medical rounds, easily two packs a day, balancing a lit cigarette butt on the edge of a hallway ashtray while she talked to a patient and retrieving it as soon as she came out of the room, so she could puff her way down the hall. She kept it up until she hit thirty and decided she was too old for such foolishness.

She took birth control pills every day to block her menstrual periods. No one was going to fault her performance in surgery because she had cramps or needed a break to change her sanitary pad. For five years she took the pills, not allowing herself the week off that was usually prescribed. She had done some research on the pill: doctors told women to take that week off because they thought their patients would feel strange without a period. Unable to find a compelling medical reason to menstruate, Love chose instead to put her reproductive system on enforced hold until her career was established.

She worked under Dr. William Silen, the chief of surgery and the man who became her mentor. Silen was singularly uninterested in the fact that she was a woman. All he cared about was that she become a decent doctor, which he defined differently than did many of his peers.

Since profit rose in direct proportion to volume, most private practice physicians kept an efficient eye on the clock. Silen instead told her to take her time and listen to her patients. It did not matter to him how many bodies she could process in an hour. What counted was her ability to care for her patients—which meant not only their physical illness but their emotional health as well.

She became the first female general surgeon on Beth Israel's clinical faculty in 1980, when she was thirty-two, and announced to anyone who cared to listen that she was far too talented to settle for the ghetto of women's medicine.

There is a pecking order among surgeons. The most invasive operations—organ transplants, heart bypass, lung surgery, gastro-intestinal procedures—were the province of an elite group of top surgeons, a fraternity Love fully intended to join. By comparison, breast surgery was relatively easy work, the removal of an enlarged sweat gland. Susan Love wasn't interested in breast surgery. It would make her a caricature, a second-level surgeon, a woman doing women's work. People would interpret it as proof that she lacked either the confidence or skill to handle more demanding procedures.

It was the second foretelling. Doctors referred breast cases to her because they assumed that a woman surgeon would be interested in women patients. Women sought her out because they felt more comfortable talking to a woman, or because word got out that she listened. Love became a breast surgeon because there were too many frightened women looking for answers. She might miss out on the high drama of the operating room, but she was suddenly indispensable—not a small satisfaction to a woman who had spent much of her life feeling like a misfit.

The Dana Farber Hospital, a cancer treatment facility, had opened the Breast Evaluation Center in 1979—and in 1982 its founder, oncologist Dr. I. Craig Henderson, recruited Dr. Love to see breast cancer patients. She had written a provocative research paper that year debunking the notion of fibrocystic disease, which she referred to as a "garbage" category for a number of benign conditions that had no causal link to breast cancer and did not require the vigilance, in terms of biopsies, surgeries, and diet, that many doctors prescribed. It sealed her fate.

She became part of a respected triumverate: Love, a surgeon; Henderson, an oncologist; and Jay Harris, a radiation therapist, who considered the trio "gadflies in our own specialities, in terms of questioning the very need for our own specialty." He knew that Love had a tendency to polarize issues along gender lines—to silence her critics with a dismissive, "That's what men doctors will tell you." But Harris was more than willing to put up with the rhetoric, for he believed that Love was ahead of her time. Someday what she had to say about how to treat breast cancer would become the standard line.

She was successful, respected, and restless. Her determination to be more substantial than her mother turned into a love of challenge for its own sake.

Love came to breast surgery well trained in the limits of modern medicine—not because of what she learned as a medical student but because of what she discovered outside of school. Breast cancer was all about exasperation and ignorance, but she lost nothing to surprise. That had happened some years before.

She spent part of the 1978–1979 academic year as a surgical resident at Guy's Hospital in London, and invited her parents to join her for a vacation. James and Peggy Love spent two weeks with their daughter, which Love hoped was the beginning of a reconciliation with her mother. They got on well; Love allowed herself to think that they might embark on a more equal relationship now that Love was an adult.

A few weeks later her fifty-six-year-old mother started to have problems with balance. She had complained of deafness in one ear for a while, and a CAT scan revealed a large acoustic neuroma, a benign tumor, behind her ear. Benign or not, it still had to come out, for it was pressing on her brain.

Love insisted that her mother travel to Beth Israel for the surgery, which she had in July of that year—or rather, she had most of the surgery. When Peggy Love learned that the surgeon might inadvertently damage her facial nerve and cause the features on one side of her face to droop she instructed him to leave a rim of tumor rather than jeopardize her appearance. Love was exasperated with her mother, but there was no changing her mind. Peggy was not prepared to endure that kind of disfigurement. The doctor agreed, inserted a shunt to prevent postoperative swelling, and sent his patient back to Mexico City.

Three months later Love was on early morning rounds in the intensive care unit at Beth Israel when she got a long-distance phone call from her father. She walked to the phone expecting to hear that something was wrong with her mother.

But James Love was calling with news about Susan's sister, twenty-six-year-old Debbie. That morning she had climbed onto a couch to open a large window in her Mexico City apartment. She reached high for the clasp and, as her husband and two small children watched, lost her balance and fell out of the window. She plunged ten floors to her death.

Love hung up the phone, dazed. Debbie was a delight to Susan, who had always admired her younger sister's ability to enjoy her life. She had been the first to fall in love, the first to have babies. What kind of madness was this, for someone so good to die in such a bizarre way?

She looked around the crowded hallway, wondering where she could go to get away from everyone. The last thing she wanted was for the others on rounds to make a fuss over her. She preferred to handle sorrow alone.

Helen Cooksey, her intern, came over to find out what had happened. "You need a hug," she said when she heard the news.

"No, I don't," Love snarled. "Get away from me, goddammit."

Nine months later Love's mother began to have terrible headaches. Another scan showed that the tumor was again pressing on the brain, but this time Peggy Love insisted on staying in Mexico City. A second surgery for the condition was extremely dangerous—it had a mortality rate of fifty percent—and she wanted to be at home. Love flew down for the surgery and hovered in her mother's room.

Peggy Love continued to complain of headaches after the operation—and of drowsiness, which Love attributed to the pain medication her mother was receiving. During the surgery Peggy had worn what the doctors called a "halo" around her head, a ring attached at her temples and neck to make sure her head remained in a fixed position, and Love noticed that her mother was bleeding at the two points where the contraption had touched her temples, but she thought the skin was bruised, nothing more.

Later she would say that she was thinking with her daughter heart, not her doctor head. It was only when her mother went into cardiac arrest that she realized what had been going on: Peggy Love was bleeding from hypertension or increased intercranial pressure.

They were alone in the room when it happened. Love grabbed the phone to report the cardiac arrest, but it was too late. Peggy slipped into a coma and developed pneumonia. While Love wrestled privately with her own culpability, her father and siblings asked her what they should do. They wanted her to make the decision.

Love weighed the options. The doctors could keep her mother alive, treat the pneumonia with antibiotics, and insert a feeding tube to nourish her. But that was not living to Susan. That was some horrid stasis, proof that medical technology had outpaced sense. She could refuse to allow her mother's doctor to administer the antibiotics, in which case Peggy would surely die. That seemed the appropriate thing to do.

She withheld her permission, and a few days later, after ten days in a coma, her mother died. Susan Love went back to work at Beth Israel treating women who were older than her dead mother, all the while thinking bitterly: I couldn't even take care of my own mom.

Her education in life's capriciousness was complete by the time she was thirty-two. She understood firsthand the finite benefits of medicine, which could keep a woman alive but not wake her up. She had had a nasty glimpse of the fragility of seemingly invincible good health, lost to as unlikely a foe as gravity. Along the way she had lost any notion of justice. Susan Love was well equipped to handle breast cancer patients.

5

A BATTLESHIP THAT
TURNS ON A DIME

HISTORY SERVED ONLY TO INFURIATE HER. WHEN SUSAN LOVE CONsidered the past she saw ignorance, a dogged resistance to change, and a perverse, resilient adversary: these were the elements that defined more than a century's effort against breast cancer.

Until the 1850s doctors simply sent breast cancer patients home to die. Most of them presented with locally advanced metastatic disease, since self-examination was hardly a proper activity for a lady, and surgery without antiseptics or antibiotics was as likely to kill as the disease was.

It was only the development of anesthesia and antibiotics that made intervention a possibility. After years of helpless watching, surgeons responded with a dramatic alternative—the radical mastectomy, introduced in England in 1857 and further developed during the 1890s by Dr. William Halsted at Johns Hopkins University. The idea was to rid the patient of any risk by dismantling the path that breast cancer supposedly took, which meant removing the breast, all the nearby lymph nodes, the muscles of the chest wall, and often the lymph nodes above the collarbone or behind the breastbone and ribs.

Love occasionally saw a patient who had had a radical mastectomy, most of them elderly women now, their chests concave, their arms weak, numb at the armpit and swollen. She found it hard to look at them, for she could see their hearts beating beneath the thin layer of skin that stretched over their bones.

One third of the patients who had the surgery died, in all likelihood because the disease had spread before it was caught, but most surgeons did not think to question the effectiveness of the procedure. They believed they needed to operate even more quickly, before the cancer escaped.

A few British doctors explored less mutilating forms of surgery in the 1930s and 1940s, and two American surgeons, Oliver Cope and George Crile, Jr., followed their lead. In the late 1950s Cope and his Harvard Medical School colleagues treated twelve patients with surgical excision of their breast tumors and lymph nodes, followed by heavy doses of radiation, and found that their survival rate—four were alive nineteen years later—was consistent with the results they would have expected with mastectomies. Crile later suggested that doctors who insisted on performing mastectomies did so not for the patients' welfare, but because it inflated their egos or their bank accounts. They both were ostracized by their colleagues, while most women continued to endure what was then standard treatment: In the 1950s and 1960s, a woman with breast cancer faced major surgery, radiation if it recurred, and chemotherapy when those two treatments failed.

In 1958 a young Pittsburgh surgical oncologist, Dr. Bernard Fisher, began to study the relationship between host and tumor in experimental animals. In 1963 he analyzed research on metastatic disease—his own data, as well as data compiled by doctors elsewhere in the country and in Europe—looking at how quickly breast cancer grew once it had spread. He calculated the time it took for one cancer cell to turn into two, two into four, and so on—and determined that the average doubling time for breast cancer cells was about one hundred days. Since it takes about ten billion cancer cells to form a one-centimeter mass, most cancers had been in the body between eight and ten years before they were detected. A mammogram might catch the process at eight years, but a palpable tumor was already about ten years old.

Fisher proposed what was then a radical thesis, that the mass in a woman's breast was a manifestation of systemic disease, not the disease itself. Cancer could spread through the bloodstream and lymphatic system long before there was a detectable lump. So surgery was not a sufficient response, since all it did was remove the most obvious symptom of illness. A woman's survival depended on how well her immune system battled the cancer cells that circulated in her bloodstream. Medicine needed a new, systemic treatment to eradicate the underlying cause.

Fisher was already involved in randomized clinical trials of adjuvant chemotherapy—in which drugs were used along with surgery and radiation as part of the initial treatment, not as a last-ditch response to obstinate disease. He also agreed with the maverick surgeons who endorsed less mutilating procedures. Patients with small, well-circumscribed tumors would likely do as well with a lumpectomy that removed the offending tissue, and radiation, as they would with more extensive surgery.

It was a wildly unpopular notion, resisted by a surgical community trained to believe that more was better. The only way to convince them was with clinical data. Eight years later, in 1971, Fisher was able to organize a team of two hundred doctors for a clinical trial, as part of the National Surgical Adjuvant Breast and Bowel Project.

The NSABP, founded in 1957, was a government-funded cooperative group that tested new cancer therapies in clinical settings, under the supervision of the federal government's National Cancer Institute. Bernie Fisher had become its chairman in 1967. The women who signed up for the 1971 study were randomly assigned to one of three groups: they had either a radical mastectomy, or a simple mastectomy (removal of only the breast, leaving lymph nodes intact) with or without radiation. The National Cancer Institute held similar trials.

Fisher would come to be known as the father of the clinical trial, since the NSABP went on to launch twenty-nine protocols that studied various breast cancer regimens. An Italian team of doctors began the first study of breast-conserving surgery in 1973, comparing radical mastectomy to quadrantectomy, in which one-quarter of the breast is removed, the less aggressive surgery accompanied by radiation. The NSABP followed in 1981 with its study of lumpectomy alone, lumpectomy with radiation, and mastectomy. The results, published in 1985, were similar to those of the Italian study. Breast-conserving surgery with radiation had almost the same success rate as mastectomy—a ten percent local recurrence rate, compared to eight percent for mastectomy.

Fisher had engineered a new era in breast cancer treatment. Twenty-two years after he began his work on cell doubling time, he and his colleagues cemented the shift from radical surgery to breast conservation, from localized treatment to a systemic approach. It was both good news and bad. A woman could save her breast; she did not yet have any better hope of saving her life.

Love opened the Faulkner Breast Center in Boston in 1988, just as a right-to-choose movement began to build among women who wanted a lumpectomy. By 1983 the number of radical mastectomies had slipped to five thousand, down from forty-six thousand only thirteen years earlier, but most women, over seventy percent, continued to choose a modified radical mastectomy over lumpectomy. The ones who opted for the newer surgery considered it a political issue—a symbol of liberation from a male-dominated medical establishment they increasingly regarded as being more interested in heroics than in a woman's self-image. Love became a crusader for breast-conserving surgery, even though the trend toward lumpectomy further diminished the status of the breast surgeon, since a patient could be in and out of the operating room in a half hour, and home the same day.

It hardly seemed a revolutionary stance, given the data that supported it, but she liked to recall the day she went to hear a lecture at Wellesley College by Dr. Cushman Haagenson, a pioneer in breast surgery, a surgeon and pathologist who had written the first medical text about the breast. At the end of Haagenson's speech he called for questions, and Love rose to challenge his continued endorsement of more extensive surgery.

When he realized who she was he brandished his pointer at her and loudly accused her of killing women.

* * *

S he had managed to alienate herself from the medical establishment, which raised a skeptical eyebrow at both her professional
and personal life. Sister Ines had taught Susan that God did not
want her to be crazy. Her mother and sister had taught her that
time runs out too soon. Those lessons combined bred in Love a
voracious desire to shake things up—to transform her early rejection of Peggy's teachings into a more principled rebellion.

In 1982 Helen Cooksey, the woman whose comfort Love had
spurned on the morning her sister died, invited Love to spend Labor
Day weekend at her family cabin in New Hampshire. Cooksey was
gay. Love had made a few failed attempts to find a man to fall in
love with—and by the end of the weekend decided that the reason
she had not had a lasting romance with a man was because she did
not really want one. She and Helen moved in together, and had
been with each other ever since.

Having found her life's companion, Love wanted children; it
seemed a completely natural progression to two women who had
both come from large, affectionate families. Susan Love gave birth
to Katie Love-Cooksey on April 30, 1988, having gotten pregnant
with sperm donated by a cousin of Helen's. It was the American
dream, tweaked just enough to accommodate Susan Love: a professional couple, both of whom happened to be women, a healthy
baby with two mothers and a father, and a successful career demol-
ishing accepted medical practice.

She had decided that part of the reason treatment was at a
standstill was because women were too terrified to question a doctor who might hold survival in his hands. In 1986 she had begun to
compile materials for what would become *Dr. Susan Love's Breast
Book,* cowritten with Karen Lindsey, which was published in the
spring of 1990.

The book tour was a revelation to her. No matter where Love
went there were dozens of women waiting to talk to her, not just
about their medical plight but about what they could do to get
more money for research, to get the government to pay attention.
They wanted change. All they needed was a framework.

In Salt Lake City she jokingly suggested to six hundred women,
"Maybe we ought to march topless on the White House. That

should get President Bush's attention." After the speech a group of women rushed to the podium to ask if there was a date set for the march.

And Love thought: If the proper ladies of Salt Lake City are ready to march through the streets of the nation's capitol with their shirts off, it is time to organize.

The idea percolated for a few months. Love was driving up to the New Hampshire cabin for a weekend with Helen and Katie, in the summer of 1990, when she felt a tap on her shoulder. God was giving her another chance. It was so clear: the time had come to politicize breast cancer. Rather than complain, she could lead the way out.

A few patients had formed local advocacy groups in Boston, San Francisco, and Oakland, California. As they drove along, Love explained to Helen that she was in the perfect position to turn those little pockets of action into a national advocacy network. The book had established her as an authority, the media had turned her into a celebrity, and the advocates needed a doctor to lend credibility to their efforts.

It was, she told Helen, like "spontaneous combustion."

Helen Cooksey was one year older than Susan Love, but she had a serene, quiet demeanor that made her seem older than that. A tall, big-boned woman with prematurely gray hair, she often wore a bemused expression as she listened to her animated companion. When Love finished her explanation Helen sighed in helpless resignation. She could see how badly Love wanted to get involved in political work. There was no point in trying to reason with her about being overcommitted.

"You're never going to be home again," Cooksey said.

"I know," Love replied. "The whole idea just makes me exhausted."

Love was always trying to make up for lost time and lost chances. She was forever busy; Katie would come to think of Helen as the parent she went to for calm, quiet time, and Susan the one she depended on for endless, antic play. It was the defense of a woman who feared that she had too little time—and given that, was always happy to cram more experience into it.

She would transform her personal concerns into public issues—

expand the universe in which she had an impact. For fifteen years the breast cancer advocacy movement, born in 1975 when patient activist Rose Kushner wrote *Breast Cancer: A Personal History and Investigative Report,* had focused primarily on the patient's need for information and access to services. The major advocacy group in 1990 was NABCO, the National Alliance of Breast Cancer Organizations, an umbrella group run by Amy Langer, a breast cancer survivor, to serve as a resource for patients around the country. Women depended on NABCO for everything from information on clinical trials to advice on where to buy a wig. What was lacking, though, was a national organization that challenged the government's research agenda. That required a shift in focus, from the patient community outward.

AIDS activists had done it. They had no time for the gentlemanly pursuit of scientific knowledge, and had forced the government to respond to their demands for research dollars. They opened a door for a new generation of activists, each a graduate of a crash course in their particular affliction. The government would have to pay attention again: Breast cancer killed more women in a single year than did AIDS, which would claim 40,000 lives in 1993. It was time to make noise.

Love, Susan Hester, and Amy Langer founded the National Breast Cancer Coalition in May 1991, and Coalition members quickly became fixtures in Washington, testifying before any committee that wanted to talk about women's health and research dollars. Love spoke to patients, to advocate groups, to newspaper reporters and TV journalists and talk-show hosts. The NBCC held its own hearings in February 1992 to figure out just what a reasonable budget for breast cancer research might be.

They came away with a daunting reply: an increase of at least $300 million above the current allocation of $155 million, for a total that would almost triple the existing research budget. The most newsworthy event in breast cancer research in recent years had been the cancellation of an ambitious study of the role of dietary fat in breast cancer risk, a mysterious relationship that had confounded researchers for decades. In 1983 the National Cancer Institute had approved the Women's Health Trial in an attempt to retire the issue: six thousand women for ten years, half on a diet of no more than twenty percent fat, half on the foods they usually ate, which in the United States meant over thirty percent fat. It was canceled in 1988 because the NCI decided that thirty-two thousand women would have to participate to get solid data, which would increase the price tag from $25 million to $100 million.

The ensuing row divided researchers, who complained that there were not enough research dollars to spend so much on a prevention study, and advocates, who said that far more than the cost of the study would be saved if lowering dietary fat did in fact reduce the incidence of breast cancer.

The lesson was clear: the key to change was not only money, but a voice in how it was spent.

Fran Visco first took the traditional route, and in the spring of 1992 stood in line with other health activists at a Senate appropriations committee hearing on the National Institutes of Health budget, "hat in hand," as she liked to say, listening as one after another asked for a bigger piece of the budgetary pie. The answer was always the same: If we give more money to you we have to take it away from someone else.

Since she had no intention of being turned away, she decided on a new tack. When it was Visco's turn she informed the senators that she did not want a bigger piece of the pie. She wanted a bigger pie. More money for health care. They would just have to look hard and find it.

She told them, "You managed to find the money when it was time to bail out all those white guys in suits from the savings and loan crisis. Are you saying now that you can't find money to fight breast cancer?"

They found only an additional $50 million for the NIH—so Love and Visco, still far shy of their goal, began to stalk congressional offices, looking for sympathy and imagination. There they found Iowa's Senator Tom Harkin, who for two years had been trying to shift $3 billion in defense funds to pay for domestic social programs that would benefit women and children. The Coalition, still trying to play by the rules, asked Harkin to include in his 1993 transfer amendment a $210 million appropriation for a two-year breast cancer research program, the money to be moved directly from the Defense Department into the NIH's coffers. But the proposed amendment violated a 1990 "fire wall" regulation that prevented transfers from defense to domestic programs, and overriding it required a two-thirds majority. The amendment failed, as it had twice before.

Susan Love happened to be in Washington for an NBCC board meeting, so she approached New York's Senator Alfonse D'Amato with a new idea. Perhaps senators objected to the size and scope of Harkin's amendment—and if so, they might agree to a smaller transfer solely for breast cancer research. Though there was no precedent for doing so, D'Amato introduced legislation to transfer one percent of the Defense Department research and development budget, $382 million, just to fight breast cancer. That lost too, but by a smaller margin. Clearly, politicians were prepared to endorse more money for breast cancer research—but only if the appropriation were presented in the proper legislative format.

Harkin saw an opportunity. He quickly introduced what his legislative director, Ed Long, called a "stealth amendment," appropriating $210 million of the DOD budget for breast cancer research but leaving it under DOD control. In 1992 the army had spent $25 million on mammography, as part of its health care program for enlisted men and women and their dependents, so technically he was expanding an existing program. That required only a simple majority to pass. This might be the way to earmark money, to exploit the army's extra cash without moving it.

Some senators resisted strenuously, insisting that medical research belonged at the NIH and domestic programs belonged anywhere but the DOD. They did not prevail. There were plenty of senators who supported the cause—and another, practical contingent that realized what the fallout of a "no" vote could be. It would seem predictably bad male behavior, a selfish slap in the face to over fifty percent of the voting public. They voted for the appropriation, but grudgingly, as a matter of pragmatism in an election year.

The House of Representatives passed the amendment on July 2, 1992, by a vote of 328 to 94, as did the Senate on September 23, by a vote of 86 to 10. President Clinton signed the budget on October 6. Afterward Ed Long had the final Senate vote tally framed and hung on the wall of his office. He liked to show visitors how many senators first voted "no," and then shifted over to "yes" when it became clear the amendment was going to pass. No one wanted to be singled out as voting against breast cancer in an election year. Harkin had found a way around the fire wall. The NIH breast cancer research budget had been increased by $80 million, not $50 million, for a fiscal 1993 budget of $228.9 million. Visco and Love had their money. What was supposed to have been a lesson in humility had backfired. They had the heady sense that they could do anything.

It almost did not happen. Visco, Love, and the congressmen who pushed the army appropriation through had managed in one single legislative act to alienate not only the Defense Department but just about everyone involved in carrying out the national health agenda.

Although $210 million represented only a tiny fraction of the total $277.4 billion military budget, it was a big headache for the army. Failure to properly launch and administer the program would make the military look incompetent, but success was an invitation to other hungry lobbyists to storm the walls of the Pentagon. The army had little idea how to spend $210 million on breast cancer, and even less enthusiasm for finding a way to do so.

In odd tandem, the Defense Department and the National Institutes of Health did what they could to make sure the rogue program did not get under way: the NIH sped up, eager to find a way to take over administration of the funds. The army slowed down, in the hope that obstinacy would give someone a chance to step in to rectify the mistake.

The National Cancer Institute, the largest of the NIH's seventeen divisions, twice made overtures about adopting the program, only to be rebuffed by Visco and her colleagues, who threatened to make noisy public objection if anyone tried to change the way the money was allocated. Congress represented the people; scientists could not simply decide that they knew better.

For despite the army's resistance, Visco saw endless possibility. There were no rules, no tradition, no history to buck at the DOD. No chance that an existing bureaucracy would dilute the funds by investing them in basic research. At a meeting with NCI director Dr. Samuel Broder, Visco, made cocky by her victory, challenged him to prove that he would spend the money the way the activists thought it ought to be spent. She was in no hurry to share her windfall unless the NCI promised a wholesale change in the way it awarded grants.

"We feel we have for the first time ever gotten a significant amount of money for breast cancer research," she said. "What are you now going to do differently?"

Broder was a twenty-two-year veteran at the NCI, the head of the research team that in 1985 had discovered the therapeutic effects of the drug AZT in treating AIDS patients. He had been the NCI's director since 1988, and as a loyalist believed that the $210 million appropriation rightfully belonged within the NIH. This was the second time activists had challenged the NCI's commitment to research—the AIDS activists were the first—and he despaired of convincing Visco of his position. He said nothing for a long moment, and then explained that the NCI was like a huge battleship. He could not turn it on a dime.

Broder's comment about the battleship haunted Visco for months. The DOD contracted with the Institute of Medicine (IOM), a division of the National Academy of Sciences, to create an advisory committee that would structure a framework for the army program, and in February 1993, Visco got to speak to the IOM group. Its members ran the philosophical gamut, from Mary-Claire King, who had spent most of her professional life searching for a breast cancer gene, to Dr. Harold Varmus, who believed in the value of more basic research. She did not want another generation of researchers to grow up in what she considered an ivory-tower environment. They had to understand the radical opportunity at hand.

So she told them about her conversation with Broder. "This is our chance," she said. "We get to design a whole new battleship— and now we can make certain it *can* turn on a dime."

The twelve members of the IOM committee published a report in May 1993, having managed to agree on three priorities, down to proposed dollar amounts: training of new doctors and scientists (up

to $27 million), infrastructure enhancement to establish a founda-
tion for future research (up to $21 million), and investigator-
initiated research projects (at least $151.5 million). Of that last
allocation, about $15 million would go to new researchers, and was
intended, according to the IOM, "to level the playing field," to
make it possible for tyros to compete with established scientists.
Another $4.5 million went to Innovative Developmental and Ex-
ploratory Awards—IDEA grants for more speculative projects.

The report was an indictment of the past. Thirty-six years after
the NSABP was founded to study breast and bowel cancers, the
United States still did not have certain fundamentals in place for
ongoing breast cancer research—tumor registries, DNA resources
for research, computerized information systems. Established researchers needed more money, new researchers had to be wooed to
the field and the next generation, recruited and trained.

The army finally released the appropriated funds to the program's administrators, the Army Medical Research and Materiel
Command (AMRMC), in July 1993, just fourteen months before
the spending deadline. It typically took eighteen months to properly
solicit, evaluate, and issue contracts for grants. The AMRMC
scrambled into action. It contracted with an outside agency to conduct the standard scientific review, and established an Integration
Panel, made up of doctors, scientists, and patients, to judge the
survivors of that process. On September 15, 1993, the AMRMC
issued a Broad Agency Announcement, soliciting grant applications.

The NIH traditionally funded its grants based on the scientific
review—funding from the top of the list on down until the money
ran out. The Defense Department intended instead to determine
which grants best responded to the needs of the community. It
could recommend skipping past three grants on the scientific review
list, if they seemed to duplicate effort, to reward an applicant with a
lower qualifying score and what looked like a fresh idea.

Visco, as a member of the Integration Panel, had won herself
the chance to rewrite history. Love, after less than four years at the
Faulkner Breast Center, had taken on an ambitious new challenge:
she had accepted a job as director of a new breast program at

UCLA. She moved west over the summer of 1992 and intended to unveil her signature project, the multidisciplinary clinic, in December of that year. It was a chance to extend her reach—to prove that what she had done in private practice was not an isolated experiment, but a practical model for improved medical care. UCLA had no existing program, so it provided what she called a "nice void." No bad habits to break, just an open space where a program ought to be.

The university setting had everything she lacked. A teaching hospital offered an endless supply of medical students, interns, and residents to help doctors with mundane tasks like taking medical histories. UCLA had a brand-new medical center right across the street from the main hospital, surrounded by the offices of other doctors who could provide referrals. The position gave her credibility in the academic community—a chance to be an insider on her own terms.

It also rescued her from the reality of private practice under managed care. When she first began seeing patients she could expect to be reimbursed for eighty percent of what she billed. That figure had slipped to about fifty percent, which jeopardized her ability to provide the kind of care that had become her trademark. She had already heard a little voice in her brain urging her to recommend a surgical biopsy rather than follow a patient for six months—because surgery paid the bills and waiting six months did not. She was determined not to give in to it, but that seemed impossible when her overhead was so high. UCLA's offer of a guaranteed salary and a subsidized operation for two years was an irresistible lure.

She thought about the academic model she was familiar with from her years as a resident. The professors had a great deal. They saw some patients, but the younger doctors handled the bulk of the load. Senior faculty ran their programs, did some research, gave talks, wrote articles. The way she saw it, UCLA was offering her the chance to mentor and to pontificate, two of her favorite activities.

She had less enthusiasm for the realities of daily medical practice. A wearing truth chafed at Love always: she provided better care than the norm—she was convinced of it—but there was nothing in her bag of tricks that guaranteed a better outcome.

One of the diagrams Love drew for her patients was of ten women with node-negative cancer. Seven would survive without chemotherapy, two would die in spite of it, and only one who would otherwise have died would live because of the treatment. There was no way to tell who was who. Doctors had a ludicrous choice: give toxic drugs to a majority of women who did not need them, or withhold the drugs and sentence one woman to death.

Love believed in Bernie Fisher's systemic model. What she no longer believed in were the accepted therapeutic solutions. She had stood too long at the intersection of frustration—her own, and medicine's. If her private hunch was right—that she, too, might die young like her mother, and her grandmother, who had died of breast cancer in her fifties—then she could not afford to stand still. UCLA offered her autonomy, power, and economic stability. It was a worthy pulpit from which to preach.

REAL TIME

6

THE PARADIGM SHIFT

WHEN LOVE WAS ESPECIALLY TIRED SHE ALLOWED HERSELF ONE indulgence: she let herself speculate. Maybe this life was in fact the preparation for paradise, the hard work before the reward. Maybe the women who died too soon were the lucky ones, already enjoying celestial happiness. Her maternal grandmother, her mom, the patients who died despite her stubborn efforts to keep them alive—Love believed that God had chosen them for early bliss.

This life? This was premed. This was trying to get pregnant. The one thing Susan Love was prepared to accept without data was an afterlife. Happy compensation for enduring the random cruelties of this one.

She prayed all the time—not just to God on a Sunday in church, but to her late mother or a favorite patient, any kindred spirit who might be able to help her out.

Otherwise it was all one-liners and outrage. By the end of 1993 she had become an increasingly strident voice of complaint. If sound bites and slogans got the public's attention, then she would sling them with enthusiasm—anything, even a little excess, to make sure that people knew what a mess breast cancer treatment was. She began to refer to the standard treatment regimen as "slash, burn, and poison," which offended many of her colleagues, who pointed out that patients with other types of cancer had to endure the same assault.

Her reply was curt. The treatment did not work well enough on breast cancer. There had to be another way.

She encouraged her patients to ask questions, to challenge received wisdom—and too often the data backed up her doubts. In December 1993 the National Cancer Institute started a furor by announcing the results of an eighteen-month review of new mammography studies. While mammography undeniably reduced mortality among postmenopausal women, it did not seem to help younger ones:

> There is general consensus among experts that routine screening every one to two years with mammography and clinical breast examination can reduce breast cancer mortality by about one-third for women ages 50 and over. Experts do not agree on the role of routine screening mammography for women ages 40 to 49. To date, randomized clinical trials have not shown a statistically significant reduction in mortality for women under the age of fifty.

Twenty-two percent of all breast cancer cases occur in women under fifty. In 1992, 10.2 million women under the age of fifty had screening mammograms. Now the preeminent medical research facility in the country, arguably in the world, had reviewed the data and relieved those women of the only security they had. The NCI would continue to endorse mammography for women over fifty. For women between 40 and 49 who had no symptoms, the NCI suggested an annual clinical exam and a discussion about "the appropriateness of screening mammography with their physician, taking into account individual risk factors."

Mammography might enable a young woman to have breast-conserving surgery instead of a mastectomy, but according to the NCI it was not going to save her life.

It was time for a third paradigm, and Love pinned her hopes on genetics—specifically on her friend, Berkeley geneticist Dr. Mary-Claire King, who since 1976 had sought a gene for heritable breast cancer. Refinements in existing therapies were not the answer. Love looked instead to molecular biology, to researchers who would someday comprehend the complicated workings of the human cell—why it functioned properly, and how it went awry. In 1990 King announced that her small team had successfully narrowed the search for the gene from all twenty-three pairs of human chromosomes to a stretch of the seventeenth chromosome—an accomplishment Love likened to limiting a city-wide house-to-house search for a criminal to a single block. In August 1993, King held a press conference at a British genetics conference to announce that she was close to discovering the exact location of the gene, dubbed BRCA-1, on that chromosome.

Researchers believed that one in two hundred women had inherited a mutated copy of BRCA-1, which dramatically raised the lifetime risk of breast or ovarian cancer. Five percent of women with a healthy copy of the gene developed breast cancer by age forty, compared to sixteen percent of women who had a mutated copy of the gene. Over their lifetime, ten percent of women with normal BRCA-1 developed breast cancer—but eighty-six percent of women with a mutated gene got the disease.

Several other researchers had joined the hunt since King's 1990 announcement, including Dr. Francis Collins, head of the government's ambitious National Center for Human Genome Research, which that same year had begun a fifteen-year effort to map the three billion units that comprise the human genome, and Dr. Mark Skolnick, who in 1979 had helped devise a technique for gene mapping and had since been involved in the search for several disease genes.

Love and many of her colleagues held out hope that King, the sentimental favorite, would be the one to make the discovery. She was in her own way as much of an outsider as was Love—a single mother in a predominantly male field, a politically outspoken woman who in 1973 stood in front of the Nixon White House on the day the newspapers announced the coup that overthrew Chilean President Salvador Allende, screaming, "You bastards," because of that administration's South American policy. King had vowed not to set foot in the White House until its occupant was someone she deemed worthy of her respect, a promise she kept until Clinton was elected. In 1984 she used her science to help *las Abuelas de Plaza de Mayo*—the Grandmothers of the Plaza of May—determine the identities of the Argentine children whose parents, *los desaparacidos*—the ones who disappeared—had been murdered or kidnapped by the Argentine military junta, leaving behind a small society of anonymous children too young to know who their parents were.

King had great moral ambition, but little interest in the vertical climb. She did not allow her name to be placed in contention for NIH director when Dr. Bernadine Healy resigned, since her passion for research was matched by a lack of interest in administration—and then signed a letter in support of Dr. Harold Varmus for the job, despite the breast cancer advocates' fear that his vocal faith in basic research would shortchange them. King was less wary than they of basic researchers like Varmus, a University of California, San Francisco microbiologist and Nobel laureate, and judged her colleagues more on their commitment to their work than on their philosophical bent. All King wanted was progress, and as far as she was concerned Varmus more than matched her obsessive level of dedication.

Love waited for King to make surgeons obsolete. Every day she put women on the surgery schedule, commiserated about the side effects of their chemotherapy, gingerly inspected their radiation-burned skin—sure that one day the combination of surgery, radiation, and chemotherapy would seem as primitive as Halsted's radical surgery now did. Genetics were the first step toward early intervention.

Over the last few years a strange, coincidental momentum had begun to build—based not on a collective devotion to task but on individual enterprise, tangential motives, and the simple passage of time. If the landscape seemed bleak to the patient, to scientists and doctors it was a remarkable terrain, exasperating and luxurious, treacherous and full of promise.

Money for medical research came from four sources—the government, private philanthropists, corporate sponsors, and cost-sharing with patients—but the balance had been upset. The federal government had less money to spend. Managed care meant dwindling profits from patients. Private and corporate money became more important; the government's disregard and the size of the demographic group at risk opened the field to entrepreneurial interests eager to invest in what suddenly seemed a promising future.

When Mary-Claire King started hunting for the gene, the government was the dominant source of research money. It still was—but in an era of dwindling research budgets researchers had to look for ancillary sources of cash. Two of King's postdoctoral fellows depended on the Susan G. Komen Foundation for sustenance. Eli Lilly & Co., the Indianapolis-based pharmaceutical giant, had already bought licensing rights to future gene tests and therapies from Myriad Genetics, Inc., the biotechnology company Mark Skolnick had founded in Salt Lake City, Utah—a $1.8 million wager on his ability to find the gene first.

There had been a time when researchers were reluctant to accept money from drug companies—it branded a scientist as a second-string researcher, one who had to go begging for funds because his own government did not consider him qualified for a grant. The funds were tainted; it looked like the researcher was working for the company whose drug or equipment he was testing, rather than working for the truth. It was hard to tell the company that wrote the checks that its medicine did not work.

Those old prejudices had fallen away, casualties of financial need. If anything, the researchers who had private money seemed clever, even progressive, for having figured out a way around a strangled federal budget.

Medicine was prepared to ignore even the most blatant ironies in the name of progress, for there was no other way to survive. The British chemical company Imperial Chemical Industries and its United States subsidiary, Zeneca Pharmaceuticals, were great friends of breast cancer research: I.C.I. had founded Breast Cancer Awareness Month nine years earlier, along with the American Academy of Family Physicians and Cancer Care Inc., a support network. Zeneca had discovered and developed tamoxifen citrate, a synthetic hormone used to prevent breast cancer recurrences and currently the focus of a government-funded NSABP prevention trial for high-risk women. The company donated the drug to that trial.

But I.C.I. also produced an array of chlorine-based products that included pesticides, paint, and plastics. In 1990 the federal government filed a major chemical dumping lawsuit against six defendants, including I.C.I. American Holdings Inc., accusing them of dumping millions of pounds of DDT and PCBs into the Pacific Ocean between 1947 and 1971—organochlorine chemicals that some researchers suspected of increasing breast cancer risk. The lawsuit would later be dismissed not on its merits but on technical grounds, by a judge who referred to environmentalists as "do-gooders and pointy-heads."

Annual sales of Zeneca's Nolvadex, its trade name for tamoxifen, were almost $400 million annually; of its carcinogenic herbicide, acetochlor, about $300 million.

Zeneca, which split off from I.C.I. in 1993, was in impressive company: Du Pont and General Electric, both with high numbers of EPA Superfund hazardous waste sites, quite literally made early detection possible; GE by selling mammography machines; Du Pont, by making much of the film those machines used. Anyone was welcome to help, even if they were on the suspects' list as contributors to environmental risk: both patients and researchers had waited for answers too long to stand on ceremony.

There was money as well from companies that had nothing to do with medicine, and everything to do with women. Revlon's Ronald Perelman had made a five-year commitment to Denny Slamon's research in 1990, and was a major sponsor of the National Breast Cancer Coalition. Evelyn Lauder, daughter-in-law of the founder of the Estee Lauder cosmetics empire, helped raise $20 million to underwrite the Evelyn Lauder Breast Center, which opened at New York's Memorial Sloan-Kettering Cancer Center in October 1992—the same month that Lauder and *Self* magazine launched the pink ribbon as a symbol of breast cancer awareness. Designer Ralph Lauren, who had known *The Washington Post* fashion editor Nina Hyde for seventeen years, led a fund-raising effort for a center at that city's Georgetown University when Hyde, who was diagnosed in 1985, complained that it was difficult to figure out how to acquire the best care.

It was a diverse community, full of competitive suspicion and energy, distrust and hope. From "bench to bedside," from laboratory and examining room, came talk of progress and speculation about how soon change might come.

Everyone wanted to have his name connected to the next big discovery, or on the signature line of the check that helped pay for it. New science and new money bred action—but an ongoing government commitment was essential to play out the dizzying array of hunches that was starting to emerge. Ten million dollars was a large private endowment, while ten times that for an annual federal government breast cancer research budget was considered an insult. The Department of Defense had received 2,700 breast cancer research applications totaling $2 billion, and by the beginning of 1994 the scientific review of those applications was under way. Since the DOD budget was only one-tenth the size of the response, some qualified applicants would have to abandon promising ideas.

Still, the ideas flew. Perhaps adding soy to the Western diet would help bring the breast cancer rate in the United States down to something nearer the low rates of Asian countries. Exercise might help. Maybe birth-control pills that lowered a woman's estrogen levels, since that hormone seemed to contribute to the growth of certain tumors. Love hoped to identify early changes in the ductal system so that someone could develop a pill to keep those changes from becoming a malignancy. And DCIS developed into invasive cancer in only thirty percent of cases: It was time to figure out how to distinguish that group from the seventy percent who did not require a mastectomy to ensure a healthy future.

No one yet knew which theories, if any, would turn out to be right—but for the first time the medical community's frustration was mixed with a bewildered excitement: someone, sooner than not, was going to make a breakthrough.

It made the patients crazy.

* * *

Every time Shirley Barber got on a plane she wondered, Is this the flight where I become a statistic? It was part of her job to anticipate the worst and have a plan for surviving it. She checked the emergency slide pressure gauge to make sure the slide nearest her station would inflate. She reviewed the evacuation procedure— reminded herself of how the exit handles worked on the particular plane she was flying and where the flotation equipment was. She tried the exit doors to make sure they opened and closed. Were the fire extinguishers where they were supposed to be?

Once she had gone through her checklist she played a grim game of pretend and imagined various escape routes depending on the type of crash. She always felt good when she was finished. The knowledge that everything worked was like insulation against the inescapable fact that some planes did go down.

Shirley had not planned on becoming a flight attendant. She had dreamed of being an actress, but she was a practical woman: her dark skin and hazel eyes, the genetic legacy of a biracial romance, would keep her from getting the big parts, and her yearning for stability made the specter of rejection unacceptable. Shirley spent one summer stock season as a prop mistress and thought about work as a stage manager, but in the end she decided that standing six feet away from actresses who were doing what she wanted to do was worse than not being in the theater at all.

So one Sunday morning she picked up the classified ads and found a new stage on which she could perform. In 1972 she signed on with United Airlines, based at Los Angeles International Airport, and had played the cool, calm professional to thousands of anxious airline passengers ever since, a member of the first generation of women not forced to retire at thirty-two or when they got pregnant, whichever came first. Shirley Barber was the stranger passengers trusted to lead them right past death to safety. She was a convincing player, and she had come to believe her own act. Shirley knew how to dodge trouble—or at least, how to face it down.

She had learned early in life to shield herself from a world that conspired to make her feel unwanted and unsafe. Shirley had been put up for adoption when she was eighteen months old, but being given away did not bother her as much as the lag time between her birth and the decision. To this day she wondered what could have possessed a woman to abandon a child she had known for that long. But she never allowed herself to look for her birth parents. She could cope with the postponed decision, dispense with it with wisecracks. The truth might be too upsetting to be so easily contained.

She met Tracy Barber in 1973 on a Los Angeles to New York flight she was working, and Tracy was so smitten that two days later he broke a cardinal rule and allowed her to smoke in his brand-new brown Datsun 240Z sports car. They married on June 1, 1974, and moved south of Los Angeles to Irvine, a liberal enclave within conservative Orange County—forty minutes south of Los Angeles International Airport, down the clotted San Diego Freeway, but a quick commute to Technicolor, where Tracy worked. Their son, Mitch, was born in 1976, and their daughter, Kimberly, in 1980.

Tracy doted on Shirley. A big, burly man, Tracy loved the idea that he could stand between her and any more emotional pain. He would protect Shirley, and she, with her barbed jokes, would keep him from being smug about it.

She had a zinger for every occasion. Shirley was saucy about her appearance, and when she wasn't working, her hip-length brown hair cascaded down her back in thick, soft waves that swung back and forth as she walked. She favored skimpy T-shirts like the one that read SHE WHO MUST BE OBEYED, cut low enough to expose a gold chain with a charm that looked like the emblem on Superman's shirt.

Over time, she had figured out how to make everything work. After flying east she indulged a working mother's yearning for a little downtime, with a postflight regimen that always included a hot bath, a room service dinner and a glass of beer, and either a novel or whatever movie was on television. When she flew back home she stopped at a coffee shop at one of the slab hotels that lined Century Boulevard, just outside the airport, and ordered a cup of coffee, a Coke, a hot fudge sundae—or if she was really tired, all three. Suitably caffeinated, she buzzed down the freeway to have dinner with her family.

She smoked a pack and a half a day and wasn't worried enough to stop. Shirley was used to playing the odds.

She came to Susan Love because two doctors had spent more than a year trying—and failing—to clear up a persistent infection in a sebaceous gland in her left breast. She was possessed by what she knew was an irrational fear—that the infection would some- how turn inward, enter her bloodstream and kill her. She an- nounced that she was going to find a doctor to perform a mastec- tomy just to be done with the damned thing.

Dr. Love noted that it had been two years since Shirley had a full set of films taken. So she ordered a mammogram—which showed a cluster of microcalcifications in the right breast, tiny pin- dots that looked like dandruff. If the spots were large and distinct a doctor might choose to monitor them rather than perform a surgi- cal biopsy. The troublesome ones, the ones that might signal DCIS, were tiny enough to fit inside a breast duct, and often clustered together. That was what Shirley had.

Love operated on Shirley's left breast for the infection and per- formed a surgical biopsy on the calcifications on the right. The pathologist came back with what Shirley called a "half-empty, half-full diagnosis, like a wart inside the duct that either was or wasn't something," and she incorporated the news into her comedy repertoire. She told people she had "intraductal papillomatosis, or something like that—it sounds like butterflies with bad breath."

No bad news was not quite the same as getting good news, but Shirley was happy. Dr. Love's surgery seemed to work. For the first time in a year she was symptom-free on the left side. The right side? Beneath worry. Shirley Barber grew up watching Ben Casey and Dr. Kildare on television, and those guys always operated on tumors. A tumor was trouble. Flecks on the film were God's little prank.

A month later, when the symptoms of infection returned, Love asked Shirley for permission to operate on both breasts again. Cal- cifications are invisible to the surgeon, who removes tissue guided only by a wire inserted in the breast by a technician who uses the mammogram as a map. Dr. Love saw a few specks remaining at the original site on Shirley's post-biopsy mammogram, and she wanted to remove them.

Always eager for a clean slate, Shirley agreed. Three days later she got the phone call that started her on the road to insomnia. This time the diagnosis was clear. Shirley Barber had breast cancer in her right breast—kind of. She had DCIS, ductal carcinoma in situ, the kind that might never turn into invasive cancer but had to be treated anyway.

The diagnosis was only the first step down a bewildering path. The tissue sample Love removed had dirty margins, malignant cells so close to the edge of the sample that there might still be DCIS left in the breast. Laura Wilcox was facing a mastectomy for DCIS—the therapy with the best success rate—because she had extensive DCIS and invasive cancer as well. Since Shirley seemed to have only a discrete area of DCIS, she could choose from a list of options.

She did not get the closure she so yearned for. Instead, she got percentages and options. Shirley could have a mastectomy with or without radiation, which gave her a five percent chance of recurrence—half the time more DCIS, half the time invasive cancer. She could have a wide excision, a lumpectomy, in which the surgeon removed an even larger segment of the breast and hoped for clean margins, with or without radiation. With the surgery and radiation she had a ten percent chance of recurrence, two percent DCIS and eight percent invasive cancer; with surgery alone the chance of recurrence jumped to twenty percent, evenly split between DCIS and invasive cancer.

She could join a five-year national clinical trial of the drug tamoxifen with radiation, conducted by the National Surgical Adjuvant Breast and Bowel Project, the cooperative group run by Dr. Bernard Fisher at the University of Pittsburgh. Tamoxifen blocked estrogen receptors on cancer cells that were estrogen-receptor positive—it locked into the space on the receptor where estrogen was supposed to fit and denied the cell the estrogen that fed its malignant growth. It was milder than chemotherapy, and comparably effective for postmenopausal women who were estrogen-receptor positive; research showed that it decreased the recurrence rate by as much as forty percent. But there were side effects, including an increased risk of uterine cancer, blood clots, and for younger women, premature menopause. The NSABP had tamoxifen protocols for women who already had breast cancer, like Shirley, and another for high-risk women, to see if tamoxifen acted as a preventive.

The treatment trial that was open to Shirley, Protocol B-24, was intended as a randomized control study, in which women were assigned to receive either tamoxifen or a placebo, with no one, not the patients nor the researchers, knowing who got what. It had opened in May 1991, with a target accrual of eighteen hundred patients nationwide, but so far only eight hundred women had been randomly assigned.

Or Shirley could go home and do nothing and hope that she was one of the lucky seventy percent whose precancer never turned into invasive disease. None of the treatments was a guaranteed cure. Each one was a hedged bet.

She chose the clinical trial of tamoxifen and radiation. For all her frustrated threats during the year she had an infection, Shirley was not ready for a mastectomy—nor was anyone in her family. Her son, Mitch, was in a panic that she was going to die before she met her grandchildren. Her daughter, Kim, said she just wanted her mother well. Tracy could barely tolerate the idea of his wife having to endure more surgery. As far as he was concerned, mastectomy was something to consider only if the other approaches failed.

A wide excision made no sense. Shirley had small breasts. If Love were going to take a sizeable piece of tissue she might as well perform a mastectomy. Doing nothing was hardly an option for a woman who had fashioned a substantial, middle-class life out of dead-ends and disappointment. The trial appealed to Shirley. With luck the radiation alone would kill off any malingering cancer cells. And testing the drug made her feel that she was doing something for Kim, making a contribution to the health of the next generation.

That was why she welcomed the night sweats that often woke her up, even though they guaranteed another exhausted day. Shirley Barber had already gone through early menopause. She knew what a hot flash felt like and hadn't had one in a couple of years. She ticked off every sweat as evidence that the little pills she got in registered bottles of two hundred were the real thing. Maybe it would make a difference.

For she had a new goal, a small one, granted, but one that would make her feel a little bit safer. All Shirley Barber wanted was a clean mammogram the next time around. No specks. No shadows. Just a nice, clean, regular mammogram like most women her age. It would buy her a break until the next mammogram, a chance to act like a healthy person and maybe get some sleep.

She took her pills and waited for a reprieve.

Jerilyn Goodman knew, at thirty-eight, that she had breast cancer, though with a clean mammogram she had only a groundless hunch to support her claim. The great frustration of her life was how long it took—five years—to convince the doctors that they and their physical exams and their mammograms were wrong about the mass in her breast, and she was right.

A small, athletic woman with short, light brown hair and limpid, hazel eyes, Goodman took a perverse pleasure in telling people her saga. She had first felt a thickening in her left breast back in 1988, when she was living in Madison, Wisconsin, and immediately went in for a mammogram. The radiologist saw nothing. Goodman consulted two surgeons, who examined her and said it was nothing. An ultrasound showed nothing. Jerilyn never stopped worrying, but she did stop going to specialists about it.

In 1991 she moved to Los Angeles and went to work as a freelance television producer. Two years later she got a summer job at CBS's Los Angeles news bureau. It was a great summer: Goodman was made the interim weekend evening news producer, and there was talk of a job in either New York or Washington in the fall, which would allow her to be closer to her lover, a woman who worked in New York as a television news producer. At the end of the summer, in September—because her fear nagged at her—she went to a doctor for a physical and mentioned the mass in her breast. This time her internist suggested that she have a biopsy.

She called her lover, who luckily was coming out from New York for work. She chose a surgeon at Cedars-Sinai, a private hospital in West Hollywood, to perform a needle aspiration, in which a thin needle is inserted into a suspicious lump to extract cells. As soon as it was over the couple left town for a long weekend.

On Monday morning Jerilyn called the surgeon's office for her results, and an assistant she did not know told her there were atypical cells. She needed to schedule a surgical biopsy.

Suddenly Jerilyn could not remember how to breathe. She looked around the room at the bed-and-breakfast inn where they were staying and thought about how strange it was not to recognize anything. She thought about the words *atypical cells* and realized she had not a clue about how much trouble she was in.

"What does that mean?" she managed to get out.

"Well, there were just some atypical cells and we couldn't tell," said the assistant, "and he wants to take a closer look at it."

It was only after she hung up that Goodman realized the doctor had not offered to talk to her. She walked into the other room and told her lover what had happened, and they sat down together and traded reassurances. It didn't mean anything, necessarily. No need to jump ahead and assume the worst.

All the while Goodman thought about her grandmother, who had had breast cancer, and her aunt, who had a mastectomy in the 1950s, and her great-grandmother, who had succumbed to what everyone in the family assumed was breast cancer. In the last years of her grandmother's life the Goodman family had traveled from New Jersey to California every winter, and one of Jerilyn's responsibilities was to help the frail Mary in and out of the bathtub. She was used to the sight of a woman with one breast and a scar—and now she remembered the eerie sense she used to have that she was destined to end up that way as well.

Goodman had a surgical biopsy on a Friday and was told to come in to get the results the following Monday. The surgeon's office called the afternoon of her appointment to recommend that she come in with a friend.

"Why?"

"Well, good news or bad, it's better to have somebody with you because it's so emotional."

Goodman had planned to go alone because she did not want to think she had cancer, and if she did not have cancer she hardly needed a companion to hold her hand. She went through a list of people in her head. Her lover was back in New York, and Jerilyn was not sure their relationship could bear the weight of more trouble. Jerilyn had few close friends in Los Angeles. She had not yet told her family, and anyway, they were all on the East Coast. She called a new friend who agreed to meet her at the doctor's, only to tell her, as they headed up to his office, that she had news of her own: she was pregnant.

Goodman congratulated her and thought, That's it. Even the person who is supposed to be here to support me isn't really here. I am all alone.

They waited an hour to see the doctor and Goodman told herself that was because he was giving someone else bad news, not because he was reluctant to face her. When he finally did appear he insisted on examining the biopsy scar—and as he did Goodman decided she must be all right because he had not yet said otherwise. Then he straightened up.

"Why don't you get dressed and come into my office to talk?" he said. "This is not a life-threatening situation, but we do have to talk. We have a problem."

She got through the next hour in a stupor. Goodman and her friend sat in the surgeon's office while he drew pictures of the ways cells changed, and after each drawing Jerilyn asked, "Is this it? Am I at this point?" and the doctor said, "No." Finally he got to what he called "microscopic invasive cancer." Goodman had a small tumor and extensive DCIS, so he wanted to perform a mastectomy as soon as possible—right after he got back from vacation in ten days. If she picked an oncologist and a plastic surgeon in the meantime, they could get to work.

An hour later she was in her car with a handful of the surgeon's business cards bearing the names of doctors he had referred her to for treatment and reconstructive surgery. Just like that.

She could not eat or sleep for three days. Her stomach was in revolt, and if she did eat she had diarrhea. All she could think about was that she was going to die.

But she quickly snapped into her producer mode: she had to think of this not as a personal crisis, but as an assignment that she had ten days to complete. Jerilyn started making calls as though she were arranging appointments for someone else, for some poor sad woman with breast cancer who was the subject of the story she was working on.

The plastic surgeon's office was unbelievable to her—filled with antique furniture, the way she imagined a mansion in Beverly Hills must look. There was a tray with water glasses and a crystal decanter, and floating in the water were little slices of lemon. She told the nurse she wasn't sure if she was ready to consider plastic surgery, but the nurse reassured her.

"They'll do a wonderful job," she said, "and no one will ever know."

She put Goodman into the examining room, and moments later a tall, imposing man in surgical scrubs came in. He told her he could make a breast that was so lifelike no one who touched her would ever know the difference, and Goodman thought, I will. He asked to examine her and told her she had beautiful breasts, and Goodman thought, I can't believe you're telling me this. This is 1993. Wake up.

The doctor told her that there was no medical evidence that silicone implants would cause problems, and Goodman thought, You guys must be crazy.

"To tell the truth," she said, "I'm not even sure I want reconstructive surgery."

The surgeon and nurse replied, almost in unison, "Why not?"

"Look at me," said Goodman. "I don't do anything with my hair. I don't wear any makeup." She was trying to explain that beyond being clean and neat, physical appearance was not a major concern of hers. The surgeon replied that if she got dressed his assistant in the next room would review the options with her in detail.

Goodman dutifully accepted a packet of information about the surgeon and his services and started to drive home, thinking that none of this felt right to her. She detoured to a friend's house because she could not handle being home alone, broke into sobs as soon as she got in the door, and announced, "I have to see Susan Love."

7

THE ELUSIVE CURE

JERILYN HAD SEEN A PUBLIC TELEVISION DOCUMENTARY ON LOVE A FEW weeks before, and the next morning she called to make an appointment. The facilitator told her that Love did not make private appointments with newly diagnosed cancer patients. They attended the multidisciplinary clinic, where they were seen either by Love or one of the other surgeons on the team. Jerilyn was not interested. To her the word *clinic* meant thirty women waiting for their number to be called.

She decided to try again. "Somebody I know," she told her friend, "has to know somebody who knows somebody who knows her and will get me in." Jerilyn tried everything she could think of to get a guaranteed appointment with Love—an academic connection, a lesbian connection, a medical connection—until she found a friend whose father was a trustee on the board of the UCLA School of Medicine. He called the dean's office, the dean's office called the Breast Center, and Jerilyn got an appointment for the following day. She would have to go through the multi process and see the other specialists, but Susan Love would probably be the surgeon on her case.

Love told her things she did not want to hear in a way she could stand to hear them. The tumor was not microscopic, although it was small, probably between 1 and 1.5 centimeters. She did have to have a mastectomy because of the DCIS. Love could do nothing about the *ifs* that had followed Jerilyn every day since her internist sent her for the biopsy, pesky little insect thoughts that buzzed around her brain and kept her from finding any peace. They would never know if there was a tumor back in 1988, or only precancer. There was no way to tell if the years since had bought the disease a better chance to kill her. Love told Jerilyn what she had told Shirley and countless other patients. She would know for a certainty that she was cured when she died of something else.

But Love could treat her—and saw no reason for her to have plastic surgery if she didn't want to. Jerilyn had a friend take black-and-white photographs of her, naked from the waist up, so she would remember what she looked like, and arranged to have her surgery on November 19, 1993. When a facilitator from the Breast Center called to move it up to the eighteenth Jerilyn, a devout Jew, heard the angels singing. The eighteenth letter of the Hebrew alphabet was *ch'ai,* which was the symbol for life.

The day of the surgery divided itself into two parts: when Susan Love was around Jerilyn felt safe; when she wasn't, Jerilyn didn't. Jerilyn arrived at the UCLA main hospital, a sprawling old building whose side entrance was across the street from the Breast Center, at six o'clock in the morning, accompanied by her mother, her father, and an eighteen-inch teddy bear in a Wisconsin T-shirt. A Valium the night before and another when she woke up had enforced an outward calm.

She checked in and was directed to the waiting room upstairs. When the orderly arrived and uttered those fateful words—"It's time to go"—she felt her heart flop.

Jerilyn climbed onto the bed to be rolled away. Her father had gone back down to the lobby because patients could have only one person with them in the surgery waiting room. Her mother leaned over, gave her a kiss and a hug, and said, "I wish it could have been me instead of you."

Jerilyn knew it was only the drugs that kept her from bursting into tears. All she could think was, No parent should have to say that.

"It'll be all right, Mom," she said, and the orderly maneuvered the bed into the hall. She believed that the operation would go well; as for the long-term, that was anyone's guess. What frightened her at the moment were two things—that she might die of the anesthesia or wake up puking.

She carried her attitude into the operating room. When Love entered with a cheery, "Hello, beautiful," Jerilyn thought to herself, She must use that because she cannot remember all her patients' names. When Love started chatting with her, Jerilyn thought, I have read too much about her shtick. We ought to be focused on what is about to happen. I am not at all swayed by her performance.

Ten seconds later Jerilyn was asleep, and her last conscious thought was that Love had done a nice job of distracting her while the anesthesiologist put the intravenous line in her hand.

She woke up freezing cold, no sensation in her left arm, swathed in bandages, with an oxygen mask on her face. All she wanted in the world was for one of the strangers who worked in that room to come over to her. The woman in the next bed was screaming. The two nurses who were standing nearby had not noticed that Jerilyn was awake. She tried to raise her right arm to get someone's attention, and finally a nurse came over, checked her vital signs, took the mask off her face, and walked away again. The man in the bed on Jerilyn's other side began to call out, "I'm going to be sick." She could not recall ever having been so afraid.

When the nurse returned, Jerilyn mustered her courage and asked weakly, "Would you hold my hand?" She was so cold and so scared. He took her hand, and his was warm, and so comforting, but after just a minute he begged off. He had other patients to look after.

A little while later an orderly took her back up to her room. She looked around the crowded elevator and said to herself, This is just like a movie. Here I am in an elevator, and these other people are looking at me, thinking, "She's just had an operation." Her anxious parents were waiting for her, but by then all Jerilyn wanted was to sleep it off.

*   *   *

She awoke at dinnertime feeling much better, and sent her parents out to eat. In the aftermath of the surgery Jerilyn was woozy with delight. Here she was in a private room on the ninth floor, where the meals were like room service in a swank hotel— lobster, red wine if she wanted it, chocolate mousse for dessert. She could not help but laugh. She had spent the last ten days learning everything she could about dietary restrictions and the prevention of breast cancer, and the hospital was plying her with rich food.

She was almost cocky when the nurse came in and told her it was time to pee. She brought Jerilyn a bedpan, but nothing happened. They both waited, to no avail. The nurse told her that if she did not urinate by eight o'clock they would have to insert a catheter. The deadline did not make it any easier.

At that moment Love strode in.

"Hi, beautiful," she boomed. "How are you?"

This time Jerilyn welcomed the familiar greeting.

"I'm okay," she said, in a tremulous voice, "but I can't pee." She did not want a catheter; she did not want anyone doing anything else to her body, but she felt as though she had temporarily lost the ability to defend herself.

"You can get up," said Love, as though the bedpan were an insult. "Just get up."

The nurse was flabbergasted at the suggestion, and it turned out not to be all that easy. The two surgical drains that had been inserted to siphon off fluid hurt when Jerilyn stood up, each one attached to a plastic bottle whose weight tugged at her chest. She felt shaky and afraid to walk, and she worried about the portable intravenous stand that dripped fluid into her arm. The nurse helped her slowly shuffle into the bathroom and sit on the toilet.

Jerilyn anxiously reported, "Nothing's happening."

The nurse instructed her to press with one finger on either side of her bladder. She did. It worked. She was back in charge of her body, at least in a small way, and it made her feel much better. Love had left while Jerilyn was in the bathroom, but the effect of her visit was obvious. Jerilyn's parents took one look at her when they returned and announced that they had their old girl back again.

They were sitting around the following evening when Love showed up again and flopped down on the floor, rather than ask either of Jerilyn's parents to give up their chairs. Jerilyn's lymph nodes looked fine; Love was there to visit. So they talked about nothing much at all.

Afterward, Jerilyn often thought about that night. She called it a "defining moment." Love was sitting on the floor in her hospital room acting as though there was no place else in the world she wanted to be, as though she was not in a hurry to get home to her own family. She was not just a surgeon who had performed a mastectomy; she was taking care of Jerilyn in a much broader sense, and Jerilyn gave in to her completely. No more wiseass defenses. She believed fully in Susan Love.

The next morning, when Love had the audacity to suggest that Jerilyn take off the big bandages and start getting used to how she looked, Jerilyn did so.

In the two months since her operation, Jerilyn had devoted herself to learning everything she could about her cancer. She was stuck on one issue: UCLA did not administer chemotherapy to women whose tumors were under one centimeter in diameter, and if a mass was between one and two centimeters the decision was based on other prognostic factors.

Jerilyn's tumor was about 1.5 centimeters. Her other indicators were positive—she was particularly proud of her S-phase, which was very low—but still she worried. Some studies suggested that all patients would benefit from chemotherapy. Jerilyn was having a hard time deciding what to do.

She came in for her January 14 appointment ready to debate, all bluster and purpose. She carried *The New York Times* and her file of medical records under her arm, and wore the uniform of the Westside media crowd—a T-shirt, wool blazer, blue jeans, and running shoes.

It was armor, all of it, and not quite enough to silence the suspicious, superstitious imp Jerilyn carried around inside her. Other women might ask, Why me? Jerilyn's response to her plight was, Of course it's me. I've been telling you all along it was me. She needed help getting the voice of doom to shut up.

But there was no right answer. It was, Love told her, one of those times when all a doctor could do was have "a balanced discussion with the patient, meaning we don't know what the fuck to do." None of the doctors Jerilyn had seen before coming to UCLA had recommended chemotherapy. Love did not think she needed it. The only dissenter had suggested tamoxifen, the drug Shirley Barber hoped she was taking as part of the clinical trial.

That one suggestion, and the reading she had done since her surgery, ate at Jerilyn's precarious confidence. One of the hardest things for many patients to accept was that there was nothing more they could or should do. If a single doctor thought that more treatment might help, a woman was hard-pressed to disagree. Jerilyn had already had a long conversation with Love about chemotherapy, and she knew the odds for node-negative patients—seven would survive without drugs, two died despite treatment, and only one survived because of chemotherapy.

Jerilyn had decided instinctively that she was not that one. She wanted to believe she was one of the seven, worried that she was one of the two, but somehow never imagined herself as the woman whose life depended on chemicals.

Mostly she wanted to be able to stop thinking about it. Today her first question was about tamoxifen, and she was relieved when Love brusquely dismissed it. "A 2.5 percent chance it'll help," she said. She had little patience for doctors who prescribed young drugs like tamoxifen outside of clinical trials. There wasn't enough data yet to show that it was useful in a case like this, and as long as doctors in private practice kept prescribing it outside of the trials there would continue to be insufficient data. It was a vicious cycle: What they learned was lost to the public, reduced to individual anecdotes within the confines of one doctor's office, and Love believed that some doctors prescribed it incorrectly precisely because they were not bound by the discipline of research—raising a dose when they ought to lower it, misunderstanding what tamoxifen could and could not do.

Love agreed with Dr. Glaspy, who as head of the Oncology Center was the court of last resort on systemic treatment issues. If there was reason to believe that any cancer remained after the surgery, they administered chemotherapy. Some doctors liked to prescribe tamoxifen as an alternative because it was less harsh a regimen than chemotherapy, but Love disliked that approach. Either you fought cancer in the way that was best for the patient—and premenopausal women responded best to chemotherapy—or you did nothing. You did not pick a halfway measure because it was easier to tolerate.

"But there are still women with all these results, like mine, who still get metastatic disease, right?" asked Jerilyn.

"Five percent," replied Love. "It's always possible. There's no one hundred percent. But you're as close as we get."

"I just want to be sure I don't need further treatment."

Love spoke in round, measured tones, like a priest uttering a benediction. But she chose her words as carefully as a lawyer: "I do not believe you need further treatment," she said, which did not mean that Jerilyn would never be back, only that the facts, which often lied, said she was pretty safe.

"Okay," said Jerilyn. "I needed to hear you say that."

Love reminded her that several oncologists had told her she did not need chemotherapy, even though they stood to make money if she had it. That was Love's standard measure of a doctor's honesty. If he would have made a profit but still advised against a particular treatment, it must really be unnecessary.

Jerilyn was prepared not to have chemotherapy as long as someone helped her with the attendant anxiety. "I'm totally paranoid," she confessed. "I need some hand-holding." She wanted to believe her surgeon, but she had seen too many doctors who had told her not to worry and been wrong.

It was the kind of reckless mistake people made when they were conned by their own bad news into thinking that nothing worse can happen. Laura had a friend, a man in his twenties, and though they had never been lovers she let him spend the night, just once, about a week after her diagnosis, because she couldn't think of any reason not to. She was lonely. It was easier being with him than with someone new, and certainly better than being alone. He didn't even live in Los Angeles anymore. One night's intimacy and no repercussions.

Except now she was pregnant and loath to have an abortion. He had returned to New York before she had gone to UCLA the first time, and had no idea what had happened. She was not inclined to tell him. She was back in an examining room a week after her initial appointment to find out if she could protect her health and keep the baby.

Laura sat on one of the chairs in chic workday black and listened as Love explained her options. Laura could not have the mastectomy in her first trimester because general anesthesia increased the chance of miscarriages, and she could not have it in the third trimester because of the possibility of premature birth. She ought to avoid general anesthesia altogether if she could. Love felt that the most reasonable compromise was to perform a wide excision right away under a local anesthetic to get rid of the rest of the invasive cancer, and wait until after the child was born to have the mastectomy for the DCIS, with simultaneous reconstruction.

Love knew that many surgeons would tell a patient like Laura to have surgery as soon as she was past her first trimester, but she disagreed. As long as the margins were clean, and the systemic threat eradicated, there was no need to risk sacrificing the pregnancy to a condition that might never become life-threatening.

But she felt compelled to remind Laura of one other variable. Women with negative nodes had a thirty percent chance of recurrence in the first five years. Women with between one and four positive nodes had a fifty percent chance. With one positive node in 1988, Laura had, by Love's estimate, a thirty-five to forty percent chance of recurrence. Chemotherapy had decreased that risk by one-third, but it was still possible. She had to decide if she wanted to have a child, knowing that she might not live to raise it.

"People either say 'No, if I'm not going to be here I don't want anyone else to raise my kid,' or they say 'Yes, whatever time I have, it's worth it,' " said Love.

Laura said she wanted to keep the baby—although even as the

words came out of her mouth she wondered if she ought to have an abortion. If she kept the child she would eventually have to tell the father. She wasn't sure she wanted a long-term relationship with him, nor was she sure she could handle the pressure of being a single working mom. But at the moment feelings overrode logic. This was the only bit of good news she had heard about herself in months. She had conceived a child.

Love offered to try the wide excision, and teased Laura about the benefits of having the mastectomy and reconstruction after childbirth.

"At that point," she said, with a sly smile, "you might welcome a tummy tuck." But if the margins were dirty, if she was unable to excise all the invasive cancer, Laura would have to have the mastectomy in her second trimester, and wait four or five months for the plastic surgery.

At that Laura began to clench and unclench her fists, and she nervously pursed her lips. Love tried to cheer her up: there was no point in having reconstruction while she was pregnant, even if it were possible. Her healthy breast would be swollen. Dr. Shaw would not be able to make one to match its normal size.

Laura studied her worrying fingers. She blamed the 1988 chemotherapy for screwing up her periods and making it impossible to tell when she was ovulating. Laura's situation was trickier than early menopause. She ovulated. She just couldn't predict when. The month before, she'd had two periods, two weeks apart.

She could have used a diaphragm and didn't. She had to admit the truth.

"I have been trying, in my own way, to get pregnant the last couple of years," she said with a sigh.

So they decided on the wide excision in three weeks, once Love returned from a week's vacation in Hawaii. At the last moment, as the surgeon was about to walk out the door, Laura stopped her. She was already on the schedule for a mastectomy and reconstruction the following Thursday—a difficult bit of scheduling, given the crammed calendars of Dr. Love and Dr. Shaw. Could Love leave her on the surgery schedule just for one more day, so she could think it over?

"It was a bitch to find a day when you and Dr. Shaw were

both available," she said. "I'll go home tonight and do my soul-searching."

Love walked out to the desk and asked Shannon, one of the facilitators, to keep Laura on the schedule overnight. This was a hard call. A recent study showed that pregnancy did not make cancer grow more quickly, despite earlier concerns that it did, but it wasn't a sure thing.

Love had just had a call from Dr. Jeanne Petrek, a colleague at Manhattan's Memorial Sloan-Kettering who specialized in women who were diagnosed while pregnant, or became pregnant after they had been treated—not because she chose the specialty but, like Dr. Love, because the specialty chose her. Petrek thought there was a causal link between pregnancy and recurrence—and that finding it was only a matter of following enough women for a sufficient amount of time. Estrogen levels rose dramatically during pregnancy, and some researchers believed that the increase fueled malignant growth. Love held back from agreeing with her, not because she thought Petrek was wrong, but only because she tried not to endorse even educated hunches. To her mind there was not enough data to decide.

On that point, the two women agreed. Petrek was writing a grant proposal for an ambitious ten-year study of about one thousand breast cancer patients under the age of forty-four, to see who got pregnant, who suffered a recurrence, and whether there was in fact a connection. If doctors knew that pregnancy made recurrence likelier, women like Laura might choose not to have children; if they knew it had no effect they could eliminate a layer of anxiety.

Without the data, doctors were reduced to instinct and informed guesswork. Some argued for immediate abortion simply because there was no guarantee that the pregnancy, and the spurt in estrogen that accompanied it, would not cause the cancer to grow more quickly. Laura did have one positive lymph node, which increased the possibility that there were malignant cells elsewhere in her body. Love wanted to be less doctrinaire—to take a woman's desire for a family into account—but it was hard to know what to do.

She yearned for hard numbers, but they did not exist and would not for years. Love stomped down the hall, late to a meeting with two other doctors, Dr. Charles Haskell, a medical oncologist, and Dr. Robert Parker, a radiation therapist, with whom she was writing a chapter on breast disease for a medical textbook. They were older men who had had time to become accustomed to uncertainty, but today Love was in no mood for their detached, scholarly air. She was spoiling for a fight, cranky about how much they still did not know.

No matter what they said she interrupted to set them straight, as though it were her job to bring them into the here and now.

Haskell chided her gently. If they disagreed they would work to arrive at a consensus, and that was the best they could do.

He asked her for her definition of "cure." It was a controversial term. Patients talked about being five years out as though that were an absolute demarcation; before it you were still at risk and the day after your anniversary you were cured. Doctors knew it was not necessarily so. Love had seen too many women recur at seven, eight, even ten years to buy that definition, much as she might want to. She thought that the five-year marker worked for some fast-growing cancers, like certain lymphomas—and she knew that doctors wanted to believe the same was true of breast cancer. But it was irresponsible to tell women they were cured at five years. Breast cancer grew slowly. She had seen too many bleak surprises.

Love did not believe in the notion of a "cure." The best she could offer Haskell was a churlish, "You die of a stroke at ninety-five." This time she did not mean it as a joke.

Haskell attempted a dignified reply. "Mine? There is personal cure and statistical cure. Personal cure is very difficult to come to terms with unless it leaves a marker." But breast cancer never announced it was gone. Love was right: the only way to determine if a woman was cured was if something else got her first.

Haskell went on. "For almost everything it's statistical, and it's the point where other factors act on the population at large and the patient with breast cancer in the same way—the survival curves are parallel." He was talking about the point at which breast cancer patients succumbed to other illnesses as often as members of the rest of the population. "You don't get that in breast cancer until fifteen years."

Love refused to rise above her despondency.

"Or maybe never," she muttered.

8

PATRONAGE

I T WAS FRIDAY, FEBRUARY 4, FIVE DAYS BEFORE LOVE'S FORTY-SIXTH
birthday, a date she often ignored because it fell so close to her
late sister Debbie's birthday. This year she had forgotten it because Monday was the first day of a week's vacation, a much more
important event in her overextended life than the beginning of another year. But her staff remembered, ordering a cake from a shop
that specialized in erotic pastries, and surprised her at the regular
Friday morning staff meeting.

HAPPY BIRTHDAY AND BREAST WISHES, read the frosting inscription at
the base of the cake, which was shaped like two large, perfectly
shaped breasts, their rosy nipples pointing heavenward. Love
hacked away gleefully and pressed a large piece on everyone, even
though it was only eight in the morning.

Sherry Goldman began to chuckle. "Look at what she's doing,"
she said. "She's cutting around the nipple."

Love lit her own candles and hesitated. "Shall I wish for the
Barbra Streisand Breast Center, and all our problems will be over?"

The West Coast viewing of Streisand's $4 million Art Deco and
Art Nouveau collection was scheduled for February 16—and the
UCLA Breast Center was going to receive the proceeds from ticket
sales. One of Streisand's staff members had called UCLA to inquire
about a rumor that breast cancer was more prevalent among afflu-

ent Westside Jewish women. Sherry Goldman had taken the call and asked Susan, who said the rumor was true.

The next thing they knew, Streisand had decided to give them money—perhaps as much as $200,000, according to the people who were organizing the $250-per-ticket event.

More important, Love would have a chance to speak with Streisand at the viewing. She was sure that if she could just get the entertainer alone for a few minutes she could convince Streisand of the need for a more significant contribution. Love wanted $10 million to finance a dedicated center that offered more programs, including a clinic for women with breast implants and expanded services for women with benign breast problems, as well as research projects and an educational program for the primary care providers who sat at the hub of the managed care system. As February 16 drew closer she began to think of Streisand as her savior.

"I have high hopes," she confessed, passing plates of cake around. "High hopes. We'll see. She could write the check without blinking."

They joked about what the $10 million would buy. A secret tunnel directly to the garage so the staff could avoid bumping into difficult patients. A special button to make the floor open up and whoosh a patient downstairs for a mammogram. A phone machine message that Love had wanted for years: "All our facilitators are busy. While you are waiting, please do a breast exam. If the lump is larger than five centimeters, press one. If it is smaller but there is redness, press two. If the lump has disappeared, please hang up."

But Streisand represented serious opportunity, and Love intended to make a good impression. She made an appointment with her Nordstrom's shopper for eight o'clock in the morning on her first day back from vacation. She might not care about clothes, but Streisand and the other guests did.

Dr. Dennis Slamon, chief of the Division of Hematology-Oncology and director of clinical research at UCLA's Jonsson Comprehensive Cancer Center, had not focused on the fact that Love was on vacation, so he showed up at the multidisciplinary conference on the following Friday, February 11, expecting to find her there. What he found instead was confusion. There was no surgeon at the conference because of a scheduling mistake. No one could quite figure out how to proceed, and the patients were due back in an hour.

Slamon was furious. He had helped to conceive this project, and his department contributed $50,000 annually to keep it afloat. Love was supposed to be his clinical counterpart, running the patient programs while he supervised the research effort—but Denny had begun to think that what Susan really needed was a boss to keep her in line. He stormed over to Sherry Goldman and, in front of all the others, demanded, "Where's Susan?"

"On vacation."

"How can she ask surgeons to work here?" he demanded, wondering how she could expect other doctors to be disciplined when she was sitting on a beach somewhere. Love took six weeks of vacation annually, which seemed excessive to Denny, and he took this occasion to make his grievance public. "She's gone too often. *Tell her that.*"

Goldman was trembling with rage. She was sure that Slamon would never talk to another doctor or another man like that. He was yelling at her only because she was a woman and a nurse, two steps down the ladder. She took a step forward so she was standing right in front of him and bit off the only words she could manage without bursting into tears.

"*You* tell her," she said, and stormed out of the room.

Denny Slamon was in thrall to his work. He and John Glaspy agreed that the only way to make progress was to stick to it, long hours, every day, all year. Anyone who did not keep up risked falling behind—and the one thing Denny Slamon was determined not to do was falter. It had taken too much effort to get where he was.

He had done everything in his power to make sure that life took notice of him. Denny was supposed to go to work in the coal mines of New Castle, Pennsylvania, like the other men in his family, except that the family pediatrician, a noble, dignified man, gave him an idea: He could be something else.

He was the first person in his family to go to college, let alone medical school. Having escaped, he was driven by an outsize ambition, as though he feared he would be sucked back into that dead-end coal town unless he pushed forward harder than anyone else. He did not want to be a clinician—to spend his days eliciting symptoms from patients and using other men's discoveries to treat them. He wanted to explore. He wanted a big specialty, one where he would have the chance to make a dramatic discovery. Denny Slamon was not interested in dedicated anonymity.

In 1982 he got involved with a group at UCLA that was looking for molecular changes in common human cancers. Researchers before them had done work on rare cancers—on retinoblastoma, a malignancy of the eye, or on certain leukemias, or on lymphoma, a cancer of the lymph system. Slamon wanted to work on common tumors like breast cancer, in the hope of finding genetic mutations that would contribute to a greater basic understanding of the disease.

In 1986 he and a research technician located an alteration in the HER-2/neu gene that seemed to occur in about one quarter of all breast cancer cases. In healthy women, HER-2/neu was an "accelerator" gene that regulated normal cell growth. It worked properly in most breast cancer patients, as well. But sometimes a mutation made a woman produce too many copies of the gene—she "overexpressed" HER-2/neu, and developed an aggressive form of the disease. If researchers could develop an antibody to attack the HER-2/neu oncogene, they might be able to help a group of patients who too often did not respond to traditional chemotherapy.

Slamon published his findings in 1987, and from that moment his attention shifted entirely to breast cancer. It was a medical backwater, but that was fine with him. Where others saw a bleak horizon, Slamon saw the chance to accomplish something.

Though he rarely saw patients, Slamon had agreed in 1982 to see television executive Brandon Tartikoff, who had been referred by a mutual friend. Tartikoff had been treated for Hodgkin's disease in 1974 and pronounced cured, but lately he had been feeling listless and weak. Slamon reexamined all of his tissue samples and concluded that Tartikoff either had had a recurrence or had never been free of the cancer in the first place. Either way, he was extremely ill. Slamon subjected him to a grueling dual regimen, both the standard treatment and an experimental program, harvesting Tartikoff's bone marrow in case the treatments caused him eventually to develop leukemia.

When Tartikoff came out the other end in remission, his wife, Lilly, was determined to show Slamon the extent of their gratitude. A slender, elegant woman who had once danced for George Balanchine at the New York City Ballet, Lilly Tartikoff knew about diligence and discipline. She asked Slamon if she could raise private research money on his behalf—and when he demurred, insisting that all he asked of grateful patients was that they pay their bills on time, she refused to go away. She called him a couple of times a year until 1989, when she came up with a new approach. Lilly Tartikoff was determined to raise money for cancer research, and if Slamon was not going to let her she was going to work instead for Armand Hammer's group, Stop Cancer.

Slamon, by then eager to speed up his search for an antibody, decided it was time to change his mind. Tartikoff knocked on corporate doors on his behalf until she convinced Revlon's Ronald Perelman that paying for research was a greater contribution than paying for a more public treatment center. Perelman spent $600,000 on Denny Slamon's work in 1990, and had spent $800,000 every year since.

The Revlon money enabled Slamon to complete animal testing of a promising antibody, which in turn allowed him to progress to a Food and Drug Administration Phase I trial, in which he determined toxicity levels of the drug on human subjects with advanced metastatic disease who had failed to respond to other treatments. He was on the fast track, thanks to the infusion of private funds, and he worked as though there was not a moment to spare. Slamon was at his office, a monastic cubicle on a chilly laboratory floor in a building tucked behind the main hospital, by five thirty every morning, and he rarely got home before ten or eleven at night. He essentially worked two jobs: chairman of the Department of Hematology-Oncology during normal working hours, and HER-2/neu researcher before and after everyone else was at work.

Everything about him betrayed his preoccupation. His wardrobe, an endless array of pale oxford button-down shirts and khaki slacks, punctuated by plain dark suits that all looked alike, allowed him to get dressed without thinking. He wore what was left of his salt-and-pepper hair short; trimming his mustache was probably the greatest concession he made to grooming. He was a tall, muscular man prone to abrupt gestures and interruptions, who always seemed to be looking at his watch.

When UCLA decided in 1991 to establish a breast center, he was determined to recruit a clinician who matched his passion and had the proper respect for the researcher's role. It was the logical next step for him: to ally himself with a high-profile clinical program that would draw more patients to UCLA, and so provide a larger pool of potential subjects for his and other trials. One day the researchers would return the favor and supply clinicians with better therapeutic tools, based on those studies.

Dr. Michael Zinner, executive chairman of the Department of Surgery and chief of the Division of General Surgery within it, was officially in charge of the search committee, but Slamon was in the field, actively looking for candidates.

The University of California, Los Angeles, was an unlikely place for such a project. When the UCLA School of Medicine held its first classes in the fall of 1951, the university faced a dilemma: how to build a national reputation against prestigious East Coast medical schools like Harvard University's, which had been in operation for almost two hundred years.

The university was located in west Los Angeles, adjacent to the wealthy neighborhoods of Bel-Air, Beverly Hills, and Brentwood, the campus surrounded by the offices of successful private-practice doctors who catered to the residents of those affluent suburbs. The doctors represented a tremendous potential resource—instant credibility in the community as well as professional respect, both of which would reflect well on the fledgling medical school—but they were used to an entrepreneurial approach to medicine. They made money on medical initiative, and the only limit to their profits was the number of hours they were prepared to put in.

University medical schools historically had required a distinctly different outlook, one that called for a fiscal commitment to the collective good. Medical schools paid their full-time faculty members salaries. The revenues from their clinical practice went to fund that operation and then, when those costs were met, to support the department's growth.

Local doctors saw no advantage to that arrangement, which fairly guaranteed them smaller profits and a larger workload. So the university tried a hybrid approach and brought in doctors as though they were independent contractors. A physician was allowed to relocate his practice to the UCLA campus, his financial autonomy and profit structure secure, with the promise of endless medical students, interns, and residents to help him with his work.

There would be teaching responsibilities, but no real disadvantages in terms of either time or money. Doctors accepted the offer, and UCLA was able to invent an established medical school almost overnight. By 1991 the university's hospital was tied with Massachusetts General for third place in *U.S. News & World Report*'s annual survey of "America's Best Hospitals," behind Johns Hopkins Hospital and the Mayo Clinic. The medical school was ranked ninth in the nation.

Dr. Michael Zinner left Johns Hopkins in 1988 to run the second largest department in the UCLA School of Medicine, the Department of Surgery. Zinner, then forty-three, was a gastrointestinal surgeon and kingdom builder, a man who tackled big, difficult surgeries and the chance to rebuild a stagnant institution with equal relish. UCLA had maintained its national reputation for excellence, but had suffered in recent years from increasing local competition and the stigma of being a teaching hospital.

Zinner had found patients on the East Coast eager to come to a teaching hospital because they wanted the benefits of the latest research, but he now encountered a certain wariness about becoming a guinea pig. Some patients stayed away because they thought they had to participate in a study to see the doctors at UCLA—not true, but it might as well have been. UCLA had a reputation as a big laboratory, while private hospitals like St. Johns and Cedars-Sinai offered one-on-one care in a more exclusive setting. The university was trying to compete in what one medical center employee laughingly referred to as "a last bastion of beeper service medicine," where patients were used to lots of attention and specialized care. UCLA needed administrators who could restore its standing.

Zinner was a deceptively unassuming man, whose quiet manner belied a fierce determination. He came to UCLA with a radical agenda: he intended to turn a loose collection of programs into a dynamic set of cooperative departments. He had been part of a multidisciplinary gastroenterology group at Johns Hopkins, and it made sense to him. He wanted to restructure several UCLA programs in that image—to dismantle the old order and create a new one.

Breast cancer was a logical candidate, since specialists so often disagreed on the proper course of treatment and their options changed so rapidly—there was always speculation about new drugs, new combinations, new lifestyle changes that might help. He knew that Memorial Sloan-Kettering, among others, was talking about combining breast cancer services in a single facility, but Zinner wanted to take the concept one step further. He wanted to force debate by having the doctors sit down together on a regular basis to discuss their patients. As far as he was concerned, that caucus—which he envisioned as a challenging exchange of ideas, not a meeting defined by a single person's point of view—was even more important than the convenience such a program would offer.

The breast program was his first priority, and he had formidable support. The core group of planners included Zinner and Slamon, whose own division, hematology-oncology, was one of only two in the Department of Medicine that had always set an income ceiling and invested profits back into the division, as well as radiation oncologist Dr. Robert Parker and radiologist Dr. Larry Bassett.

He did not have the support of the university's preeminent breast surgeon, though. Dr. Armando Giuliano had been at UCLA since 1976, and was widely regarded as a superb surgeon. Giuliano had been pursuing a private donor for a $3 million endowment for his idea of a breast center, which differed dramatically from Zinner's. He believed in the weekly conference, but he saw no reason to corral a team of specialists to spend two afternoons a week seeing patients. He wanted what he considered to be a more efficient program, in which a woman saw all her specialists within a few day's time, at a single location, and they met weekly to review the cases.

Giuliano felt he was simply being practical, but his colleagues were determined to try their approach—which involved hiring at least one other breast surgeon to work alongside him. Giuliano turned them down and departed for St. John's, along with a few of his colleagues. Slamon was not surprised. Giuliano had always struck him as a brilliant surgeon, but something of a loner, not the type to get involved in a collaborative endeavor.

As a result, he and Zinner faced a more difficult challenge—not only to build a breast center, but to create a program that compensated for the departure of a very visible doctor. They decided to go outside the university to recruit a replacement, someone who could lend the program credibility in much the same way that those first doctors, in 1951, had endowed the School of Medicine with a reputation.

They needed a surgeon who had a high profile, preferably a woman and a breast specialist. That narrowed the field rather drastically, and put Dr. Susan Love at the top of the list. She was a provocative choice, a controversial woman who seemed to collect enemies every time she opened her mouth, but there was no denying that she would be a powerful asset. Slamon had met her when they both testified before a congressional subcommittee on the need for increased research funding, and was convinced that she was worth the attendant risk. It was hard to find a clinician who understood the importance of research as she did. Zinner had seen her on public television's *MacNeil/Lehrer NewsHour,* and was very impressed with her outspoken energy.

They began to make inquiries in Boston, and found that opinions about Susan Love were distressingly contradictory. Her detractors complained that she stole patients, flaunted her gay lifestyle, and subverted their best efforts by complaining about the poor state of breast cancer treatment. Her admirers said she got patients because she treated them well, was appropriately frank about her private life, and raised her voice in complaint because current treatment was, in fact, little more than habit injected with wishful thinking. Either the Faulkner Center was a progressive experiment in multidisciplinary care or it was the exile to which Love had retreated because she could not get along. Either she was a visionary who deserved support or a bad administrator who required help.

Zinner and Slamon were left with the question of whom they ought to believe. They decided that the benefits outweighed the possible problems—and to further dignify the choice they convinced themselves that UCLA was the one place where Love would mature and reach her full potential. They began a courtship. Michael Zinner, a lifelong academician, told Love that an affiliation with UCLA would give her the one thing she lacked, a substantial platform within the academic community. This was an opportunity for her to broaden the scope of her activities immensely—to bridge the academic and advocacy communities. Slamon appealed to her ambition and told her she could build a bigger, better center than she had in Boston.

They did not have a big donor to back the center, which was the traditional way to launch a new program, but that would come. When she said yes they were elated—and determined to keep close watch, to make sure that she succeeded. Susan Love would run the center. A steering committee, made up of the members of the selection committee and an administrator, would oversee her efforts.

Slamon and Love had argued about vacations before. She dismissed what she considered his "male model" of proper behavior and took short breaks every three to four months. She told anyone who wanted to listen that it was the only way to guarantee that she was at her best with her patients, fresh and full of energy.

As far as Slamon was concerned, that was patent nonsense. He couldn't believe she had gone to Hawaii, particularly when the center was floundering, which was how he saw it. The first year had been a nightmare of bad administration and confusion, of high-ticket programs that still did not draw enough patients to justify the cost. He had given Love more authority than he now thought was proper, and she had convinced him only that she needed a keeper.

"Slamon's Folly" was how some of his colleagues snidely referred to Dr. Love. Susan teased about going back to private practice if the center didn't work out, but Denny was a UCLA lifer. He had to make the program work.

His future depended on it. Slamon and Lilly Tartikoff had decided it was time to ask Ronald Perelman to make an even greater commitment to UCLA, and recently had submitted a formal proposal for a women's health center that would incorporate the breast program but also offer general health care. The Revlon/UCLA Women's Health Center would cost $7.5 million over the next seven years, including Slamon's annual research stipend.

Perelman was a businessman as well as a philanthropist. If the Breast Center was a healthy, growing operation he might well want to invest in it, but if there were two patients on a Wednesday afternoon and the director was on holiday he might reasonably think his money could be better spent elsewhere.

The only remedy Slamon could think of was to keep even closer tabs on Love—to make sure he dropped by the multi, to check in frequently with the new administrator who would arrive the following week, and to remind Susan exactly how important the next few months were. He could imagine a dark scenario in which Perelman decided not to fund a center and Zinner was pressured to pull the plug, and breast cancer care at UCLA reverted to individual surgeons seeing private patients. Slamon could not understand why Love refused to worry like he did. He despaired of getting her to take the threat seriously.

He had come to distrust her, believing that she oversimplified complex issues and warped the truth in the process. Denny shared Susan's feelings about the often slipshod nature of breast cancer care—unnecessary procedures, belligerent loyalty to the mastectomy, inappropriate optimism that only made the patient feel twice as bad when her treatment did not work. What upset him was the way Love talked about it. He hated her line about "slash, burn, and poison," because he thought it frightened patients and demoralized the decent doctors who were doing their best with limited resources. And he resented her barbs about how the government had managed to fund research that resulted in a test for prostate cancer, but not breast cancer.

No one had decided that prostate cancer was a political priority and breast cancer was not. Prostate cancer just happened to be easier to nab; Mother Nature was the one to blame for that.

He told Love again and again that she had a good enough case without resorting to slogans—and if she raised the level of her game she could have the respect of the medical community, as well as the patients' loyalty. Denny admired and depended on discipline, strict discourse, and long hours as proof of his colleagues' commitment. Anything else was a waste of time.

He heard a clock ticking, always. He had told Susan that they had twenty more years of their working lives to give to breast cancer. This was their turn at the wheel. He could not stand the notion that it might not work out the way he wanted it to.

Celebrity was relative. On February 16 Susan Love arrived unnoticed at the St. James Club, a restored Art Deco tower on Sunset Boulevard in West Hollywood. The shadowy bar was full of tastefully dressed people, most of them in minimalist black, who had paid $250 to catch a glimpse of a Tiffany lamp valued at between $800,000 and $1 million, or perhaps of its owner, Barbra Streisand. The good deed they were doing by contributing to the Breast Center was an ancillary pleasure. People who did not know Susan Love were perfectly prepared to ignore her.

She plunged in gamely, introducing herself left and right, answering questions and touting the center until the crowd began to move toward an adjacent room where the Streisand collection was on display.

It was there, after forty-five minutes of small talk and glances toward the door, that the atmosphere suddenly changed. The paparazzi, as though catching a scent, began to line up on the far side of the doorway. A phalanx of young men with receiver wire curling out of one ear marched into the room in two parallel lines, sliced the crowd in half, and then began to create a path by standing arm to arm and backing up.

Finally, fifteen minutes before the evening was supposed to end, Streisand came in, strode over to Susan Love, kissed her and chatted as though they had met many times before, and made sure the photographers got what they needed. With a practiced hand on Love's shoulder she guided the surgeon toward one of the Tiffany lamps. They posed with someone from Christie's. They posed with Margery Tabankin, who ran Streisand's foundation and was executive director of the Hollywood Women's Political Committee. They made their way back into the bar, where a microphone had been set up.

Streisand, skittish, leaned over and whispered to Love that she hated speaking in public, so Love decided to shorten her already brief comments rather than alienate the woman she perceived as her patron. Streisand thanked everyone for coming, introduced Dr. Love, and stepped aside. Dr. Love thanked everyone for coming, told them a bit about the Breast Center, and then it was over. Streisand was out the door before the applause died down.

"I didn't get the $10 million check," Love told her expectant staff early the next morning. "But I decided to wait to ask for that for the second date."

Later that morning Denny Slamon called Susan to ask her why the numbers were down—only two women at yesterday's multidisciplinary clinic. She tried to tell him how well the Christie's viewing had gone, but he wasn't interested. The Breast Center had to be popular before they could expect anyone to invest in it.

Neither of them brought up her vacation, although Love had heard about Slamon's outburst from Goldman. There was no point in arguing; the only thing that would change his mind was numbers.

Love knew nothing about getting research grants—except that Slamon was breathing down her neck, and she was drowning in paperwork. Grants were essential to the health of the program— they paid for research and attracted new researchers and students to the university. Studies also drew patients who were looking for the latest treatment. The field was fiercely competitive, and tightening up all the time. To Love it seemed an almost insurmountable challenge; a first-time applicant for NIH money had only a twenty percent chance of success, while researchers who already had NIH funds had a fifty percent success rate.

Slamon was all too familiar with what he called the catch-22 of federal funding: to get a grant a researcher had to present preliminary data, but to get preliminary data a researcher needed a grant. This year was the odd, probably temporary, exception. The infusion of money from the DOD meant that people who might not get funded by the NIH, like Susan, could still hope for a grant. He felt that Love ought to get a big grant from the Defense Department, if for no other reason than that she had been instrumental in getting that money earmarked for breast cancer. He knew that wasn't the way decisions got made, but this was her chance. He wanted her to exploit her position as much as possible.

Love was perfectly willing to do so. She disliked the process of writing applications, the endless details, the formal requests for federal Food and Drug Administration approval or a blessing from the university's Human Subjects Protection Committee. But she understood opportunity. She had three grants pending at the DOD—two large ones, for a statewide tissue bank and a registry of high-risk patients, and a smaller IDEA grant application involving a duct endoscope, a hair's-breadth scope that she wanted to insert through the nipple to study the ductal system of the breast. She had declined an invitation to serve on the Integration Panel, the review committee Visco was on that would evaluate DOD grant applications for relevance. It would have been a great honor—and a thrill, to be part of the first grant review committee that included advocates in the process. It was more important to stand in line for the money.

9

VISIBLE DAMAGE, INVISIBLE THREAT

NO MATTER WHAT A WOMAN DID ABOUT HER BREAST CANCER, there was always the other issue: how she felt about her breasts. They were her vanity, her sex life, her motherhood, an outward symbol of an attractive and useful self.

When a woman lost a breast the most mundane fact of life became an effort. She could no longer get up and get dressed in the morning without thinking about it. She could not bathe or make love without being reminded of it. Even when she did forget, others—fashion designers, lingerie companies, Hollywood, the media, plastic surgeons offering to augment her breasts and enhance her appeal—were quick to insist that she remember.

A healthy woman faced endless public analysis of her form. *Playboy* magazine said her breasts had to be large. Couture designers said they had to be small and the following season changed their minds. Whatever the size, they ought to be high and firm: in her 1991 book *The Beauty Myth,* Naomi Wolf wrote about the "Official Breast," promoted by a culture that valued the illusion of youth above the endless variety of the real world.

In the spring of 1994 tilt as well as size became an issue, as the manufacturer of the Wonderbra, a push-up bra that had been wildly successful in Great Britain, prepared to introduce to the United States its antidote to gravity.

A woman's breasts were cultural currency. Her decisions about treatment, and what to do in the wake of it, were all bound up in image.

Laura saw plastic surgery as her salvation, the way to cope with what had happened to her without having to face it every day when she looked in the mirror. Scars would fade. Health, to her, meant being able to toss on a T-shirt without first positioning a prosthesis inside her bra.

She decided that she wanted to keep her baby—and was suddenly in a rush to have the lumpectomy, to free herself of any concerns except a healthy pregnancy. Love refused to do what she called "hit and run" surgery, to operate on a patient and leave her postoperative care to someone else, so on Thursday, February 3, another surgeon on the multi team performed a wide excision and removed Laura's right breast implant. Laura had managed to convince herself that she could handle having one breast smaller than the other as long as she could look forward to reconstruction once the baby was born.

Bad luck was not finished with her, though. She came in for an appointment with Love on February 17 bearing a new surprise. Laura had just been given two weeks' notice; she had been fired on Valentine's Day. She would be out of work at the end of the month, and her severance pay and health insurance would run out at the end of September. She wondered if she ought to have the mastectomy for the DCIS right away. Was it likelier to turn into invasive cancer because she was pregnant? And what about the reconstruction? She had to have that before her insurance ran out.

Love tried to calm her down. She wanted Laura to appreciate exactly where she stood. There were no dirty margins on the re-excision—all the invasive cancer was gone—so she could wait until the end of the pregnancy for the mastectomy. She could start the insurance preapproval process now for the simultaneous reconstruction, to avoid any problems later on.

Laura was skeptical, but Love insisted that she was "comfy waiting." She told Laura to go home, take it easy, and try to get used to being lopsided for seven more months. Her body was going to change so much with the pregnancy that no one would even notice.

There would be plenty of time to be beautiful after the baby was born.

Dee Wieman was standing in an underground parking garage when she opened the envelope, unfolded the pathology report, and read, "Labelled 'right axillary node' is a 4.5 x 3.5 x 1.5 cm apparent lymph node completely replaced by white-gray glistening tumor." Her knees buckled. Her surgeon at St. John's, Dr. Armando Giuliano, had warned her that he had not done the excisional biopsy he had planned to do. He said it looked like she had more than one tumor, so he had to take several tissue samples from different parts of her breast. He performed a lymph node dissection as well. She remembered him saying to her, "It's not good," but she had refused to allow herself to think that it would be very bad.

He had promised to sit down with her to talk over the pathology report, but Dee had not been able to wait. She drove over to St. John's even though she knew it was one of Giuliano's surgery days, and managed to convince the nurse that she was supposed to have a copy of the report.

Giuliano would be furious when he found out. He always discussed the pathologist's findings with the patient for exactly this reason: Dee was not supposed to find out how desperately ill she was standing alone in a parking garage.

She stumbled to her car, sank into the driver's seat, and continued to read. The pathologist had looked at six tissue samples from Dee's right breast and reported a numbing array of findings. Invasive lobular cancer. DCIS with dirty margins. Most frightening of all, twenty-six out of twenty-eight lymph nodes were positive—and anything over ten was an indication of micrometastasis, the presence of microscopic malignant cells, the precursor to full-blown metastatic disease.

"Oh my God," she whispered in her velvet, breathy voice. For a long time she sat without moving.

*   *   *

Six months earlier her gynecologist had dismissed a hard lump in her right breast as a benign fibroadenoma, a common fibrous tumor more often found in young women than in someone Dee's age. Then, in November 1993, she noticed that her right nipple had changed color a little bit. It seemed rosier than it had been, which convinced her that something strange was going on. Dee watched it for a couple of days and decided she had to show it to someone.

A bilateral mammogram showed nothing on the right, but an abnormality on the left side. Immediately Dee started calling area hospitals to see who could most quickly perform a biopsy. She went to the first one that could take her, Long Beach Memorial, a half hour south of Los Angeles near her home in Huntington Beach. The head of the breast program there ordered a stereotactic core biopsy of her left breast—a new technology that utilized a high-speed needle guided by computer to quickly remove a tissue sample without subjecting a woman to anesthesia and surgery.

The next day at one, stuck on the freeway an hour away from home, she started calling from her car phone to find out the results. She had left messages with everyone she could think of—the oncologist who ordered the biopsy, the pathologist—and then the cell phone rang.

"Where are you?" the oncologist demanded.

"In my car."

"*Where* in your car?"

"Los Angeles."

"Can you be here in an hour?"

"No," said Dee, half thinking that if she couldn't get there she could avoid hearing what he seemed so determined to say. Suddenly she was in no hurry at all.

"Can you . . . how soon *can* you be here?"

She sighed. If the oncologist wanted to see her that badly it meant trouble. She drove to his office to get the news.

Dee had a small invasive ductal carcinoma in her left breast. She needed to talk to a surgeon about having the tumor excised and a sampling of lymph nodes taken, and the doctor suggested that she also consider having a biopsy of the mass in her right breast. But he wanted Dee to understand that as cancers went, this was not a bad one.

He tried to put it in context for her. Eighty-six percent of breast cancers started in the ducts, like Dee's, and the tumor that formed was hard, often easy to detect at an early stage. It appeared in a woman's other breast in about fifteen percent of cases. The next most common invasive form, lobular cancer, was more danger-ous—it might form a subtle thickening that was harder to evaluate, and showed up bilaterally about twenty percent of the time. It was hard to think about being lucky and having breast cancer—but it looked like Dee had got off fairly easy.

The doctor suggested that she buy Susan Love's book and read only the section that pertained to her. Instead she bought Love's book and four others and spent the entire weekend devouring them. By Sunday night she had decided that at best she had eighteen months to live.

Monday morning she started calling surgeons all over town, as though a comprehensive assault would blanket the cancer and smother it. Dr. Giuliano performed two surgical biopsies at St. John's. The first confirmed the diagnosis of cancer in her left breast. The second, a biopsy of two pieces of tissue from her right breast, showed DCIS and a very small focus of invasive ductal cancer, less than .5 centimeters. But Giuliano wanted to look at her right breast again, so they scheduled another biopsy.

During one of her visits to St. John's she picked up a magazine in the waiting room. Its cover blared, "The Fifty Most Important People in L.A.," and Dr. Susan Love was on the list. Dee called UCLA from a pay phone and made an appointment for the multi-disciplinary clinic. She had already decided that what she needed was a "shepherd," a single doctor who would coordinate all the aspects of her treatment and make sure she was well looked after, and she intended to shop until she found the one best able to look after her.

Dee saw Love for the first time the day after her second biopsy, and walked out of the Breast Center confident that she could beat breast cancer. Susan Love felt something new—not the fibroade-noma that Dee's first doctor had dismissed, but a larger, hard area in the right breast that she wanted Giuliano to look at. Even with that news, Dee came away feeling that she was not under a death sentence. Giuliano had scheduled the final excision on her right breast for the following week, but Dee made another appointment with Dr. Love for a few days after that surgery.

Dee sat in her car for a long time reading the report from Giuliano's third procedure, which she dubbed "the big mean surgery." The small invasive cancer in her left breast was nothing compared to what Dr. Giuliano had found in her right, a large lobular cancer and all those positive nodes. The first doctor she had seen had told her not to worry: it was the big lobular cancers with positive nodes that were the scary ones. The pages she held in her hand were proof that she had plenty to worry about—this time, the surgeon had found all the things she thought she had been spared.

Dee's appointment with Susan Love was scheduled for later that day. She had two hours to fill, but the usual activities of her day—a quiet cup of coffee at an off hour in a deserted restaurant, browsing for crafts projects or tiny gifts for friends—seemed impossible. She drove directly to UCLA and assured the facilitator that she would happily sit and read until Dr. Love was ready. She did not want to be anywhere else.

They spent an hour and a half together reviewing the pathology report. Although Giuliano reported four distinct tumors in Dee's right breast, Love thought she felt one large tumor—the mass she had felt the first time she examined Dee. She dismissed the DCIS even though the pathology slide showed dirty margins; in context it was hardly the primary concern.

The question was how best to treat the lobular cancer—and how to address Dee's cold terror at the prospect of losing a breast. Love suggested that Dee have three cycles of chemotherapy before surgery to try to shrink the tumor.

If it decreased in size, Love was willing to perform a lumpectomy. She might not be able to get all the cancer, which meant Dee would have to have a mastectomy with reconstruction—but it might work, and Love was prepared to try. She wanted Dee to come back the next day with her husband, Gary, to talk it over.

The twenty-six positive lymph nodes were the most troubling news, but they could talk about more aggressive treatment, possibly a transplant, later.

* * *

Dee Wieman was a big, round woman, five-foot-nine, 190 pounds, at forty-five an enduring amalgam of sex and civility—a perfect blond bob and a tasteful pastel suit, or perhaps a linen sheath and blazer, over an impossibly curvy body and a pair of huge breasts that were the essence of her sexual identity. Dee liked her body. Her husband, Gary, seven years her senior, revered it and regarded anyone who wanted to tamper with it as a heartless villain. They went back to see Dr. Giuliano, who suggested a mastectomy, and Gary was appalled. When Gary and his wife arrived at UCLA, he made his position clear. "Let's not do anything," he told his wife while they waited for Dr. Love, "and we'll die together."

Giuliano had told Dee and Gary that the issue was simple. They had to save Dee's life with as little trauma as possible, which meant mastectomy followed by chemotherapy, a stem cell transplant, radiation, and finally, months later, the reconstructive surgery. Love told the Wiemans that she would suggest neo-adjuvant chemotherapy, in which the patient received chemotherapy before surgery instead of after it to get a head-start against systemic disease. Dr. Linnea Chap, a UCLA oncologist, came in to describe the stem cell transplant procedure.

Two of the leading breast surgeons in the city had looked at Dee Wieman and suggested different courses of treatment, each regimen a reflection of the doctor's personal philosophy. Giuliano treated the cancer; Love treated the woman who had cancer. Love appreciated Giuliano's position, and in fact expected that she would have to perform a mastectomy eventually, but she sensed from Dee and Gary a powerful resistance to more aggressive surgery. There was no point in insisting on a mastectomy if Dee froze up and did nothing at all.

Love was careful to let Dee know how much trouble she was in. "This is serious business," she informed her new patient. "This could kill you—but it won't kill you tomorrow. You'll get treated. It'll come back, but you'll have warning."

But Dee and her husband were happily distracted by the good news, which they immediately promoted from a probability to a surety. Dee would not have to lose a breast.

Dr. Chap gave Dee the twenty-five page transplant consent

form and told her to take it home and study it, but Dee was adamant. She wanted to sign right away and get on the schedule.

The painful truth was that the choice of surgery was almost beside the point. The threat to Dee's life was already coursing through her bloodstream, and the real challenge was to stop it before it claimed one of her organs and started to kill her.

Outside the examining room Love glanced over at the resident who was following her around. "Twenty-six of twenty-eight nodes is bad, bad, bad," she said. "The prognosis is shitty. Her only chance is a transplant."

She shook her head. "I don't like being right on something like this."

Dee sat up alone night after night and thought about metastases. She imagined little things breaking off from the large tumor in her right breast and floating through her system. But she was paralyzed by the finality of treatment, by the notion that she was about to do things to her body that would change her forever.

She got hysterical as the date for her first chemotherapy session approached. The day before she was supposed to begin she called Dr. Chap to postpone it for a week, but Chap urged her to get started. The day of the appointment she got Dr. Glaspy on the phone, who told her to come in even if she did not want her first treatment, just to talk it over.

She and Gary went to a therapist that morning and Dee said she felt as though she were at the edge of a cliff with her feet dug in, and someone was pushing and pushing at her from behind. Once the chemo started she would be over the edge. She would be putting poison into her body, and there would be no way to ever again be the person she used to be.

When their hour session ended, Gary informed his wife that they were not going to UCLA to talk to Glaspy. They were going to have lunch at a nice restaurant and resolve the issue of where Dee ought to go. She had continued to see the doctors at St. John's and Long Beach Memorial, as well as UCLA, and she had a rationale for each of the three places. Long Beach was the most convenient,

St. John's was where she had had all her surgeries, and UCLA had Dr. Love, who for the first time had given her some small hope.

Gary saw it differently. Long Beach and St. John's were run by men who wanted to mutilate his wife, and UCLA was a great bunch of women who understood how important it was to save his wife's breasts. He wanted Dee to go to UCLA for her chemotherapy.

The next day she bolted and, instead of going to UCLA, called Dr. Peter Boasberg, an oncologist who worked with Dr. Giuliano at St. John's, a quiet, soft-spoken man who assured her that he could administer the chemotherapy.

"Come in tomorrow," he said. "It will be a good experience."

So she did. Dee Wieman considered deference a virtue and hospitality a high calling; her life was built around accommodating the needs and wishes of others. When people asked her what she wanted, the answer was always the same—she wanted to know what they wanted so she could provide it. Going to Dr. Boasberg seemed to solve a lot of potential problems. It was the treatment Dr. Love and her husband wanted her to have, which would make them happy, at the hospital Dr. Giuliano was affiliated with, which enabled Dee to maintain her relationship to him as well. She had decided to switch surgeons and let Dr. Love perform the lumpectomy, but she would make that announcement in her own good time.

She could please everyone at once, and she would be able to save her breast.

The end of a woman's life began with a wicked secret, as breast cancer cells sneaked into the bloodstream and sailed for a new home. It made no difference how loudly doctors demanded to know what was going on. They had at best a clumsy array of tools—lymph nodes that signaled the likelihood of metastasis but were not proof, blood tests that could spike for reasons that had nothing to do with cancer's spread, lung and bone and liver scans that showed hot spots after the malignant cells had already landed and taken hold. The enemy at its most dangerous was invisible, silent, and always, finally, victorious.

The only hope was a transplant, but at about $100,000 the

future did not come cheap. Since it was an experimental treatment, insurance companies balked at having to pay for it.

Transplants became a dramatic, David and Goliath issue: a woman alone, facing death, fighting the big, rich insurance company. The drama obscured a difficult truth, which was that despite Dr. William Peters's data, no one yet knew how well the procedure worked. Peters's Duke University study, like the program at UCLA, allowed anyone who qualified for a transplant to have one, which meant there was no way to compare their survival to a randomized control group on a standard, less aggressive regimen. Some of the women who did well after a transplant might have lived without the treatment. The NCI had approved four randomized transplant trials in 1991—but the patients who qualified were not interested in being assigned to the traditional therapy; they wanted the stronger stuff, and enrollment was abysmally low.

In an era of cost-benefit calculations, transplants did not seem to the insurers like a wise investment. Some doctors shared their reluctance—Dee's oncologist, Dr. Boasberg, felt that women with positive nodes ought to have the procedure, but that women who already had demonstrable metastatic disease ought to settle for existing palliatives, since their cancer's resistance to standard chemotherapy made it unlikely they would respond to the high-dose regimen.

Doctors involved in the work complained that there were no rules: Duke's Bill Peters and Dr. Mark Rogers reported in the February 17, 1994, issue of the New England Journal of Medicine that insurance companies acted in an "arbitrary and capricious" manner when they considered requests for reimbursement. They said that an insurer rejected one woman's claim and then allowed another's. They said that a woman who could afford a lawyer had a better chance of getting what she wanted.

An insurance executive told The New York Times's Gina Kolata that the inconsistent industry response during the five years that Peters and Rogers tracked payments was evidence not of confusion but of a reevaluation process. In the meantime, decisions were made in the courtroom and in the headlines: In December 1993 a southern California jury had returned an $89 million verdict against Health Net, an HMO that refused to pay for a transplant for a forty-year-old woman who died before her case came to trial.

The questionable survival statistics did not deter patients—and the insurance companies' reluctance only made the treatment seem more valuable, for being just out of reach. Women wanted salvation, the medical community wanted answers, and a new, more cost-conscious insurance industry stood in the way of both.

It was one issue where the activists and federal health officials agreed. Fran Visco did not think an insurance company should pay for a transplant just because a woman hired a lawyer to press her individual case. She wanted insurance companies to pay for the procedure as part of a clinical trial, so that researchers could compile data. Dr. Bruce Chabner, director of the division of cancer treatment at the NCI, warned that insurance reimbursement was critical to the continuation of medical research.

"Without that support," he told the *Times,* "our whole clinical trials apparatus is going to collapse."

Dottie Mosk did not have breast cancer. A series of mammograms said so. The two doctors she went to about the uncomfortable bump under her arm said so. One could not feel it. The other said that it was a swollen hair follicle, and she ought to put hot compresses on it and stop worrying. She let it go and convinced herself it could not be cancer. Everything she read in magazines said that cancer did not hurt. This hurt, so it was not cancer.

If her internist had not retired after forty years she might have waited longer, but her new doctor was not satisfied by clean mammograms and theories about hair follicles. He wanted to know what that lump was. A week later the results of a fine needle aspiration told them: the cells were malignant. Dottie had what was called an "occult primary." No one could find the cancer in her breast, but it had already spread to a lymph node.

Again the doctors disagreed. The surgeon who did the needle biopsy wanted to do a surgical biopsy of the breast, because in hindsight the latest mammogram looked suspicious. An oncologist wanted to put Dottie on two cycles of chemotherapy to shrink the node and then take it out.

Dottie started calling her friends for advice, and one after another they recommended UCLA—Dr. Love, and an oncologist there, Dr. Patti Ganz. Since she was rather tired of imperious and, as it had turned out, inaccurate male doctors who told her not to worry, she made appointments and decided to let the two women devise a treatment. They tried two cycles of chemotherapy to shrink the lymph node—and did, from four centimeters to two. But the question remained of what to do about the invisible source of the swollen node.

"There's three votes," said Dr. Love. "Your vote, my vote, and Dr. Ganz's vote. If you had your choice, what would you want?"

"Take my breast off," said Dottie without hesitation. "I don't care. I'm an older woman. I want this thing out of me, period."

Dottie barely made a ripple under the thin hospital blanket, and her face, just hours after the mastectomy, was the same overwashed beige as the bed linens. She lay flat on the pillow, her white hair a frothy halo around her face, the skin on her closed eyelids thin and webbed with spidery blue veins. Her husband and daughter sat at the other end of the room, in the blue light of the basketball game they pretended to watch on television.

It was Tuesday, February 22, and that morning Love had performed a mastectomy and lymph node dissection on Dottie. She came by to check on Dottie before she went home for the night, and Joe and his daughter took their places on the other side of the bed and tried to make small talk about how nice the room was, how friendly the nurses.

There was nothing substantive Dr. Love could tell them until she got the pathology report, but any tidbit was sustenance. Sixty-four-year-old Dottie had come through the surgery well, which was enough to tide them over until the next day.

"Everything went great," said Dr. Love. She checked the incision and was about to go when Dottie called her back. She grabbed Love's arm with both her slender hands and pulled her down so that her face was an inch away. She wanted Dr. Love to know how wonderful she was—and how much it mattered to Dottie that she was looking after her.

Love kissed Dottie on the forehead. When she stood up her

voice was uncharacteristically husky. "Well," she said, trying to compose herself. "You're stuck with me. I put my mark on you. We're a team."

Dottie had lived a fairy-tale life for a long time. She and Joe grew up in the same comfortable neighborhood at the edge of Hancock Park, and started going out when she was seventeen and he was eighteen and a half. They got married three months after Dottie's eighteenth birthday. Joe embarked on a successful career in real estate, and Dottie, an only child who grew up comfortably surrounded by loving parents and doting grandparents, decided that the best thing she could do would be to create an equally happy and gracious home.

She and Joe had a son and a daughter, and moved into a handsome home on a quiet street near the neighborhood where they both had grown up. Every May the jacaranda trees formed a canopy of fluted purple blossoms over the broad street, and by June a carpet of fallen flowers lay at the curb like a frilly ruffle on a summer dress. Every winter the broad street was lined with peaceful dormant grays and browns. Dottie had an eye for flowers. She ordered dozens of plants to line the front driveway and surround the backyard and pool—and when she began to tire of a particular look she revamped the greenery. Everything was to look fresh, and just so.

Dottie had a bunch of cronies with whom she had lunch, or went shopping, and every Saturday night she and Joe went out for dinner with friends. Dottie loved to dress up, and a dozen photographs in the hallway outside her dressing room testified to that fact, as did the designer garment bags that often hung on the closet door.

It was a life of easy privilege, until it wasn't anymore. One night a drunk driver slammed into her son's car and killed him—and a month later, as though her grief had invaded her and sapped her strength, she was diagnosed with fibromyalgia, a debilitating rheumatologic condition that transformed her into an invalid who depended on a daily exercise regimen just to be able to do what she had always taken for granted—walk, stand in a fitting room for a half hour, drive five miles to have lunch with her friends.

She took steroids until she developed an ulcer. Now she got by on banked anger; she simply was not going to let the pain get the better of her.

In the ten years since her son's death she had developed a grim fortitude. When Love had asked her for her vote she thought of all the things that might have caused the breast cancer. Extensive X rays when the doctors were trying to diagnose the fibromyalgia. Fifteen years on estrogen. Her age, sixty-four, which was a risk factor itself.

It was relatively easy for Dottie to choose surgery. She waged war daily against a chronic illness that defied resolution. What a relief it was, in an odd way, to be able to rid herself of a new illness with surgery. There was a comforting finality to the act. The breast cancer would go away, as the fibromyalgia, and the woeful memory of her son's death, would not.

10

PLAYING THE ODDS

MARY-CLAIRE KING HAD A DISARMING ABILITY TO REDUCE THE SO-phistications of her work to a simple explanation: All cancer is genetic. Some of it is hereditary and some of it is acquired over time, but all of it has to do with genes run amok. A woman who inherited a mutated copy of the BRCA-1 gene would not necessarily develop breast cancer, while a woman who had radiation to the chest for severe acne when she was a teenager might be diagnosed with the disease twenty-five years later.

The notion that cancers were the result of multiple genetic insults had been put forth first in 1971, when Alfred Knudson of the Fox Chase Cancer Center in Philadelphia published what scientists called the "two-hit" hypothesis, suggesting that certain cancers were caused by damage to both copies of a particular gene.

The accumulated damage could come from the family or from the environment. What no one yet understood was the exact recipe—the sequence, cumulative number and kind of genetic mutations that combined to make a cancer patient sick.

The gene King was looking for, BRCA-1, related to the five to ten percent of breast cancer patients who inherited a predisposition—or to some of them, since researchers agreed that more than one gene might contribute to a woman's risk. King and her colleagues hoped that BRCA-1 would also teach them something about sporadic breast cancer, the type that ambushed unsuspecting women who thought they were safe because they had no risk factors.

King stood at the center of the adventure, her universe narrowed to family trees and genes that stubbornly refused to align themselves in any consistently suspicious pattern. Dr. Larry Norton stood at the edge looking in, and from his broader perspective saw a glorious revolution. Norton was an oncologist, the chief of the Breast and Gynecological Cancer Medicine Service at Memorial Sloan-Kettering Cancer Center, and the director of the Evelyn Lauder Breast Center. He was a member of the Institute of Medicine panel that had advised the army on how to allocate its breast cancer research funds. His work centered on a mathematical model for tumor growth that would help oncologists determine the most effective schedule for administering chemotherapy—but his imagination lived in the future, a world so delightful to him that his words raced past each other in a rush to get there. When he talked about it he kept interrupting himself to say, "All right? All right?" lest his listener be left behind.

A serious amateur pianist, Norton liked to tell the story of the alien from Venus who came to Earth and heard pleasant sounds.

What are those? he asked.

Music, he was told. That was the first step—the realization that there was such a thing as sound.

He walked along a street and saw a group of people standing together, each one holding a strange object—perhaps a thin metal pipe studded with push-buttons or a round tub that one of them hit with sticks.

What are those? he asked.

Musicians, playing musical instruments. Step two—sound comes from a source.

The alien glanced at the sheets of paper the musicians were studying, covered with sets of horizontal lines and little stick-and-circle figures. His escort explained that those were musical notes. Once you know how to read those notes, he said, you can play music. Take a pencil, erase one note and substitute another, and you have a new sound.

To Norton, the whole of medical history was the story of the alien who did not understand music. It was only since the middle of the nineteenth century, with the study of pathology, that doctors began to comprehend what disease was and where it came from: breast cancer came from abnormal breast cells the way music came from musicians. Understanding the notation—the DNA—was a very new skill; scientists had discovered it in 1953 and completed deciphering the genetic code in 1966. Once they determined how to alter that notation, to erase a damaged gene and jot in a new one— they would be able to orchestrate change.

The most impatient women were the ones who did not yet have breast cancer, women at high risk for the disease who hoped for any good news—a preventive strategy, a genetic intervention, a reliable cure—before it was too late for them.

Every Tuesday morning the Breast Center offered a high-risk clinic. The patients shared a forbidding genetic legacy: one first-degree relative, either a mother or sister, who had been diagnosed with premenopausal breast cancer. Some had multiple relatives with breast or ovarian cancer. Others worried about additional acquired risk—they had had their children late, or had no children at all; they had taken birth control pills or fertility drugs. One woman recalled chasing a truck that sprayed DDT when she was a little girl, and wondered if inhaling the fumes had made her more susceptible.

Love did not see any of these women. Since they only anticipated illness, there was nothing she could do for them but commiserate. The high-risk clinic was run by Dr. Patti Ganz, the director of the Division of Prevention and Control Research at UCLA's Jonsson Comprehensive Cancer Center. Ganz was Dottie's oncologist, a taciturn woman whose stern demeanor seemed to exert a forcible calm on the apprehensive women she talked to. In 1989, after a decade's research into quality-of-life issues among cancer patients, she had cut back her clinical practice from half-time to one day a week, to expand that research. She concentrated now on women at high risk for breast cancer, and on AIDS patients. Ganz had come to believe that prevention, not detection or treatment, was the road to a cure for breast cancer in her lifetime—and hoped her work might uncover common denominators that could lead to a prevention strategy.

Dr. Ganz, forty-six, favored dark tailored clothing, and wore her thick black hair in a tight bun at the nape of her neck. She spoke in an almost perfunctory manner, armed with a little diagram she called a risk thermometer. She colored it in bit by bit, as she determined a patient's risk factors. If her combined genetic and environmental risks equaled the risk level of a sixty-year-old woman, the patient was eligible for the two-year-old NSABP tamoxifen prevention trial. If not, she qualified only for comfort and advice. Women who signed up for the high-risk clinic tended to exaggerate their plight. It was up to Ganz to translate terror into more regimented categories.

At the moment the tamoxifen prevention trial seemed a decidedly mixed blessing. In January hundreds of researchers had received a letter from the National Cancer Institute, which was in turn responding to a recent report from Dr. Bernard Fisher, the director of the NSABP. Data from the tamoxifen protocol for women with breast cancer, which had begun in 1981, cast a troubling shadow on the prevention trial. The increased risk of uterine cancer—a known side effect of the drug—seemed higher than early estimates, and that disease harder to cure than initially thought.

Patients had originally been told that tamoxifen could double or triple the chance of uterine cancer, but that the disease was relatively easy to treat. New data showed that twenty-three of the 2,693 breast cancer patients who took tamoxifen had developed uterine cancer. Four died. There were only two cases of uterine cancer in the placebo group, and neither was fatal.

The new figures promised controversy. Women who had an elevated risk of breast cancer could literally make themselves sick seeking protection from a cancer they might not ever get. Still, the NCI endorsed the continuation of the trials, as did Susan Love. This was the only way to find out if the benefits of tamoxifen outweighed the risks. A clinical trial was, after all, just that: doctors tried out treatments to see if they helped, whom exactly they helped, for how long, and at what cost. Love always reminded patients who came with questions about a promising therapy that there was no such thing as a free lunch. Any medication strong enough to affect a cancer cell was going to have an effect on the rest of the body as well.

On one Tuesday morning in late February a particularly high-strung young woman sat in an examining room, her chair pushed all the way into the back corner, as though she were afraid she was about to be attacked. She clutched her backpack against her chest, her ankles twined around the leg of the chair. Her younger sister had just been diagnosed with breast cancer and her first cousin was scheduled for a surgical biopsy. She managed a quick, weak hand-shake when Patti Ganz walked into the room, and tucked her hand around her waist.

Ganz gave her a brief lesson in genetics. An altered gene pro-duced altered cells, which did not behave the way they were sup-posed to. The only question was how a woman sustained genetic damage. Five percent of breast cancer patients actually inherited a damaged gene. Another ten percent inherited characteristics, like body chemistry or hormonal function, that might cause them to start menstruating early or reach menopause late, both risk factors for breast cancer. These women had a head-start on the road to trouble. The rest of the population had to incur environmental damage to catch up.

Ganz started on her list of questions, and was pleased to learn that the woman had had her first child at twenty. Early pregnancy seemed to protect against breast cancer because mature breast tis-sue—tissue that was capable of producing milk—was less vulnera-ble to genetic mutation than immature breast tissue.

The patient cocked her head and smiled. A month ago she might have believed Dr. Ganz, but not since her sister was diag-nosed.

"Yeah," she said, "me and my sister *both* had our kids early and breast-fed. So that goes out the window."

The sigh that escaped Ganz's lips was barely audible. She re-viewed her findings. The patient probably had two to three times the usual risk. An average woman had an eleven percent chance of developing breast cancer in her lifetime. For this woman, it was about thirty-three percent. She should have a physical exam every six months as well as a mammogram.

Psychologist Dr. David Wellisch was a quiet, kindly presence at UCLA's high-risk clinic. At forty-six he had prematurely gray hair and a bushy mustache, and his slender shoulders drooped just a bit, as though from the weight of too many sad stories. His mother had died of cancer when he was a young man, and after that Wellisch made a career of working with cancer patients and their families. He talked to the patient Ganz had seen and reassured her about her "grief response" at learning of her sister's diagnosis. He found it absolutely appropriate. They talked about the various causes of stress in her life, in the hope of helping her to reduce them.

Wellisch was studying the high-risk patients to see if intervention would decrease their anxiety level, as he believed it would. It wasn't much help—he wished for something more concrete in terms of prevention—but after almost twenty years he had become philosophical. He was used to waiting.

"Hope," he admitted, "runs a little bit ahead of capacity."

Treatment kept a woman very busy, but when it was over there was a precipitous drop: she was a cancer patient with nothing to do, in terms of her disease, but wait to see if it came back. She could improve her diet and get more exercise, but there were no promises. Having worked so hard to get rid of the cancer, she now had to get used to being idle.

It was a difficult transition. Jerilyn Goodman had been trying to find her feet ever since her surgery. Newscaster Connie Chung, who had met Goodman when she was working for the network over the summer, had picked her to help track down figure skater Tonya Harding after the attack on Harding's competitor, Nancy Kerrigan. Goodman spent days holed up with Chung in a car outside various locations in Harding's hometown of Portland, Oregon. When Chung followed the skater to the Olympics at Lillehammer, Norway, and snared an interview, Goodman was at her side.

That led to more work for the CBS magazine show *Eye to Eye,* which should have made Goodman happy. Instead, she worried that her swift professional ascent would be followed by an equally rapid physical decline. She felt vulnerable and depressed. Life was back to normal—far better than normal as far as work was concerned—and yet all she could think about was the cancer and whether it was coming back.

Like many of Love's patients, Jerilyn tried to please the gods of good luck. She showed up twenty minutes early for a follow-up appointment with Sherry Goldman, and hung around Connie Long's cubicle, showing her Norway photographs to the staff and chatting aimlessly, until Love roared around the corner to grab her phone messages on the way to see a patient. Jerilyn stepped forward with an Olympic souvenir pin she had brought back for Love's daughter, Kate—and when she held it out to Love, her hand was shaking. Love let herself be a few more minutes late so she could talk with Goodman about her trip. Visibly relieved, Goodman trotted down to the examining room and studiously began to read her copy of *The New York Times*.

Sherry Goldman had been a nurse-practitioner in an obstetrics and gynecology practice for seven years, and a labor and delivery nurse for nine years before that. When the Ob-Gyn she worked for decided to retire, Sherry could have stopped working as well—her husband was a successful attorney, and her children were grown, with their own families—but Sherry loved being a nurse. She started looking for another job immediately, and when a friend told her that Susan Love wanted a nurse-practitioner at UCLA, she called for an interview.

Goldman was skeptical about her chances, since she had no experience taking care of breast cancer patients. She and Love hit it off immediately: two sarcastic, exasperated women who savored at least the illusion of independence. Love made the Breast Center sound like an all-female island of sanity within UCLA—all the fun of private practice, with the stability only a university could provide.

She asked Goldman if she wanted the job.

"I don't know how to do breast exams," said Goldman.

"I'll teach you," said Love.

It was irresistible—the chance to go to work for a famous doctor who happened to be a lot of fun, and to do something more than gynecological maintenance. Goldman said yes and became Love's unlikely sidekick—a trendy, fashionably dressed woman who favored dramatic eye makeup and French manicures, lacy body suits and platform shoes. She devoted herself to her new discipline like a missionary educating the heathens, teaching breast self-exam, debating Chinese herbs versus estrogen, trying to convince women that happiness, if not perfect health, was within their grasp. She was the medical professional as best girlfriend—equal parts information and affection.

She rushed into the room where Jerilyn was waiting, all corkscrew curls and rattling bracelets, and asked, "How are you. How are *you*, since you're paying so much attention to everyone else."

Goodman looked up, startled, as though someone had seen through her busy disguise. "I don't know," she said. "The only thing this has done is force me to realize I have to do everything I say I want to do. I don't have the luxury of lying around."

"Susan says your life is never the same," said Goldman, wanting to be helpful. "I think for people of a certain mind-set, it's better."

As she did the physical exam she reminded Jerilyn of all the services available to her—the nutritionist, the physical therapist, the support groups at the Rhonda Fleming Mann Center.

"I'm in a support group," said Goodman, who had joined right after her surgery, in November 1993. "I hate groups, but I love this one. My biggest issue right now is low-grade anxiety. I feel great, I think I look great, but . . ."

"Anxiety over what? Recurrence?"

Goodman nodded, suddenly mute.

"I can't take that away," said Goldman. "You've got to face it head-on—and I believe you will. Your prognosis is excellent. Susan's written 'good' all over your chart. But we all have to face our own mortality."

"I just have to decide what language I'm comfortable with," said Jerilyn, staring past Goldman into space. "I'm not ready to stand up and say I'm a survivor. The worst thing is when people say, 'Did they get it all?' But do I say I *had* breast cancer? I *have* breast cancer? I feel fine. I feel very optimistic. I just don't want to be surprised."

Goldman had no answer for that. She went out to look for the nutritionist, while Jerilyn dressed and decided that from now on she would have to figure out a way to see Dr. Love. Goldman was perfectly competent, but Jerilyn needed to see Susan. The same words coming from her carried a different weight.

Jerilyn tried to talk to the nutritionist, but they were at cross-purposes. The young woman who advised follow-up patients clung to the few bits of data that existed on diet and breast cancer: she wanted Jerilyn to take in enough calcium to stave off osteoporosis, since it was unlikely that she would take estrogen replacement therapy, and she wanted her fat intake down to fifteen percent. Dietary fat continued to mystify doctors. There was plenty of evidence to suggest a correlation, particularly the comparatively low breast cancer rates in countries like Japan, which had a much lower fat intake than the United States. But there was no consensus. One study where women maintained a diet of twenty-five percent fat showed no impact on incidence rates, but there were two ways to analyze that—either the fat percentage was still too high to help, or dietary fat was not a contributor to breast cancer risk. There was no data at all on its effect on recurrence rates. In the absence of answers, nutritionists pushed an even lower level of fat.

"Just tell me how much fat I should take," Jerilyn said, "because I want the whole percentage in chocolate."

The nutritionist dutifully did a computation based on Goodman's height and weight, and suggested twenty-five grams of fat per day.

Goodman shook her head and sighed. "And a bag of peanut M&M's is fifteen. I looked at a bag yesterday."

It was hard for Jerilyn to take advice about her lifestyle seriously. She had been a vegetarian in her teens, and now only occasionally ate chicken or fish. At five-foot-two, she weighed a trim 111 pounds, much of it muscle. She swam regularly, played golf, and had always been active. She already did all the things people were supposed to do to prevent breast cancer.

In her current morose frame of mind, she imagined that any day now the newspapers would trumpet a new study that showed that a low-fat diet caused some other disease. For all she knew, the pesticides in those supposedly healthy vegetables had helped to do her in.

Leaving the pin for Kate and staying in touch with Susan would probably do her as much good as a nonfat granola bar. When she went to the facilitators' office to make her next appointment they told her that Sherry would be on vacation the week she wanted to come in. She lied and said that was the only time she would be around, and so they scheduled her with Dr. Love.

"Hello, beautiful."

Susan Love had decided the first time she met Shirley Barber that what Shirley wanted more than anything was to be treated as an equal. You could not be solicitous of Shirley; she did not want kind words or a comforting hug. For Love it was a welcome release.

They shot information back and forth like a Ping-Pong ball. Both women wondered if Shirley's long-term exposure to low-level radiation as a flight attendant had contributed to her illness. Love had found an epidemiologist in Seattle, a doctor who studied disease trends in large populations, who believed he had calculated the exact amount of radiation a passenger on an airplane was exposed to. Shirley jumped at the news. She thought that the flight attendants' union had statistics on radiation that she would try to find to send to him.

Love dropped her voice to a conspiratorial whisper.

"So, how're you?"

"Okay," said Shirley. "Strange. I like the burn." She often examined her lobster-red chest in the mirror, happy to see that ten solitary seconds on a table in a lead-lined radiation therapy room was having an effect. The sunburn was a welcome sign—proof that something was happening.

Radiation was an eerie experience. Every day she took off her clothes, donned a plain cotton gown, and was positioned on what the technician called an alpha cradle—a backrest molded to Shirley's shape and covered with a plastic garbage bag, which was supposed to ensure that she was in exactly the same position each time. Once she was properly aligned, the technician left the room, and the invisible radiation entered her body. It was like science fiction. Death to the dirty margins, without any proof of battle.

One morning Shirley asked the radiologist to put nachos on her chest to see if the radiation would melt the cheese and toast the tortilla chips.

Love cringed. "They have support groups for people like you," she said. "And funny jackets."

"If they'd just turn on the light in the padded cell," said Shirley, wistfully. "But I did lie there during radiation and think, 'Is anything happening? Or is there a tape recorder just making sounds?' "

"People with chemo have the same reaction," said Love. "It's, 'Is this the placebo group?' They get pissed if their hair doesn't fall out. They worry they're getting the sugar pill."

Barber smiled. "And do they go in again to check that you've done surgery?"

Love looked abashed. "The truth is, we have no way to know if any of these treatments work."

But Barber wanted a hint. She asked how soon she could have another mammogram.

"One month. How's your nipple?" Barber had had so many surgeries on her infected left breast that there was an indentation that ran along the areola and across her nipple.

"Twin Peaks?" cracked Shirley. "Fine."

"How's your energy?"

"Up."

"Your ambition?"

"Oh, I have 133 projects to do." The banter stopped. "But I would like to sleep through the night."

"Want something?"

Barber gave her a rueful glance. "I *had* a sleeping pill. Took it with codeine, with codeine and a six-pack. I still stayed awake."

"Okay. Drugs aren't the answer."

Before Dr. Love could suggest anything else, Shirley hopped up on the examining table and loosened her gown. She did not want to dwell on the anxiety that plagued her at night.

"Okay," she said. "Let's do boobs."

Love began to palpate her breasts, and as she did she muttered, "I want you to know I'm a United Premier Executive now," referring to an exalted caste in the airline's frequent flyer program. "So I'm getting the radiation too."

There was no such fun with Dottie. The pathology report was a shock: of the thirty-five lymph nodes Love removed when she performed the mastectomy, nineteen were positive. Dottie had Stage 3 cancer even though no one could find a lump in her breast. Because of the fibromyalgia, she was too fragile to undergo a stem cell transplant. She would have radiation and two more cycles of standard chemotherapy, but that was the equivalent of two aspirin for a migraine. It wasn't enough, and yet Susan had to tell Dottie and Joe that it was all medicine had to offer her.

For all her skepticism about transplants, it pained Love not to be able to offer Dottie the most aggressive treatment available. The older woman burst into tears at the news, and Love found herself crying along with her.

11

CONSTRUCTIVE CHAOS

THE ADVOCATES MIGHT THINK THAT THE NATIONAL ACTION PLAN ON Breast Cancer was theirs—a direct result of their efforts, like the Department of Defense research program—but Health and Human Services Secretary Donna Shalala was more practical about it. She would not have a viable national plan without the scientific community, and she could not have the scientists without acknowledging their position on how best to fight the disease. Disagreement was virtually guaranteed. It was her job to make sure that everyone kept working while they argued.

She had invited Dr. Harold Varmus, the new head of the National Institutes of Health, to be the keynote speaker at the first organizational meeting for the Action Plan in December 1993. Varmus, then on the job for only one month, was an unknown commodity as far as the activists were concerned. He had won the Nobel Prize in medicine with his research partner, J. Michael Bishop, for their discovery of oncogenes, altered genes that promoted malignant growth. For over a decade Varmus's San Francisco lab had studied a gene called WINT 1, usually dormant in the breast, but when activated by a virus capable of causing breast cancer in laboratory mice. His mother and grandmother had died of breast cancer. His work and his life were defined by the disease—

and yet he was careful to say that he did not consider himself part of the "breast cancer mafia." He was instead, he said, a "student of cell biology and genetics and cancer genes."

His own work provided a cautionary example of the limits of earmarked research. Varmus still had no proof that an altered copy of the WINT 1 gene affected women in the same way it affected lab mice; it was not one of the genes implicated in human breast cancer. But he had discovered along the way that WINT 1 was "incredibly important": knock it out and a mouse was born without a cerebellum.

Varmus told this story at the National Action Plan organizational meeting for a reason—to illustrate to his audience the value of basic research, which he believed held promise for everyone, unlike directed research, which might not even help the group it was intended for.

"We should continue to devote most of our efforts to a broad understanding of cell growth and function," he said. "The alternative is to decide that we know enough about such fundamental aspects of cells—that it is time to commit ourselves to improving the diagnostic and therapeutic strategies now in use or to fashion new ones from the few pieces of the puzzle already in hand. This is our dilemma: Should we have invested in better iron lungs or in attempts to grow polio virus? Breed better leeches or work on the germ theory of disease?"

A tall, slender man who favored plaid flannel shirts and made the twelve-mile commute to his office by bicycle whenever the weather permitted, Varmus believed in what he called "creative chaos." He considered the "coordination myth" to be just that, the illusion that a more carefully orchestrated research plan would somehow yield better results. And he like the fierce competition for grants that so frustrated Susan Love. To Varmus, it was simply "survival of the fittest."

Shalala believed in management by forced cooperation: she threw disparate groups together and hoped for synergy. Shalala had named Fran Visco cochair of the National Action Plan along with Dr. Susan Blumenthal, a psychiatrist, long-time NIH employee, and congressman's wife. The lobbyist and the insider. If Fran Visco was going to get results she would have to learn to be something of an insider as well.

Shalala named twenty-three group chairs at that December meeting. They ranged from Susan Love, who had endorsed the President's controversial policy on mammograms for women under fifty, to American Cancer Society deputy executive vice president Harmon Eyre, who adamantly continued to press for annual mammograms from forty on.

On Donna Shalala's "watch," as she called it, adopting the naval term favored in political jargon, everyone got a seat at the table.

Love was a member of the National Institutes of Health's $625 million Women's Health Initiative advisory committee as well, and she eagerly took a day trip to Washington in late February for a meeting with the study's organizers. The Initiative promised to answer questions about the relationship of diet and hormones to the three greatest threats to women's health—heart disease, breast cancer, and osteoporosis. Over the course of fifteen years, researchers intended to collect data from two randomized control studies as well as an observational trial. The WHI hoped to recruit 27,500 women between the ages of 50 and 79 to compare one group, which received hormone replacement therapy, to another group, which did not. The dietary study would involve 48,000 women in that age group, half on a standard American diet, half on a low-fat regimen. One hundred thousand women would participate in the observational trial, filling out lifestyle and medical questionnaires and submitting themselves to periodic blood tests and physical examinations.

It was an ambitious plan, but it had been plagued by problems from the start, attacked by critics who charged that its emphasis on diet and nutrition was misplaced—that such a study was not adequate compensation for decades of neglect. Worse, it promised to be an expensive misstep: in July 1992 Congress had asked the Institute of Medicine to assess the program, because the cost estimate had risen from $500 million to over $600 million.

The WHI began enrolling women in September 1993. Two months later the IOM issued a blistering critique. The IOM found that the landmark study was "too expensive, will take too long, and ought to be redesigned," according to *The Washington Post*. *Science* magazine quoted a panel member who revived early skepticism about whether dietary changes after fifty had an impact on disease at all, calling the idea a "weak hypothesis." Some members of the committee wanted to cancel the study altogether.

But the WHI symbolized the government's mandate to study women's health, and it had an equally vocal group of supporters, including Love's UCLA colleague Dr. David Heber, an endocrinologist who had been studying the relationship between nutrition and disease since 1968 and was a member of the study's design analysis committee, as well as its coprincipal clinical investigator at UCLA. The $140 million contract to coordinate the WHI had been awarded to the Fred Hutchison Cancer Research Center in Seattle, Washington, and fifteen of forty-five participating centers had been chosen. Sign-ups continued.

The sheer size of the WHI gave it momentum—but it was an obvious candidate for an overhaul, which made Love excited about being involved.

She and a few other activists on the committee promoted the standard National Breast Cancer Coalition line and got consumers—women who were going to participate in the study—added to the committee, as well as some of the data monitors who would be tracking results. Everyone involved in the study, from whatever angle, would have a voice.

Then the disagreements began. The women Love referred to as "the radicals," a category that included Love and the breast cancer activists, wanted changes in the participants' questionnaire—including the addition of a question about sexual preference, since the incidence of breast cancer was higher among lesbians. They wanted to discuss the fact that seventy percent of the investigators were men. The organizers resisted. They simply wanted to move ahead with a study that had been in place months before the committee was named.

Love came home deflated, feeling as though she was nothing but a figurehead, a name added to the committee roster to curry favor with other advocates. She grudgingly agreed to attend the next meeting, only because another committee member had convinced her that the Initiative was too important to surrender without a fight.

Home was not much better. She looked at her schedule, littered with administrative meetings, and complained for the first time that a university center simply could never be as good as a private practice. There were too many distractions from the work.

What Love liked to call her "big ideas" usually erupted out of her frustration. She emerged happily from surgery on Monday, March 7, and announced to Connie that she had decided to start the Los Angeles Area Breast Cancer Research Group. Information was the key to the future, and yet doctors and researchers tended to keep to themselves, guarding their projects with a proprietary air. Love wanted to invite doctors from UCLA and the University of Southern California, as well as from private institutions—St. John's, Cedars-Sinai, and the Breast Center in the San Fernando Valley—to get together over dinner and talk. The cross-pollination might yield some interesting ideas, and she liked the idea of crashing through professional barriers.

That was as far as she got. Love was admittedly bad on implementation. Her ability to let a big idea drift into space was one of the things that irritated Denny Slamon, but details, to Love, were so much tidying up. She hated the busy work—and she liked to think her mind was meant for more important matters than logistics.

Luckily, Connie was adept at filling in the blanks. She pinned her boss down to a date far enough in the future to ensure decent attendance, and got her to draw up a list of a dozen invitees. Two days later Connie had picked a restaurant in a nearby hotel and was debating the relative merits of salmon and roast beef.

While the politicians, doctors, and advocates argued policy and moved millions of dollars around, Mary-Claire King tried to get to the end of the voyage she had at first described as "insane"—her attempt to search the twenty-three pairs of human chromosomes for a specific disease gene. When she began her postdoctoral work in Berkeley, genetics was a young science, and tracking a single gene an almost impossibly sophisticated task. In 1980 she embarked on a two-year study of 1,600 women with breast cancer, identifying 326 high-risk families in the hope that she could determine why they had more breast cancer than the others. It could be environment or heredity, and if it was heredity there might be several genes working together, or a few genes working independently—or perhaps a single gene that in an altered state greatly increased a woman's risk. Again, her desire outpaced science; though there were new methods for sampling genetic material, she did not have a large enough supply of DNA to effectively narrow the search for the gene.

It was not until 1988, once new lab procedures made it easier for King to copy and mark DNA samples, that she published a study proposing the existence of a gene for heritable breast cancer. That was when the fine work began, the endless toil in an increasingly competitive and secretive environment. Her 1990 announcement that she had narrowed the search to the seventeenth chromosome was like a call to arms; other teams rushed in hoping to build a victory on the foundation of King's work. Her instinct was to collaborate, since the goal was first to find the gene and second to be the one who found it. She found that the others were not always so interested in sharing their information.

Partisan onlookers like Love divided the competitors into two camps, the pure scientists and the entrepreneurs, those who wanted the Nobel Prize and those who wanted to get rich from the gene patent and whatever screening tests would be devised from the gene sequence. King was clearly a member of the first category, since fourteen years seemed an awfully long time to invest in a speculative payoff. On the other side were researchers like Mark Skolnick, who joined the hunt late but with resources that enabled him to catch up: the genealogical riches of Utah's Mormon families, who tended to stay put, have big families, and keep detailed health records, and as of early 1993, over $10 million in funding for his Myriad Genetics, Inc., beyond the initial Eli Lilly & Co. investment. Myriad was not a huge company, but it was richer and bigger than King's effort—a forty-four-person team at sites in the United States, Canada, and Great Britain, with twenty-two staffers in Salt Lake City, compared to King's handful of researchers at her UC

Berkeley laboratory. She had done all the preliminary work, but there was no reward for tenacity. This was a new race.

By March 1994 she was starting to tire. Her team had managed to identify almost all of the two dozen genes within a target region on chromosome seventeen, but it was grueling, repetitive work: over and over they compared the patterns of proteins in the DNA of healthy people with the DNA patterns in breast cancer patients, looking for a pattern that distinguished the two groups from each other.

Time had faded King's happy announcement of the previous August, that she was on the brink of finding the gene. Her lead had disappeared. Finding BRCA-1 was taking longer than anyone had expected.

D r. Mark Skolnick saw himself as a businessman by default; he embraced capitalism because he considered it the fastest route to progress. If anything, he had been raised to question the capitalist motive—the son of a couple committed to what was, in the fifties, a radical political agenda. Skolnick's mother was the president of the American Civil Liberties Union chapter in San Mateo, California, and a member of the League of Women Voters, and in the 1930s had been a labor organizer. The Skolnicks took black families into their home and helped them buy their own houses.

It was, he said, a "decidedly pink" household, and as a young man he embraced its ideals. In 1963, when he was seventeen, Skolnick traveled to Russia, Czechoslovakia, Poland, and the Berlin Wall, on a peace mission organized by a Quaker group. He considered himself a pacifist—and had he not been rejected for military service on a medical deferment, Skolnick would have gone to jail rather than serve in Vietnam.

But San Mateo was a comfortable suburb twenty miles outside of San Francisco, the sort of place where even a liberal Democrat stood at the fringes of society. He saw his childhood as "a community of one, in terms of my political belief. It came from my parents and not anybody else." Along with his politics, Skolnick had learned not to mind being different. He was used to being at odds with people. If anything, he had been taught to be proud of it.

He had no problem becoming an ardent capitalist, if that was what it took to find the gene. The important thing, always, was the cause. Money was just a means to an end.

The future of breast cancer treatment was large drama, mounted on a national stage, a matter for committee votes and philosophical debate. The present played out in miniature—and too often, in isolation. Doctors could tell women how to fight their disease, but no one could tell them how to go on living. The model from the previous generation was too limited: Laura was hardly ready for passive acceptance, for a life of childlessness and cautious necklines. She still wanted everything she thought she was entitled to.

Laura lived in a little wooden bungalow near the beach in Venice, the sort that locals referred to as a California cottage—one story, a small, enclosed sun porch in the front, hardwood floors. The house belonged to a friend who rented it to Laura, but she cared for it as though it were her own. The exterior was painted pale yellow with deep blue trim. The inside was ivory, a canvas for all the objects Laura loved: big heavy vases of colored glass that held sprays of fresh flowers, a squat brass pot filled with dried stems, an old flocked velvet couch covered with brocade pillows, a long dark dining room table at which she could preside over dinner for twelve.

Her home was the one place where Laura was in control. She loved to spend time there alone, the blinds drawn, the phone machine on, a nice little salad and a glass of wine for dinner in front of the television.

She went back and forth about the baby. She wanted to keep it, but she could not make a perfect husband appear, or the cancer disappear. The only thing she could manage was work. She started calling everyone she knew to see if she could find a job.

She couldn't believe how vicious people were—position's filled, click, over and over again. Laura had told herself that she would take a chance and keep the baby if she could just find a job. But the world refused to cooperate, and she did not see how she could possibly handle everything at once.

With barely four weeks left before the end of her first trimester, she called her gynecologist to schedule the abortion—and arrived at the hospital on the morning of March 10 a jittery wreck, begging for a Valium to help her calm down.

Her doctor had seen a cyst on one of her ovaries when he did an ultrasound, so Laura was scheduled for laproscopic surgery to remove it as well as the abortion. The surgery required only an inch-long incision, but Laura was already thinking about her revised future.

"Save the stomach area," she told the surgeon flatly. "Save that. That's my breast."

For a week afterward she refused to answer the phone. Finally she called the man who had spent the night and told him what had happened. He told Laura he loved her. She got off the phone and muttered, "Who cares?"

Right now the idea of intimacy seemed ludicrous to her. Every time she got in the shower she looked at her uneven breasts, one with an implant and one not, and wondered how she would ever be able to be naked with a man again. She did not want anyone to see her. Even if a man were to say that he loved her, even if he said he did not care what her breasts looked like, Laura cared. There was no way she could enjoy sex now.

The real trick was to stop caring. She thought that if she could just let go of her vanity she would love herself, and be loved, but she could not quite give it up. Three hundred sit-ups a day were as important to her as a daily meditation.

On Thursday, March 17, Laura came across a television interview with Elizabeth Glaser, the AIDS activist who had contracted the disease from a blood transfusion when her first child was born in 1981, and then unwittingly transmitted it by breast-feeding that daughter, and a son born in 1984. Her daughter, Ariel, was already dead, and she and her son were both HIV-positive.

Yet Glaser talked about never having felt more alive. Laura hung on her words and chastised herself.

I'm just this wimp who's barely alive right now, she thought. Here I am feeling sorry for myself because I'm deformed. I'm sure she'd trade circumstances with me in a minute.

Elizabeth Glaser had a disease that would kill her. Laura had a disease that might kill her. It was a huge distinction.

12

DATA AND DECEIT

S USAN AND HELEN HAD A WEEKEND CABIN IN THE MOUNTAINS ABOVE Santa Barbara, ninety minutes north of Los Angeles. It was Love's chance to swap her workday wardrobe for the comfort of Birkenstocks and broken-in T-shirts and jeans, to sit on their little stone patio with a glass of wine while Kate played with Susan's sister's kids just up the road. She always said that this was where she would come if things at UCLA did not work out.

She was shopping for a Walkman at Circuit City in Santa Barbara, when her beeper went off. Kelly Hunt, the young surgeon who had performed Laura's lumpectomy, was covering for Love on the weekend of March 11, and as Love headed for a pay phone she wondered what medical emergency could possibly require her long-distance input.

The crisis had nothing to do with her patients. Hunt was paging her because ABC News, *Good Morning America,* and a handful of other news organizations and television programs wanted her reaction to a story about falsified breast cancer research that would appear in the Sunday, March 13, edition of the *Chicago Tribune.* Five minutes later she had an early copy of the article, via one of the fax machines Circuit City had on display.

The *Tribune* disclosed the results of a three-year federal investigation of the National Surgical Adjuvant Breast and Bowel Project—including evidence of falsified data in Protocol B-06, the landmark NSABP clinical trial that compared lumpectomy and radiation to mastectomy. Investigators had found more than 100 examples of falsified data so far among 1,511 patients enrolled in various trials between 1975 and 1991 by Dr. Roger Poisson, a researcher at the University of Montreal's St. Luc Hospital. "Poisson enrolled at least 100 of his cancer patients . . ." wrote the *Tribune*'s John Crewdson, "even though they were ineligible on medical, technical or consensual grounds. Poisson and his assistants then falsified or fabricated the medical records they forwarded to NSABP headquarters at the University of Pittsburgh to make the patients appear to have been eligible."

The largest number of falsifications were made in the lumpectomy trial, where sixteen percent of the participants came from St. Luc's. In addition, Poisson submitted falsified data in three other NSABP trials—Protocol B-13, published in 1989, which compared chemotherapy to no drug treatment for women with node-negative, estrogen-receptor negative breast cancer, and two tamoxifen trials, published simultaneously in 1991—B-14, which compared tamoxifen to a placebo after surgery for patients with estrogen-receptor positive breast cancer, and B-16, which compared tamoxifen alone to a combined regimen of chemotherapy plus tamoxifen for patients over fifty.

Even more troubling, it seemed that everyone except the patients had known. The *Tribune* reported that NSABP Director Dr. Bernard Fisher's staff had stumbled over a discrepancy in the lumpectomy data more than three years earlier, in June 1990—two surgery records for the same patient, one with a date that made her eligible for the study, one whose date would have precluded her participation. Although they found other problems with the St. Luc data, they decided to wait for the results of an upcoming audit—rather than inform the National Cancer Institute or confront Poisson.

The September 1990 internal NSABP audit showed more falsifications, according to the *Tribune*, but Fisher failed to notify the NCI until five more months had passed. He finally suspended Dr.

Poisson in February 1991, and then informed the NCI of what the paper called "irregularities" in the Montreal data.

The NCI, which sponsored the NSABP trials and theoretically supervised Fisher's efforts, informed the federal Office of Research Integrity (ORI), which began its investigation. In January 1993, NCI officials twice wrote to Fisher, asking him to publish a reanalysis of the lumpectomy trial results, eliminating Poisson's data. They complained as well about an audit procedure that had allowed inconsistencies in the data to go undetected for over a decade.

Another year passed. ORI chief investigator Dr. Dorothy Mac-Farlane told the *Tribune* that she was still waiting for a final document despite the fact "that everyone was behind the strategy of trying to get out a publication as quickly as possible." She indicated that she had seen what she called a "preliminary reanalysis," but not the data upon which it was based—which made it impossible for the ORI to evaluate the revised conclusions.

One of the largest cooperative research groups in the country, which received about $16 million from the NCI annually to conduct its research, had failed to adequately police its own member doctors, or inform the public when it did uncover discrepancies. The NCI had tolerated delays from the NSABP. As a result, thousands of women would pick up their morning newspaper or turn on the television news and wonder if they had chosen the wrong therapy.

The lumpectomy study was the foundation of the breast-conservation movement—a ten-year trial involving 5,000 doctors and 2,163 patients at 484 medical centers around the country and in Canada. Susan Love had built her practice and public reputation on the efficacy of less mutilating surgery. The media wanted to know what she had to say. If a doctor who enrolled sixteen percent of the study's total population had failed to play by the rules, did that mean that women who chose lumpectomy over mastectomy had made a mistake?

That was not the issue, not as far as Love was concerned. There was still plenty of data to support lumpectomy. The real question was, what would this do to clinical trials? It was hard enough to get women to enroll, to take the chance that they might receive a placebo instead of a new treatment. This was only going to make it worse.

Shirley Barber did not care about the news that there was falsified data in some of the tamoxifen protocols, nor was she swayed by the new, higher risk figures for uterine cancer among women who took the drug. She came to see Dr. Love in March only because of the latest in a string of unwelcome surprises—what Shirley called a nipple discharge "the color of Jack Daniel's." It was coming out of her right breast, where she had had the surgery for DCIS.

"Oh, I don't care about that," said Love.

Barber shot her a droll glance and drawled, "Oh, good."

"No, really. This is nothing. Post-op."

If it happened once a week for a month they might have to investigate, but for the moment Love was not worried. She wanted instead to talk about Shirley's favorite topic, her first postoperative mammogram. Shirley wanted clean film as proof of her progress; Love told her to schedule an appointment in six weeks.

Tracy tried to match his wife's nonchalance, but events were beginning to catch up with him. He explained to Susan that in the last six months they had endured the Northridge earthquake, a fire that came dangerously close to their house, two teenagers with chicken pox, and their son's arthroscopic surgery for a benign tumor on his knee. His anxiety level about any perceived threat was pretty high. He did not like the revised statistics on tamoxifen and uterine cancer at all.

"This is great," he complained. "We can go from one cancer to another."

"No, the real issue is for healthy women on the prevention trial," insisted Love. "They don't have breast cancer. So if they die of uterine cancer you really feel bad."

Shirley chuckled. "We have good news, and we have bad news. . . ."

". . . You don't have breast cancer," said Tracy, "but we *gave* you uterine cancer."

Shirley shrugged. "I feel okay about it."

When she got out into the hallway with Tracy, though, Shirley was suddenly, visibly agitated. Sometimes being tough took a toll on her nerves, and when no one but Tracy was looking she fell apart. She hooked the fingers of one hand between the first and second button of her blouse and rattled on about her symptoms— the discharge, the lingering pain, the things she continued to worry about despite Love's lack of concern. She dug through her big purse for the bottle of Tylenol she had with her, until Tracy put his hand on her arm to stop her.

He bent down so his face was next to hers, and in a low voice reminded her that Dr. Love had suggested an anti-inflammatory pain medication. Tylenol would not help. He would buy her some Advil or aspirin in the little pharmacy downstairs. She could sit outside and smoke one of the cigarettes that he wished she wouldn't smoke. Then they could go to their favorite restaurant for his glass of Pernod, her bottle of beer, and an early dinner.

ABC News sent a camera crew to the UCLA Medical Center to interview Dr. Love on the NSABP data scandal. She had agreed to speak to them on one condition: she would not under any circumstance criticize Dr. Fisher. She believed he was about to be crucified for what had happened, and she refused to be part of it.

While the cameraman set up his equipment, Love told the producer that everyone was overreacting. The lumpectomy study was still valid, and its findings were supported by other studies, so to say that the NSABP had duped a generation of women was a gross overstatement. She could even understand Fisher's decision to hold back the information rather than needlessly frighten women.

But it was an arrogant thing to do, and he was going to pay for it. It hurt Love to see a man she so idolized compromise his reputation. The same strong, authoritarian nature that had made Fisher a leader in clinical trials had been his undoing. He could not admit a mistake—a chronic problem, as far as Love was concerned, among American doctors, who believed, as did too many of their patients, that they were God. Now he would likely be remembered not for his research, but for his pride.

When the crew was ready, the producer asked his first question: Should a woman think twice about having a lumpectomy?

Love stared him down. "It should not impact a woman's decision," she said. "It won't impact my practice." She launched into a defense of clinical trials. Women should not feel betrayed by a single clinician who falsified data. What should upset them was the appalling lack of research into women's health issues, particularly the link between estrogen replacement therapy and breast cancer.

The producer said that patients he had talked to thought there would be even more coverage if the scandal had involved a man's disease, like prostate cancer.

"It's much ado about nothing," replied Love. "We're scaring a lot of people unnecessarily." There was an Italian study of women who were fifteen years out that showed the same results. She believed the real issue was the pressure of academic medicine, which required a doctor to publish and do research to get promoted.

"What's the remedy?" asked the producer.

"Women have to stop being good little girls and start speaking up," answered Dr. Love.

Fran Visco, who had chosen to have a lumpectomy and radiation, parted company with Love on the falsified data scandal. The news confirmed her worst fear—that researchers essentially operated in secret, as members of an exclusive society whose doors were closed to the women who made their studies possible.

She was enraged at such high-handed behavior, and at the same time aware that it presented a valuable opportunity. The falsified data was a weak spot in the usually impenetrable wall that surrounded the research community. She was determined to drive a wedge in at that spot and improve her access.

The Coalition immediately issued a statement that accused the NSABP and the National Cancer Institute of having "put women's lives at risk."

"Recent events at the National Cancer Institute and the National Surgical Adjuvant Breast and Bowel Project underscore the necessity of including consumer advocates at the table. . . . The public funds biomedical research; scientists who perform this research are accountable to the public. NCI and NSABP's failure to disclose these data in a timely manner impinges upon the rights of the patient who is entitled to make her decisions with all relevant information revealed, of the scientist and physician who have a responsibility to the process and their patients, and to the public that funds the research.

". . . Diversification," she wrote, "will result in new ideas and approaches and decreased opportunities for development of a 'club-like' atmosphere among researchers."

V isco wanted better traditional therapies, a project for an optimist with a long-term perspective. Individual patients who knew the survival statistics often looked for ancillary therapies right away. It was all a matter of faith. Once a woman allowed herself the smallest doubt—and it was difficult to avoid them, given the headlines—she had to ask herself if she still believed in what she was doing. If she didn't, she looked for alternatives.

The first time Jerilyn visited Dr. Rong Zhou she took her mother along. The acupuncturist's office was pleasant enough, white walls and pale wood, but there was an unusual smell, a sour, thick scent from some unfamiliar incense, not one of the fruity ones that had been popular when Jerilyn was in college. The twangy Chinese music grated on her ears. She did not like the lighting. It took discipline—and the memory of all the Western doctors who had let her down—to keep from bolting. Surely her mom was going to read her the riot act as soon as they got out the door.

Dr. Zhou did little to reassure Jerilyn, who could not recall ever having met a doctor who spoke so quietly, and in such a diffident manner. She had none of the aggressive manner Jerilyn was so used to from Western doctors. In fact, she seemed almost childlike, her face delicate and unlined, her baby-fine black hair sitting obediently on her slender shoulders. Dr. Zhou was probably in her thirties, and she had been in practice for ten years, but she seemed timid. How could she possibly help Jerilyn fight cancer?

Dr. Zhou guided Jerilyn and her mother into a small room and began to talk about energy, and slowly the acupuncturist's manner began to make sense. The Chinese did not isolate symptoms and attack them. Dr. Zhou saw Jerilyn's breast cancer as a manifestation of an imbalance. Her *chi,* her essential energy, was stuck somewhere, and together they would figure out how to release it. But she was not going to cure Jerilyn. She was going to show Jerilyn the way to cure herself.

Suddenly Jerilyn's mother spoke up. "That's right," she said, to her daughter's amazement. "You're right. I've always noticed that Jerilyn doesn't seem to have as much energy as I do." Iris Goodman stayed with her daughter through the appointment and never uttered a critical word. When she got back to New Jersey she called often to see how Jerilyn was doing with her new treatment.

After five months Jerilyn was a believer. She swore that the slender steel needles that Dr. Zhou inserted along her mastectomy scar had revived feeling there, even though Dr. Love had told her to expect numbness. She tolerated mood swings and told herself it was her energy being freed, surging through her at unexpected moments.

Laura believed in vitamins to supplement her vegetarian diet and combat stress. She already took antioxidants—vitamins A, C, and E—to fight the free radicals that were loose in her system, trying to damage her cells. With the abortion behind her, and facing an eight-hour surgery, she decided to step up her offensive.

She had heard a lot of talk about shark cartilage, which had been featured in a 1993 *60 Minutes* segment as a possible cancer treatment. Sharks rarely got cancer, and some researchers believed that a protein in shark cartilage inhibited tumor growth by blocking the development of the tiny blood vessels that fed tumors. The NCI had decided in August 1993 not to begin clinical trials, because the data that was available was "incomplete and unimpressive," but shark cartilage was harmless, and no one could prove it did not work.

There was enough anecdotal evidence to convince a willing mind. Laura ordered pills from an 800-number telephone outlet and added them to her daily regimen.

B arbara Rubin told anyone who wanted to listen that she was living proof of the power of alternative healing. Barbara was fifty-three, the twice-divorced mother of three grown children, happily sharing her apartment with a man half her age. In 1987 Rubin had received a Ph.D. in psychology at the University of Southern California, and since then had spent most of her time seeing private therapy patients. The only remnant of her previous career as a teacher was a wall full of photos of Barbara and an array of well-known actors; from 1988 until late in 1993 she had occasionally worked as a studio teacher, tutoring child actors on the set.

When her annual mammogram showed a shadow on her right breast, she grudgingly had a fine-needle aspiration. The report came back benign, which Barbara was prepared to accept, but the radiologist insisted that the lump was malignant. He performed another needle biopsy with the same results, and recommended that Rubin have a surgical biopsy. Exasperated, she went to UCLA, where she had a stereotactic core biopsy, the same procedure Dee had had, in which she lay prone on a table and a high-speed needle removed tissue samples from her breast. Barbara finally got the answer the radiologist had expected—invasive ductal cancer, just over one centimer.

That did not mean she was going to rush to get treatment. Rubin decided to shrink the tumor herself. She spent a week at the Optimum Health Institute near San Diego, visualizing the tumor shrinking, drinking wheat grass juice to cleanse her system. She visited an eighty-five-year-old hypnotherapist who suggested to her that she had given herself cancer because her relationship with her lover was too perfect, and Jews were used to suffering. She had a fight with her boyfriend and felt better. She stopped taking Premarin, her hormone replacement medication.

After one month of diligent effort Rubin had another mammogram. The tumor did seem to be somewhat smaller, but it had not disappeared and it had to come out. Reluctantly she allowed Susan Love to perform a lumpectomy, and in March she went in to discuss the results.

The pathology report said the tumor was 9 millimeters in diameter, but since it was an invasive cancer, not DCIS, Love wanted to operate again and take a sampling of lymph nodes. She also wanted her patient to have radiation therapy, the standard complement to breast-conserving surgery.

Rubin turned her down.

"I'm going to stick with wheat grass," she said, adamantly.

Love was equally stubborn. The National Cancer Institute was going to fund several studies of alternative treatments—and as soon as there was data to support wheat grass, or shark cartilage, or whatever else people believed in, Love was prepared to embrace a new treatment. In the meantime, she thought that such things ought to be used as a supplement to traditional treatment, not a replacement.

"It's harder for me to have the courage of my convictions when you don't agree with me," said Rubin.

"I can only speak from my experience," said Love. "I provide counsel. Then you have to make the decision."

But Rubin had a theory about radiation. It might kill cancer cells. She felt certain it also diminished the effectiveness of immune cells in her scar, and increased her chance of recurrence. If she lost lymph nodes she would have a greater chance of infection. It was absolutely clear to her: What was supposed to help her would likely do her in.

Love repeated the medical statistics. If Barbara's nodes were negative and she had radiation treatment, her chance of recurrence would be between four and eight percent. If she did not it jumped to thirty percent. If her nodes were positive, her chance of recurrence was thirty percent with radiation and sixty percent without. They were compelling numbers. Love asked her to reconsider her decision.

"I'm going to heal myself," said Rubin. "The mind and body are connected."

Love gave her a hug, asked her to go home and think over her decision, and promised that she would always be Rubin's doctor, no matter what she decided.

Barbara's life since her diagnosis was defined by a new regimen of healthful habits. She had heard that soy was supposed to reduce the risk of breast cancer, so she poured soy milk in her decaffeinated coffee and ate a salad with grilled tofu for lunch. She saw a reflexologist who worked on her feet a couple of times a month, and had a standing weekly appointment with her body work masseuse. She drank wheat grass juice and ate organic produce. As far as Barbara was concerned, the world was full of opportunities for healing, as long as she remained open to suggestion.

That much choice unnerved Dee. She put her faith wholeheartedly in Western medicine. It was an extravagant relationship: once she started the neo-adjuvant chemotherapy she embraced it with the same fervor she had once invested in avoiding it, certain that three or four cycles of drugs would shrink the large mass in her right breast and knock out the small tumor in her left breast.

Visiting Dr. Boasberg, the oncologist who had succeeded in getting Dee to start chemotherapy, became a social event, glorified by lunch out afterward, even if she had no appetite, or perhaps a stroll down a nearby shopping street. Her best friend, Suzy Drawbaugh, often accompanied her. They sat in one of the little treatment rooms and nattered on about where to eat lunch while three drugs—5 fluorouracil, Adriamycin, and Cytoxan—dripped slowly from a bag into an intravenous needle inserted on the top of Dee's left hand. She got the three drugs in combination, alternating with separate doses of 5-FU, which Boasberg mixed with the vitamin leucovorin, a folic acid derivative that he believed enhanced the effectiveness of that drug.

Dee told Suzy that she had changed her mind. "Chemotherapy," she said, "is my friend." She bought a $400 blond wig even though she knew it did not look quite as good as the $700 model she had seen in another store—and then, after two weeks of primping and complaining, she bought the more expensive one as well.

The stem cell transplant held a terrifying fascination for her—a bruiser of a treatment, surely big enough to wrestle even the invisible cancer in her bloodstream into submission. She was eager and frightened. When she heard about a support group that UCLA sponsored she begged Gary to go with her.

He did not want to go, but she refused to let up.

"You need to understand how scared I am," she said. "My liver could go down. My heart can stop."

Grudgingly he agreed to accompany her. The support group was held at an Italian restaurant in the San Fernando Valley, a two-hour drive from their house if the freeways were working, so the Wiemans left early in the afternoon to make sure they arrived on time.

They were too lucky. They hit Ventura Boulevard, the main business street that ran through the valley communities, a full two hours early. There was nothing to do, so they sat in the dimly lit restaurant bar and ordered a bottle of wine, and then another. When it was time for the group to begin they made their way to a private dining room.

The organizers wore pink lapel ribbons and determined smiles. Gary quickly ordered himself another glass of wine.

There were no other men there, just a handful of women trading war stories, many of them wearing scarves to cover their baldness. One pulled hers back to proudly display errant little tufts of hair that were beginning to grow in. When they found out that Dee was about to have a transplant, they started telling her what to watch out for—the side effects that their doctors had failed to tell them about.

The worst surprise, they agreed, was that their fingernails and toenails had peeled off. They had been told about the big reactions, the nausea, the vomiting, but somehow no one had remembered to tell them about this little insult. Dee should be prepared for it to happen.

She glanced over at her husband, the man whose first instinct had been to do nothing at all. He was visibly uncomfortable listening to this kind of detail.

"I'll be right back," said Gary. "I'm going to make a phone

call." He couldn't take this. All he could think was, Here is a group of pretty women, screwed, probably, surrounded by a sea of people who don't know what they are doing, trying to help them. To Gary it felt like a death march. It was too much for him to bear.

Dee watched his retreating back and thought, He never makes phone calls from a public phone. He is either going to the bathroom or going to the bar, and he did not want to say so in front of these women.

He never returned. Dee ate dinner with the other women and listened to a speaker talk about the emotional life of the cancer patient, a soothing speech about how it was all right to cry or be angry.

"You will not think about things in the same way ever again," the woman said. "Other people will wonder, and you will wonder, 'Well, how come this didn't bother me before but it bothers me now?' It was a different time. We have to look at everything. It doesn't matter what it was before. It is a different time now.

"You're assessing things differently," she said. "You look at your children and your family differently." Dee wrote it all down. It made sense to her. She had allowed herself to wonder more than once if she would stay with Gary when this was all over. Now she worried: What if she got sicker and could not depend on him to take care of her? She had never expected to be the one who got sick. Dee had thought that her role would always be to look after others.

Two and a half hours later she went out to the car to find Gary sitting at the steering wheel. When she mentioned that she was going to see her oncologist at St. John's he got furious.

"Why are you going?" he said. "You're going to UCLA. You're not going anywhere else. You don't need to ever see him again."

Dee had no idea what to say. It seemed as though Gary wanted her to organize and carry out this project without bothering him about the details—and if it did not work, it would somehow be her fault. A failure of management.

He would not let her get a word in.

"You're going to screw it all up," he said as they barreled down the freeway in the dark toward home. "None of your doctors are going to see you because you're vacillating back and forth, back and forth."

Dee thought to herself, Screw it. I just won't have the transplant. But she did not say that. Instead she remembered what the support group speaker had said.

"Your life has changed forever when this happens," she said.

13

THE BATTLEFIELD

IRENE AURELIA MEYERS RICH BUILT A FORMIDABLE CAREER IN THE MILItary. She served one stint as a combat nurse for a NATO operation in Turkey, in 1985, but ended up devoting most of her twenty-one-year career to women—first the wives, mothers, sisters, and daughters of enlisted men, and more recently the growing number of enlisted women as well. She received a doctorate in nursing science, and was named head nurse, Gynecology, Gynecological Oncology and Plastic Surgery at Walter Reed Army Medical Center.

On the gynecological oncology service she encountered a new group of needy patients who began to haunt her—women, so many of them young women, who suffered from breast cancer. People died; she had come to accept that. What she could not stand was people dying of a disease that had so far outsmarted those who treated it. Rich judged experience by a simple, almost naive set of guidelines. It was wrong for women who wanted so badly to live to die of a disease no one understood, and that was all there was to it.

She took care of one woman who was dying of breast cancer that had metastasized to her bones. The woman had a baby, and all she cared about was finding a position where she could hold her infant without too much pain. Rich gently placed the baby in the crook of her mother's arm, and then stood by, helpless. Two years later, she could not speak of that woman without crying.

In August 1992 Rich was made assistant chief of the Nursing Research Service—and was at work on a research project on pregnancy among enlisted women when the call came, in early 1994. The general in charge of the army's new breast cancer research program had decided to retire, and Rich had been chosen to take over, as of March.

She started work just two weeks before the first meeting of the Integration Panel, which was to review the 1,280 applications that had survived the scientific review. Rich had heard that several members of the panel had a reputation for adamancy—particularly Fran Visco, one of the patient activists in the group—and she anticipated heated debate. One of her first acts as program director was to send out a letter of introduction to each member of the panel. It was accompanied by a copy of the book *Getting to Yes: The Art of Negotiation.*

Irene Rich had led a more dutiful life than the president of the National Breast Cancer Coalition had. While Fran Visco was marching against the Vietnam War in the summer of 1971, Rich, then Irene Meyers, was sitting in her dad's car waiting for him to get off work at Elmendorf Air Force Base in Anchorage, Alaska, where he was employed by the Federal Aviation Administration. She was a nursing student at the University of North Carolina, but summers she came home—and since her family had only one car, she had to pick up her dad every afternoon.

She sat in the parking lot and watched the same ritual repeat itself over and over again. A plane came in from Vietnam bearing wounded soldiers, and the ones who were too weak to make the next leg of the trip were taken off. Then a truck drove up, and men loaded the coffins of boys who had died in the base hospital onto the plane for the journey stateside.

Injured soldiers off, dead soldiers on, day after day.

Rich had always planned to be a nurse. Watching that sorry parade, she decided to be an army nurse. To the dismay of her parents, who feared for her safety, and the ridicule of her friends, who questioned her sanity, she enlisted at the end of the summer.

If there were any logic to life, she and Visco would have grown old without ever being aware of each other's existence. But Fran Visco's life abruptly stopped making sense on the autumn day in 1987 when she was diagnosed with breast cancer. Six and a half years later, Fran Visco and Irene Rich became unlikely allies, guardians of a breast cancer research program the army did not want.

Fort Detrick, Maryland, was a brooding gray compound at the bottom of a boulevard that rolled along, innocently enough, past minimalls and manicured shrubs, to a dead end at the base's gate. This was where killer viruses lived in security tombs, a landscape frighteningly devoid of any signs of human activity. It was an unsettling place. The first time Fran Visco visited she had the irrational feeling that her hosts, surely aware of her antiwar past, would not allow her to leave. A tiny yellow brick bungalow sat like an afterthought at the left edge of the base—the headquarters of the Army Medical Research and Materiel Command Research Area Directorate VI, which housed the main office of the breast cancer research program.

On March 29, 1994, the Integration Panel assembled for the first time at a somewhat friendlier venue, a conference room at a nearby hotel. The panel members were assembled around a U-shaped table, with the army representatives sitting at the edges of the room. Rich, who had never met Visco before, took a seat behind her.

They were the custodians of change, mismatched both in appearance and attitude: Visco a short, stocky brunette with a pugnacious attitude, a woman who had elevated the pointed interruption to an art form; Rich a tall, rawboned woman at home in olive drab, a dignified full-bird colonel whose one concession to vanity was a formidable set of deep-pink fingernails.

Rich hoped that the seating arrangement would communicate what she saw as the army's proper role in these proceedings—administrative support. But as soon as she sat down Visco turned to confront her.

"Colonel Rich," she said, "am I the only person you sent this book to?"

Rich assured her that she had not been singled out, and the meeting got under way. Rich was thrilled. Her colleagues' criticisms of the program did not bother her. She had weathered her parents' concern and her friends' taunts when she enlisted; surely she could survive a new round of skepticism. She was doing just what she was supposed to do, after all, obeying a government edict. It did not matter that some of her coworkers thought the appropriation was a bad idea. Congress had voted, and she was carrying out their instructions. She was a sanctioned troublemaker, and she intended to wage war.

The government gave, however grudgingly, with the DOD program—and in the name of honesty, health care reform, and prudent finance, the government took away. On the basis of the NCI's December 1993 report on mammography, the Clinton Administration had devised a proposed policy for its health care reform package: mammograms for women over fifty were covered; for women under fifty, only if a doctor specifically requested the procedure.

In March 1994, the Congressional Research Service, a government-funded Library of Congress service that provided information to Congress, published an overview of breast cancer detection, prevention, treatment, and research funding, and fully half of it was taken up by information about mammography. It provided Congress with the rationale for Clinton's position: women between forty and forty-nine whose cancer was detected by mammography saw "no benefit at 5 to 7 years after entry," in terms of improved survival, "an uncertain and marginal benefit at 10 to 12 years, and an unknown benefit thereafter."

For every one thousand women screened in that age group, only one invasive cancer and one case of DCIS would be found. Mammography was great at finding malignancies in postmenopausal women, who tended to have fatty breasts; cancer showed up as a white shadow against a dark background. Most younger women had dense breasts that themselves cast white shadows on the film.

Reading their film was harder: one study showed that mammography missed as much as forty percent of premenopausal breast cancer.

It did not reduce mortality, as it did for postmenopausal women, whose cancers tended to be slower growing and more responsive to early intervention. Mammography for premenopausal women was a bad investment, whether for private insurance companies or, if Clinton's health care reform policy passed, for the federal government. Screening five million women between the ages of 40 and 49 cost $500 million, plus $120 million to $170 million for additional mammograms and biopsies for the ten percent of women whose films showed an abnormality.

Any woman who worried about breast cancer had likely memorized the enemy's strategy: a tumor grew in size from a grain of sand, to a pea, to a walnut, to a lemon, and as long as she caught it when it was a pin dot she was safe.

The American Cancer Society had started selling annual mammograms in 1982 with a potent promise: mammograms saw cancer before a woman felt a lump—and caught early, breast cancer could be cured ninety-five percent of the time.

The truth was more convoluted; Love felt that the ACS campaign telescoped a handful of subtle truths into a saleable mantra that turned out to be right only part of the time. Love explained it over and over again to women who came in feeling cheated, demanding to know why they felt a grape-size lump three weeks after they had a clean mammogram.

"Mammograms can see eighty-five percent of breast cancers—which is true," she said. "They may already be the size of a grapefruit, but we can see them. Then we say, 'Mammograms can find cancer early,' which is also true. They can't always, but sometimes they can. Then we say, 'Early cancer is ninety-five percent curable.' Which is true"—at least according to the admittedly untrustworthy five-year survival marker. "So when you say those three sentences fast, one after another, you come away thinking, 'Mammograms can find eighty-five percent of cancers when they're ninety-five percent curable.' Which is not true at all."

There were good cancers that grew slowly, were easy to detect, and responded well to treatment. There were nasty cancers that seemed to grow up overnight, having already invaded the lymph nodes. Early detection was not possible with those cancers, because by the time they registered on film or under a finger they were already juvenile delinquents—and premenopausal women tended to have more aggressive disease, which either was detected late or showed up early but took off too quickly to be caught.

What looked like results in younger women could at least in part be what doctors called "lead-time bias"—the illusion of progress where there was none. If a forty-five-year-old woman detected a breast cancer that was destined to resist treatment and kill her when she was fifty-two, it looked as though she had survived for seven years. If she found it at fifty she lived only two years. The numbers looked better if she found it early, but the result was the same. Jerilyn Goodman might feel she had improved her chances, but vigilance was not a guarantee of success.

A n unusual alliance formed to fight the Administration on mammography: feminists, conservative politicians, the American Cancer Society, and the American Medical Association, all of them determined to protect a woman's subsidized access to mammography. Their position was that it was still the only game in town, however flawed, and insurance ought to cover it. The number of women whose cancers were found early might not be statistically significant—but mammography seemed a lifesaver to those women, regardless of new doubts about its impact on mortality.

To critics, Clinton's position looked like the worst sort of economizing, with no consideration given to the long-term consequences—or to the fact that poor women would suffer more than wealthy women, who could choose to pay for their annual mammograms out-of-pocket. Dr. Bernadine Healy, now a Republican senatorial candidate from Ohio, attacked the Administration for making a "cost-based decision to limit women's health care choices," sacrificing early detection to the god of frugality.

Others dismissed the data. Dr. Daniel Kopans, the director of breast imaging at Massachusetts General Hospital and an outspoken proponent of mammography, insisted that the new studies were wrong; *The Wall Street Journal* reported his contention that "about thirty-five percent of the cancers detected in his radiology practice are in women under fifty." He complained that the NCI had been "influenced by political and health-care cost containment pressures," at the expense of women's health. The American Cancer Society said that the data was based on mammography done with outmoded equipment, and asked the NCI to reinstate its old recommendations for women under fifty, lest those women be confused by the conflicting reports.

Susan Love had an annual mammogram for two reasons: she had what she said were "the breasts of a seventy-year-old—fatty tissue, not dense, perfect for mammography," and she had risk factors that increased her chances of someday developing breast cancer. Both of her grandmothers had had the disease; she had taken birth control pills; and she was gay, which alone might raise her risk threefold, although the increased risk was usually attributed to gay women's tendency not to have children and to drink alcohol. If she were her own patient, she would have recommended screening.

But she believed the National Cancer Institute review, and because she did, Love found herself in an unlikely and unpopular position on mammograms: she did not think the government ought to pay for them for women under fifty. Mammography simply was not reliable. A woman with a false negative mammogram went home deceived and happy; a woman with a false positive endured all the anxiety associated with breast cancer until she found out, at additional expense and after more procedures, that she did not have the disease. The few younger women who did have a breast cancer that showed up on a mammogram might not live any longer than they would have otherwise. Buying that group the chance for less extensive surgery was not enough of a reason to spend the money involved in ferreting them out.

Love found all the concern about younger patients to be dangerously misplaced. The real problem was that only one third of older women had mammograms on a regular basis, compared to seventy percent of women under fifty. Love blamed the imbalance on the media, which seemed to her obsessed with a marketable minority subset, the young, attractive patient, usually with a husband and kids. That was the tearjerker story that landed on television talk shows and in magazines, while the majority of patients—women fifty and over—were invisible.

On March 13, 1994, Love's article, "The Untold Truth Behind the Mammogram Dispute," appeared on the Opinion page of the *Los Angeles Times*. She wrote:

> This change in policy was not prompted by a desire to save money in President Bill Clinton's health-care reform. . . . Nor was it an "insult" to women. . . . Rather, it was about telling the truth: We simply do not have the answers.
>
> In 1982, the American Cancer Society, on the basis of a few inconclusive studies, decided that mammography screening might save younger women's lives. . . . Over the years, these guidelines, although more the product of wishful thinking than good science, became etched in stone. Women believed they were rooted in established fact. Many professional organizations uncritically echoed the guidelines.
>
> Eight major studies of mammography screening, however, have failed to demonstrate a single benefit for women 40 to 49 five to seven years after their first mammogram. Ten to 12 years later, the benefit is marginal, at best.
>
> Mammography can detect small or early cancers in some women. But that is not the issue. Rather, it is whether finding such lesions early can actually save lives. The answer is consistently no. In some women, cancer is so slow growing that it doesn't matter whether it is found this year or next; they will live, either way. In others, the cancer is so aggressive they will die no matter when diagnosed.

Squabbling over mammography was beside the point. Love was fed up with what did not work. She wanted a better effort to find tools that did. She wrote:

True prevention of breast cancer requires that women be given the truth about medical tests, and that means better-funded studies rather than fiery rhetoric.

The question of whether mammograms improved mortality for women under fifty flitted at the edge of Larry Bassett's consciousness. He was not yet sure. The Canadian study that had started all the controversy suggested that mammograms in that age group yielded an expensive mess of false readings, unnecessary biopsies, and only a few cancers. But Bassett had heard about a large, well-designed Swedish study that said just the opposite: mammograms definitely improved mortality for women under fifty. Diametrically different conclusions—with ardent supporters for each one.

As chief of the Breast Imaging Section of UCLA's Department of Radiology and chair of the Breast Task Force of the American College of Radiology, Bassett was all too familiar with the two camps in this debate, and was often caught between them. On one side he had Susan, who said that the government's health care reform program ought not to pay for mammograms for women under fifty. On the other side were his colleagues, many of whom believed mammography was valuable for younger women, and something they were entitled to.

Susan liked to tease him. Of course radiologists supported more mammography. That was how they paid their bills.

His professional peers liked to hector him. Wasn't there some way he could put a gag on Dr. Love?

But Bassett liked Susan, and was prepared for the time being to tolerate what others considered her outrageous position. He thought she brought a new sense of community to the breast program at UCLA. Before she came the breast surgeons had treated him like some glorified technician who was incapable of discussing a mammogram with a patient. Radiologists were not to tell patients about anything abnormal they saw on the film, only to send the film on to the specialist, who would then divulge its contents. Love was different. She encouraged the radiologists to develop a relationship with the patients. Her primary intention was to make women feel less isolated, but the pleasant consequence for Bassett was that he and his staff felt less cut off. She respected him. The least he could do was defend her until he was ready to make up his mind.

Privately, Bassett thought that much of what Love said about mammography in younger women was true, but he was in no hurry to take a public stand. He was a methodical man who for fifteen years had juggled two specialties, bone and breast imaging. He published in both disciplines, taught, attended meetings of the Society of Breast Imaging with one group of cronies and made another set of friends in the International Skeletal Society.

When he finally began to feel schizophrenic, he chose breast imaging. Bassett liked the bone people, the surgeons, the sports medicine folks well enough, but he saw the chance to make a difference as a breast specialist. He could have a way of life instead of a job—and in the two years since he made the decision, he had come to refer to his work as "a campaign."

He took great satisfaction in doing his job well. Every cancer that his staff found early was a victory for him. What came after that was an issue for the others—the surgeons, the oncologists, and the radiation oncologists who fought systemic disease. His job was early detection, as early as possible, as many patients as possible. If he could not promise the younger women longer life, he might be able to spare them the more aggressive treatments. A lumpectomy instead of a mastectomy, or the chance to avoid chemotherapy altogether. That was certainly something.

Among all the people who worked at the Breast Center, Bassett was the only one who seemed immune to anger and frustration. He was a youthful fifty-one, a cheerful man who always looked as though someone had just shared a pleasant surprise with him, with a shock of prematurely white hair, pale eyes behind oversize clear plastic eyeglass frames, and a rounded baby face to which a slight smile was permanently affixed. He was patient and optimistic, an unusual combination among breast cancer specialists. He wanted more, but he acknowledged that he had a wily adversary.

Rather than bemoan the uphill struggle, he set modulated goals for himself, the kind of practical ambitions a man could reasonably hope to achieve. First, he wanted more women to come in more often. Sixty percent of all women over forty had had a mammogram, but only half of them returned for the kind of regular screening that kept women over fifty alive. Annual mammograms allowed a good radiologist to find a cancer early. The woman who came in once and never came back until she felt something did not improve her odds at all.

Second, he wanted more kinds of women to have screening mammograms. Well-to-do white women could afford to be diligent, but with fees as high as $165 at some private facilities, poor and minority women tended to stay away. Bassett had brought the cost at UCLA down to $89 by having technicians take the mammograms, which were read in a batch at the end of the day by two radiologists; a woman did not get her results immediately, but she also did not have to pay for the radiologist's time.

He hoped in the coming year to expand his reach even farther. Bassett's pet project was a mobile mammogram unit that was being outfitted by a mobile coach manufacturer in the Midwest. His benefactor, Iris Cantor, had staged a fund-raising event at which Hillary Clinton had appeared, and raised $500,000 to reach what Bassett called the "underserved" populations—working women whose schedules did not allow them to take off time for a mammogram, and poor women who could not pay for it. The coach might be the answer. He hoped also to do some research on new digital mammography technology, to see if it was possible to send clear images from the coach back to UCLA, via telephone lines.

Last, he wanted the quality to improve. Women frequently came to the multi with poor quality film from other facilities. Bassett was cochair of the U.S. Department of Health and Human Services' Agency for Health Care Policy and Research, involved in defining clinical practice guidelines for mammography. He also sat on the National Mammography Quality Assurance Advisory Committee, charged with defining the national standards that were the basis of the Mammography Quality Standards Act, which had been signed in December 1992 and would go into effect October 1, 1994. The sad fact was that mammography was only as good as the equipment, the technician who used it, and the radiologist who read the results—and too many women were victims of poorly maintained equipment, shoddy technique, or an imprecise eye.

There was much work to be done. Bassett estimated that at

least twenty percent of mammography machines did not yet meet the American College of Radiology criteria for accreditation. Before the passage of the MQSA, only about forty percent of the nation's mammography facilities even participated in the voluntary accreditation program. Starting in October, all facilities would have to meet federal standards similar to the American College of Radiology's guidelines. The act required all mammography facilities to undergo annual on-site inspections as well as reviews of staff and sample films, for certification by the Food and Drug Administration.

Bassett's fond hope was that improved technology would someday obliterate the gap between good intention and useful results—that perhaps digital mammography or computerized images might help identify early cancers in young women with dense breast tissue. For all the talk about finding the gene and developing a blood test, Bassett saw a long future for breast imaging. What if someone did find BRCA-1 and developed a test for it? There still had to be a way to find the cancer and look at it.

Larry Bassett expected to retire as a breast imaging specialist— and if someone could figure out a way to prove him wrong, he could always go back to sports medicine.

14

ILLUSION

T HERE WERE DAYS WHEN SEEING PATIENTS SEEMED A PROLONGED GAME of Beat the Clock, of processing bodies in just the way Bill Silen had taught Love not to, but teaching was happily exempt from profit considerations. She adored the few classes she taught. She was happier with what she called "the baby docs"—the medical students, residents and fellows—than she was with her peers, most of whom lacked her affinity for tumult. The baby docs were likelier to listen to her ideas without demanding footnotes.

Every Tuesday Love held an informal teaching conference to acquaint the younger members of the staff with some aspect of breast cancer treatment. Most of them would end up in another discipline—there was only a handful who wanted to be full-time breast surgeons. The newest member of the crew, Brooke Herndon, had announced on her first day that she intended to go into family practice, but she wanted to have a basic understanding of breast cancer.

As managed care grew, general practitioners would be the gatekeepers who sanctioned a referral to a specialist, so it was important that they know what to look for. Love was happy to have Herndon—family doctors had to be better trained if they were going to properly supervise a patient's medical future.

The conference on March 15 was a basic lesson in breast cancer pathology conducted by Love and Dr. Sanford Barsky, a medical school classmate of Love's who was on the multidisciplinary team. A shy, rumpled man who viewed the world from behind thick eyeglasses, Barsky existed in an isolated universe, where language was turned upside down. A bad cancer was "exciting" or "impressive," while a tumor that offered a decent prognosis was "unremarkable."

The easiest way to make sense of it, Love explained, was to remember that any cancer that had a special name was too languid to be killing someone. Medullary, tubal, and mucosal cancer might sound terrifying, but they usually had a better prognosis than run-of-the-mill invasive cancer, which had a more linear intent. These cancers dallied, creating odd designs and by-products, while invasive cancer existed to live up to its name—to inhabit the body's outposts.

"In my crude surgeon's mind," she said, "if they have all the time in the world, they sit around making tubes or mucus. If they're really aggressive, they don't bother. They just head out."

Barsky began a molecular explanation of the various types of breast cancer, but that was more information than overtaxed minds could absorb; one of the young men in the room almost instantly fell asleep, and a few others had to work hard not to. Love abruptly changed the subject. The mammography debate was still on her mind—and the more she thought about it, the more potential problems she saw. The congressional report quoted a statistic that bothered her: If one thousand women between the ages of forty and forty-nine had a screening mammogram, about fifty would have an abnormal finding, and thirteen of those would require excisional biopsies—to find one cancer and one DCIS. Women in that age group had 2.5 as many biopsies for every diagnosed cancer as women over fifty did.

A biopsy was minor surgery, but surgery nonetheless. Surgery depressed the immune system. Love thought that the healing process from a biopsy bore an unnerving resemblance to the malignant growth process, with white blood cells rushing to the site of the wound and an excessive level of cell activity. She found what she considered to be "lots" of cancer in wounds and scars. When she put those two truths together, she had to wonder: Did the very act of performing a surgical biopsy encourage the cancer it was designed to ferret out? In the 1960s Bernie Fisher had observed that it was possible to trigger cancers "that otherwise lived in peaceful coexistence with the host" and had not developed into life-threatening disease. If surgery could set off a malignancy that might otherwise lay dormant, then that was a damning argument against mammogram under fifty, which was where she saw most of the unnecessary biopsies.

To most oncologists this was an outlandish notion. The growth factors that accompanied the healing process could conceivably encourage a malignant cell to grow, as well as a healthy one. But if there was cancer, the surgeon was supposed to take enough tissue to guarantee clean margins—and if the patient was free of malignancy, how could the surgery spark its growth? Skeptics refused to dwell on the possibility that a single cell left behind could thrive on a procedure meant to eradicate disease. Susan, exasperated with existing treatments, was more willing to give in to her imagination, however farfetched her colleagues might find an idea.

Barsky did not like the idea, but he could not reject it entirely. He had to admit that cutting promoted cell change and growth. It was reasonable to ask whether a surgical biopsy might speed the development of an existing malignancy.

It was all too awful to consider. One resident glumly tried for safer ground, and asked how they could learn more about high-risk women.

"With my ductoscope," muttered Love, who had just received a third request for information from the FDA. "If I ever get it. If it ever works."

She let them go with a brief warning, that the only dependable thing about cancer was its unpredictability. "That's my sermon for the day," she said, glancing at her watch.

Dr. Michael Racenstein attended Love's teaching conference when he could, despite the fact that he had been a radiologist for two years. There was always something new to learn—or unlearn. The congressional report on mammography troubled him, since he spent much of his time reading mammograms for women under fifty.

He caught up with Love as she pawed through the day's phone

messages at Connie's desk. He had read her essay in the *Los Angeles Times,* and he wondered, just theoretically, what she thought would happen if there was no screening at all for women under fifty. If nobody even looked for breast cancer until a woman hit that age, what would happen to the mortality figures? Did detection before then have any impact at all on outcome?

When he put it that way, she was trapped. Much as she hated to say so, she did not think it made any difference. "If a cancer is meant to kill you in year ten," she said, "it will do so whether it is detected or not."

She had a question of her own for Racenstein. Love was always on the lookout for environmental and lifestyle clues as to why women got breast cancer. As the baby boom population blip headed for middle age and menopause, she worried most about estrogen replacement therapy. The Women's Health Initiative promised answers about its link to breast cancer risk, but that was at least ten years away. In the meantime there was not a single randomized control study on hormone use—no way to know if the women who took it got breast cancer more often than women who did not. Pharmaceutical companies touted its beneficial effect against heart disease and osteoporosis, in pamphlets illustrated with pictures of vibrant, happy women. To Love it was nothing more than a marketing campaign planted in sand. No one knew for sure what the long-term consequences would be.

She liked to describe what estrogen did as "tricking" the body into thinking it was still premenopausal. What if the trick worked too well? If more and more menopausal women took estrogen, and if the drug delayed changes in breast tissue, Love worried that mammography would start missing cancer in older women as well. In her darkest imagination she saw women taking hormones to make themselves look young—to the point where they fooled even a mammography machine.

She asked Racenstein if Premarin, the most popular hormone replacement medication, made it harder for radiologists to evaluate older patients.

"When we see menopausal women with dense breasts," said Racenstein, "that's the first question we ask."

Young women had a ritual mammogram for no good medical

reason; it was habit, and they needed to feel they were doing something, and that was it. Older women, seeking a defense against osteoporosis, heart disease, and the signs of aging, took hormones for decades—and so might decrease the odds that mammography would detect their cancers early enough to make a difference.

Dee Wieman loved all of it—the drugs, the scans, the bimonthly mammograms, anything that made her feel she was aware of the most minute change in her condition. She refused to accept that doctors did not understand her disease and treatments might not work. To her it was all a matter of research and organization. The answer was out there somewhere, and if the doctors were too busy to look, she would find it for them.

She still had to decide what to do when she was finished with her fourth cycle of chemotherapy, whether to have the transplant or the surgery first, but after two cycles she felt like she could handle anything. She was in control—being a responsible patient while she continued her quest for enlightenment.

She started carrying a large tote bag that she dubbed her "bag o'breast cancer," and the fuller it got the better she felt. Everything went into it—dozens of mammogram films, pathology slides, articles she clipped from magazines, books she found at the bookstore, copies of articles from UCLA's Louise M. Darling Biomedical Research Library. She had a calendar to keep all her medical appointments straight, and a couple of legal pads and red pens to take notes whenever she saw a doctor.

She still made parallel appointments with Dr. Love and Dr. Giuliano, despite her vow to switch over to Love exclusively. On the morning of March 16 she got ready to drive up to St. John's Hospital, intending to issue Dr. Giuliano a challenge. Dee wanted a new mammogram to see if two cycles of chemotherapy had done anything. If he did not agree she would never go back.

"That'll be the deal breaker," she promised her husband. But she was unable to say good-bye, even when Giuliano reiterated his position—that Dee needed aggressive therapy, a mastectomy and a transplant, the sooner the better. She wanted the two surgeons to reach a consensus.

Besides, she was looking for something to do. The time between appointments stretched out interminably. In addition to her private therapist, Dee decided to attend a support group at St. John's—not to talk, she insisted, but to listen. When she was finished with Dr. Giuliano she made her way to a conference room where a dozen women were assembled for a low-fat buffet lunch and an introductory session.

She left with another project to occupy her time. One of the women at the support group had said that her insurance paid for a $1,000 wig. Dee had never thought to bill her insurance for what seemed a cosmetic purchase, but it turned out that any of her doctors could write her a prescription for a better wig than the one she was wearing. She could keep that one for backup. She could take the first wig she had bought out of the bathroom sink cabinet where she had stashed it and donate it to some cancer group. That one, she had complained to Gary, made her look like Edie Adams in the old Tiparillo cigar ads. Now, at least, she could improve the illusion.

On March 21 she was at UCLA at Love's insistence. Dee wasn't scheduled to come in until April 6, but the process was dragging on too long. Love told women with smaller tumors and no lymph node involvement to take their time. "Breast cancer is not an emergency," she liked to say; they could shop doctors, read, think it over, and then decide what to do. Dee acted as though she had that luxury. Someone had to disabuse her of the notion.

Love had a single goal for the appointment—to get Dee to agree either to the transplant or the lumpectomy. She had one or two more cycles of chemotherapy to go, so it was time to commit. The whole debate about which surgery to have—Giuliano's mastectomy or Love's lumpectomy—was beside the point. She had to get Dee to decide to do something, whatever it was.

Just before the appointment she darted into Dee's examining room and said, "Hello, beautiful. I'm going to see you second, after this other woman, because I want to take a long time with you. So it's not that I don't love you, it's that I do."

Ten minutes later she was back. She breezed in and repeated her standard greeting.

"Hello, beautiful."

Dee fingered the parenthetical curves of her pageboy and replied, "Actually I'm not looking so good today, but thank you."

"So give me an update. Where are we in the scheme of life?"

Dee studied her lap. "Actually, I'm not sure yet." And she was off, a vortex of facts, fears, and rumor. She had heard that she would have to take baths or sponge baths, not showers, if she had a transplant at UCLA, and she did not like that idea. She worried that BCNU, one of the drugs UCLA used, would damage her lungs. She had a new pain under her right breast that was so bad she had sent Gary out to buy her a copy of *Gray's Anatomy,* but she could not find an explanation there. She had to be out of this appointment on time because she was booked on the three forty-five flight to Seattle, where her invalid mother, who suffered from emphysema, and her sister lived. Dee wanted to talk to doctors at the Fred Hutchison Cancer Research Center there about their transplant program.

Hutchison used a different drug regimen than they did at UCLA; maybe it was the perfect answer she was looking for. She was an incurable romantic—always ready to fall in love with a bright, shiny alternative.

She told Love that she wanted a new mammogram.

The more she talked, the quieter Love became. Since November, Dee had had thirty-two mammograms, the last one on February 15, but she wanted another, because perhaps it would show that the tumors had shrunk and a lumpectomy would work.

That opened another worry. What if she had a lumpectomy, and then the DCIS that was left led to metastasis?

Susan spoke slowly, in the hope that what she had to say would sink in. It was a long road from DCIS to invasive cancer to metastatic disease, but it was a very short hop from twenty-six positive lymph nodes to mortal danger. Dee had to stop thinking about her breasts and start thinking about her life.

"The risk of metastasis is already there," Love said. "It's already happened. It has to do with the nodes. The fact that you had it in all those nodes means there's a high chance that there are microscopic cells elsewhere. That's why you're getting the chemo and the bone marrow transplant and all that stuff. Whatever we do to the breast is not going to change that one way or another. What we do to the breast is just clean-up. That's all it is.

"You can do clean-up either with lumpectomy and radiation or with mastectomy," Love said. "But it doesn't affect living or dying. Okay? What affects living or dying is what you're going through now."

"Okay," said Dee. "This is where I get totally nuts." She told Love about a woman who had a lumpectomy and came to the bone marrow transplant support group to decide whether to have high-dose chemotherapy. She had three children. She already had metastatic disease in her shoulder bone. Dee was horrified to hear what they told her: she had only a ten percent greater chance of survival with high-dose chemotherapy. Dee still wanted to believe that the reward for enduring a transplant was a clean slate.

"My question is," said Dee, "these are women who have been through the scare of cancer, who obviously are taking care of themselves. How the hell—doesn't the high-dose stuff kill everything and you start all over again?"

Love wondered for a moment how many times she would have to explain the same information. Dee simply refused to accept the painful truth, which was that not everyone responded to a transplant.

Dee saw the tired look on Love's face.

"Okay, so you've got to worry about it forever," Dee said. She went on in a staccato panic. How could breast cancer grab someone just two years after a transplant? How come there were no reliable tests to confirm metastatic disease? How come the high-dose chemotherapy did not carry a warranty?

Love reviewed the statistics they had discussed before. Women with more than ten positive lymph nodes did not do well with standard chemotherapy—the cure rate was thirty, maybe forty percent. No one knew how much of a difference the transplant would make for this group, because the early research had all been done on women who already had demonstrable metastatic disease. With women like Dee it was simply too soon to tell.

"In some of the cells, the chemotherapy may stun them and not kill them," Love said. "In some of them, it may not do anything."

Dee was quiet for a moment. Then she said, "Okay. So we just don't know."

"We don't know," said Love. "Therefore we've got to try. Our plan is to cure you. So we've got to try the best we can to do that." She wanted to move quickly to try to wipe out the cancer before Dee showed signs of demonstrable disease.

"It's sort of like the Vietnam War," Love told Dee, "one of the first wars where the enemy was hiding behind the bushes. You never really saw him. You assumed he was there. You shot the hell out of the bushes and you never really went back to check because it was too scary. So you may have killed him and you may not have.

"We assume that the metastatic cells are there because, statistically speaking, there's a high chance that they should be. So we give you something and assume we've killed them, because we shoot the hell out of you. Then we wait and see. They either come back out again and say nyah-nyah-nyah-nyah-nyah, or they don't."

Love asked her patients to make a difficult leap, to move forward knowing just how uncertain the outcome was. That was why some patients left her. Ignorance—or a little blind faith—was a comforting buffer. She needed a decision from Dee. John Glaspy preferred surgery first and then the transplant, to reduce what the doctors called the "tumor burden," and allow the drugs to work on systemic disease. But UCLA was prepared to accommodate Dee. If she wanted the transplant first, in the hope of sparing herself extensive surgery, she could have it.

She promised to talk it over with Gary. In the meantime, she gave Love her newest blood workups and films, just in case Love saw something promising that the others had missed.

Love left the room with the resident who had observed her hour-long tussle with Dee. "It's interesting what people hear," she said to him as they walked over to copy some of Dee's records from other doctors. " 'If the chemotherapy kills all the cells, why does it come back?' " She could not in good conscience let Dee have a transplant thinking it would kill all her cancer, even though it would have been easier for both of them.

*   *   *

In addition to her infiltrating cancer, Dee Wieman, like Shirley Barber, Laura Wilcox, and Jerilyn Goodman, had what Love called "precancer," or DCIS, ductal carcinoma in situ. Had she come in with that as her only diagnosis, she would have heard the same thing those women had been told: mastectomy was the only way to get rid of a condition that developed into invasive cancer just thirty percent of the time.

Dr. Boasberg was beginning to think that a bilateral mastectomy would be a good idea for Dee, to get rid of all the localized cancer at once, but he left that conversation to the surgeons. Love's strategy of starting with a small surgery for the most dangerous of Dee's cancers could turn out to be best. He could imagine that Dee might refuse to do anything if her doctors suggested too radical a treatment.

Dee was obsessively concerned with the size of the tumor. She asked every doctor who examined her to measure it and compare the measurement to earlier figures, and she monitored it herself, feeling for the lump, trying to determine whether it felt smaller or softer from one day to the next. Her life so revolved around her looks that she could not yet grasp what it would be like to survive in a different body.

The tasteful, tailored clothes she now wore were a recent charade, an odd stab at decency, as though a matronly appearance would make her seem more deserving of a cure. Before she was diagnosed, Dee Wieman dressed to show off her cleavage—not to flaunt it, but to enhance what she and her husband considered her most seductive feature. She favored a sundress with a plunging neckline or a form-fitting top. She liked lounging in a bathing suit at the water's edge with a bottle of wine and a group of good friends. Dee and Gary were always entertaining. Everyone who knew her considered her the perfect hostess—generous, gracious, always ready to have a good time.

It was all twisted up together, being sexy and being alive. Life was allure.

No more. Gary had stopped touching her, confused by his wife's reluctance to do any of the things they used to do. He dated the change from the day her hair had begun to fall out. Suddenly she was terrified. They stopped enjoying dinner together or going to the movies. Even sitting at home at night watching television was a strain. Intimacy seemed to him out of the question.

But all the decisions were unspoken, which only served to confuse things. Gary might feel that his wife shunned everyone's company, including his own; Dee, for her part, wondered silently if Gary realized how distant he had become. He blew her kisses now instead of kissing her on the lips, and what had once been an embrace was now a wave from the door as he left for work.

She started wearing heavy socks and sweat clothes to bed, because the chemotherapy made her cold, but the chill breeze off the water penetrated, and most nights she gave up and headed for the living room couch. But she never complained about the bedroom's sliding door being open. They had always slept that way, for a bit of ocean breeze. Gary thought she slept alone because being jostled in bed caused her pain.

The results were the same, whatever the explanation. Once Gary went to bed, around seven, Dee was all alone—no one to talk to, no one to cuddle. Even if she tried the master bedroom, it usually did not last.

Dee's stepmother and her stepmother's mother had died of breast cancer, and one relative swore the younger woman succumbed because she thought about the disease too much. Dee worried that she, too, would think herself into trouble. She also believed the inverse: that she could think herself out of trouble if she just did more research.

If the doctors did not agree among themselves, or if they pushed her to decide before she was ready, it was because they had a different goal in mind. The doctors were trying to save her life. Dee Wieman was trying to salvage the way she lived.

The fact that no one had as yet found BRCA-1 did not stop the government from spending money in anticipation of its discovery. The combined resources of the NIH and the DOD had forced the research community to broaden its definition of breast cancer research—so the NIH issued an announcement that $2.6 million was available to pay for eight to ten three-year grants, to study how best to counsel women who had the gene for heritable breast cancer. Once there was a gene, and a blood test to detect it, medicine was going to run into a brick wall. It had nothing to offer women beyond good intentions and frequent exams.

Love and a dozen other doctors gathered in the Breast Center conference room to figure out how to help patients endure the high-stakes waiting game. Dr. Wayne Grody, the medical geneticist who ran the university's molecular diagnostics laboratory, wanted to go after the new NIH grant because he saw great similarities between BRCA-1 and a gene for cystic fibrosis which he was studying. They were both big genes, with hundreds of possible mutations, and it was unlikely that any early test would be able to detect them all. Love got involved because she was always on the lookout for research projects she could hook up with, grants where she would be named one of the principal investigators because she was able to supply either patients or clinical data. The Breast Center's high-risk clinic could provide subjects for this study, women whose family histories made them likely carriers of the gene.

The group had to figure out what kind of intervention and counseling would be productive. Psychologist David Wellisch anticipated that women would fall naturally into one of three groups—those who investigated and decided not to take the screening test, those who took the test and had the gene, and those who took the test and did not. What he could not yet predict was who among those three groups would be most in need of help, or what kind of help they would need.

"How do we counsel them?" Love asked. "What do we say medically? About nutrition? We don't exactly have a preventive answer. What we have are these quasi-preventions that may or may not work. You have to standardize what you're going to offer, and how you do it, before you can study how these women do. The way you present it is crucial. You say, 'Have your breasts cut off if you have the gene,' and women are going to have their breasts cut off." Any recommendation was going to come off sounding like a rule—not because the doctor meant it that way, but because women were so eager for a definitive answer.

One of the other doctors suggested that they might do a more "naturalistic" intervention, and Love groaned defensively. They were getting uncomfortably close to an emperor's new clothes grant—pretending that nothing was something, just to get the funds.

Dr. David Heber looked up from the papers in front of him as though he had just awakened, and announced, "You have to have a study outline."

No one was more successful at getting government money than Heber, a slender, preoccupied man known in the halls at UCLA as the doctor who intended to turn wealthy west side women into rural Chinese peasants. Heber, an endocrinologist, had the previous year received his second $2 million grant from the NIH to study the relationship between nutrition and cancer, and had a new thesis he was very excited about—that soy and particular kinds of fats, not the total amount of fat, combined to explain the lower breast cancer rate in Asian women.

Heber believed that a combination of low-fat diet, soy products, and strenuous physical exercise would diminish the amount of estrogen a woman produced—a powerful preventive against developing breast cancer later in life. He intended to write a new grant proposal for a clinical study just to look at that possibility.

He attended the meeting about the counseling grant primarily as a financial advisor, to counsel the group how to put together a proposal that would sell. Ideas were fine, as long as there was an outline full of practical details to support them. The government liked plans, one for spending the funds and a contingency plan if the original idea did not work out. And the group had to define what Heber called a "primary outcome variable," the goal they hoped to attain.

"Acceptance," said Grody. Until someone could devise a medical response to a positive gene test, the best a woman could hope for was to come to terms with the verdict.

Love grabbed a grease pencil and began to write a diagram on the board. They needed three groups of high-risk women—those who decided not to have the gene test, those who had it, and those who received information before and after they took the test. The last group would be divided in two, to see which helped more, educational literature or counseling.

The researchers would look for behavioral changes in the various groups. Did the women continue to come in for clinical exams? Did they continue to get mammograms?

Dr. Ganz chuckled. "And," she said with a dark grin, "are they denied health insurance?"

The longer the medical community had to wait for BRCA-1, the more opportunity they had to contemplate the fallout from its discovery. The only benefit to the delay was that it enabled the government to prepare. A federal advisory council from the National Center for Human Genome Research had studied the social and personal consequences of genetic testing for heritable breast cancer and concluded, "It is premature to offer testing of either high-risk families or the general population as part of a general medical practice." Testing on demand would only lead to abuses of the sort that AIDS patients or those who tested positive for HIV had encountered.

One woman in the room reported that the location of the gene would be announced "momentarily."

Love gnawed on her thumbnail.

"We've been saying 'a year or two' for a year or two," she said.

15

THE ECONOMICS OF COMPASSION

ONLY TWO WOMEN SIGNED UP FOR THE MULTIDISCIPLINARY CLINIC on Friday, March 25. Susan Love loitered in the hallway outside the examining rooms with Sherry Goldman and Leslie Laudeman, her new administrator, wondering how she was going to face the doctors who had volunteered their afternoon and stood little chance of making a dime off the investment. On days like this it was hard to ask for their altruism, when she received a guaranteed salary no matter how many patients showed up.

She was full of bravado, determined not to let Sherry or Leslie see how concerned she was. Like many of her patients, Love was adept at denial.

"Here's my alternate plan," she said in a conspiratorial tone. "If we go up in smoke—if we go up in smoke at UCLA—then we open the Santa Barbara Breast Center and Spa."

Her grin widened. "We charge a flat fee for food and lodging," she said, "and that way we save a lot of money. Everybody's too busy throwing up to eat. And we don't need a beautician on staff because their hair is falling out. Maybe a wig person."

Goldman was red in the face from trying not to laugh too loud and rattle the waiting patients.

"It'll have to be on the beach," said Love. "I think we could make a killing, so to speak."

"And you go into a cabana for radiation," said Goldman.

"Yeah," said Love. "You wouldn't take long to get undressed because you'd be in a bikini."

The first patient that afternoon was a young woman whose pathology report showed nine positive lymph nodes. Her lawyer husband had neatly organized all her paperwork in a notebook with colored subject dividers, in the hope that the ritual his profession demanded would buy his wife justice, but the cutoff for transplant eligibility was ten nodes. He and his wife were frantic. The doctors they had seen so far had given them no hope. They felt as though they had been sent home to wait for her to die.

Love asked the woman if she could show the pathology slides to Dr. Barsky. If he looked hard enough, perhaps he could find evidence of cancer in a tenth node.

"Don't worry," she told the anxious patient. "We're not looking for a tenth to be able to say that you're sicker." She just wanted the patient to qualify for a transplant. Love instinctively agreed with John Glaspy's position: while she had questions about the efficacy of the treatment, she preferred doing something to doing nothing, and she would be happy to be proven wrong.

The woman agreed. This was the first time anyone had suggested that there was more she could do. "But please," she said, a bit superstitious about being in worse trouble than she was already in, "don't make it more than ten."

The next morning Sherry reported that the patient had called to say that she was thrilled with the way Love had dealt with her. "She nearly jumped out of her chair when you said, 'I think there's hope for you,'" Sherry said. "Today she said that was the first time anyone had said that to her."

It all came down, too often, to attitude. The patient had the same disease she had had when she visited the other doctors. All Love had done was to suggest she might not die—not hope, exactly, but not hopelessness, either. For all her skepticism about the treatments she provided, she was loath to give up possibility.

*   *   *

In UCLA slang, Leslie Laudeman came from "the other side of the street"—the inpatient hospital, where she had been a nurse administrator for oncology and bone marrow transplants, as opposed to the outpatient medical plaza where the Breast Center had its offices. Barely six weeks into her new job, she was already painfully aware of how different her perspective was from the rest of Love's staff. She told her husband, himself a cancer survivor, that she felt like the devil's advocate—a conservative among liberals, a woman who was supposed to talk about responsibility and priorities to a group of rebels.

She had worked over the past ten years with John Glaspy and Denny Slamon, which did little to enhance her credibility. Whenever she disagreed with Love she sensed resistance, to the point where she felt compelled to reassure Susan: She was not some mouthpiece installed by Slamon and Michael Zinner to enforce their point of view.

"You need to understand," she told Love. "I really am here for you and the Center." But Laudeman made a distinction between unquestioning support, which she would not provide, and informed advice, which she could. There were some problems Love could do nothing about, even if she were so inclined. UCLA had always had a reputation for elitism—for seeing itself as "the mecca," as Leslie put it, not as part of a larger community. Even if Susan were diligent about medical etiquette, which she was not, many private practice doctors simply preferred to work with competing area hospitals.

And Love would never be on equal footing with Slamon and Glaspy, UCLA lifers, men who had status in the academic community. Patients might perceive the Center as Love's program. The men behind it were never going to hand it over and walk away.

There were plenty of things she could do, though. When Love approached Laudeman about the Physicians' Referral Service, which continued to follow university policy and refer new breast cancer patients to its roster of surgeons, the new administrator was firm: It was not a plot to deprive the Center of patients. There were other surgeons at UCLA who made part of their living performing breast surgery, and the referral service had a responsibility to send patients to them as well as to Susan. Rather than complain about something she could not change, Laudeman suggested that Susan try harder to improve her standing at UCLA, which in turn would lead to referrals from other faculty doctors.

Susan might be a celebrity, but she had to learn not to act like one. Even the smallest misstep had ramifications. She had drafted a form letter to go to the referring doctors for all multidisciplinary patients, to go out over her signature. Laudeman gently suggested a correction—that the lead doctor on the specific case sign the letter, since that doctor undoubtedly had an ego just as Susan did.

On the little things Love usually acquiesced, glad to have someone around who could tend to the bureaucratic details she found so distasteful. Laudeman had not yet worked up the courage to broach what she considered the largest issue. She felt that Love could spend less time with her patients and still provide the quality care she talked about. Less time would mean more volume, more revenues, an important consideration for a program that was about to enter its third year in the red.

Laudeman prided herself on what she called a "holistic" approach to medicine. It was what separated oncology nurses from surgery nurses, who never saw the patient before or after a procedure, or emergency room nurses, who got someone stable and sent him on his way. Leslie had seen people recover and go back to their lives, but she also had stood by while a patient received treatment, faltered, and died. She had spent long hours talking to family members, trying to get them, and the patient, to accept what was happening. So she shared Susan's feelings about the importance of quality care. She just thought there had to be a cutoff point.

She rehearsed her comments as she went about her day. As Leslie saw it, the minimum level of care gave a patient what she needed to get better, and no more. The ideal level of care, the maximum, was the hour-long appointment with Susan Love herself, a nice idea, but impractical. If the Center did not survive and Love made good her threat to decamp, then no one in Los Angeles would get to see her at all. That was hardly progress. The solution? Maybe forty-five minutes, tops, instead of an hour. Maybe a tight fifteen minutes for someone who really did not have a problem. Not surrender, but a reasonable compromise.

Whenever Laudeman had to evaluate a service or program she

asked herself, "Whose need is this?" She had seen how happy Love was when seeing even the most difficult of patients. Yes, the patients had needs—but perhaps Dr. Love did, too, and Leslie wondered if she sometimes lingered with a patient because it made her feel better.

Whatever the reason, it had to change. The university could not afford to give away time. The patient could not realistically afford to pay for it. More to the point, fifteen extra minutes holding a nervous patient's hand did not make a difference in the outcome. The new administrator put it on the agenda for the next meeting of the Breast Cancer Steering Committee; this was not a battle she could win without help.

Dr. Michael Zinner, the ambitious executive chairman of UCLA's Department of Surgery and Chief of the Division of General Surgery within it, liked to quote Sister Mary Madeleine, the CEO of St. John's Hospital. "No margin," Sister Mary had once told him, "no mission."

He might have alienated some of his staff early in his tenure by suggesting that there was such a thing as making too much money. There was also such a thing as making too little. He had rigorous expectations of his surgeons. Medicine was business. Susan Love could talk about quality care as much as she liked. If the Center did not start to show a profit, he was not going to be able to protect her.

The Breast Center was one of the few General Surgery programs that was losing money—at a time when the Division was reeling from the loss of over ten percent of its $8 million to $10 million operating budget. The Sepulveda Veterans' Administration Hospital contributed $1 million annually to faculty and resident salaries—but the VA had collapsed in the January 17, 1994, Northridge earthquake and was to be shut down permanently and replaced with an ambulatory care center. Zinner had to figure out how to pay salaries for the upcoming 1994–1995 academic year without that money, and the first question anyone asked him in a discussion of the deficit was which programs were not making money. The Breast Center always headed the list.

As chairman of the department he was in a position to buy the

Center a little more time. He was as stubborn as Love, if quieter in his determination, and still convinced that he would prevail. He could wean her from public life, and once she devoted all her energies to UCLA the program would flourish. At the end of March he made a unilateral decision to underwrite the program for a third and final year, regardless of how the numbers looked in July. He had the authority to do so, and saw no reason to submit the issue to the faculty—better to risk their resentment than to allow them a say in the matter. Perhaps in the next year Slamon would have the Revlon money in place, to fill the gap between Love's university budget and what she needed to survive—or less likely, Love would start making money on her own.

This was not charity. In return for his generosity he expected certain sacrifices. As he saw it, any decent doctor had long since abandoned hope of a regular life, no matter what their job description said. On the wall of his office Zinner had proudly hung a photograph of himself holding an impressively large fish. He had gone to Cabo San Lucas for five days earlier in the year—the only vacation he gave himself, although officially he was allowed two weeks. He stayed late on Wednesdays and came in early on Saturday mornings for the M & M—the mortality and morbidity conference, where doctors presented unusual cases from the preceding week and discussed them with their peers. A normal vacation and reasonable hours were for other professions.

Zinner believed in hiring good people and then leaving them alone, but that strategy was not working at the Breast Center. Unlike Laudeman, he did not care if Love spent a long time with her patients. His complaint was that she spent too much time doing everything else—that her political work and an endless stream of public appearances and interviews got in her way. He also thought she was beginning to believe her own publicity, running the multi conference as though her point of view was a given, expecting the other doctors to prove their case if they disagreed.

He believed that people judged a facility by the amount of attention they received, not by quantifiable criteria like survival statistics. But he defined attention differently than Susan did. She thought that spending an hour with a patient was good work; Zinner wanted her to be at the Center more often, so that patients and prospective patients felt she was a dependable presence. And he wanted her to give her colleagues a bit more respect.

It was time for her to stop acting like she ran a boutique. The university, as Zinner perceived it, was not unlike the convent. One was expected to be faithful and selfless, and leave worldly concerns to others.

Love was mystified at the demands that were being made of her, and suspicious of anyone who asked her to alter her behavior. It always sounded like they were trying to lure her back into the fold—to make her look right, ever the good daughter. Why on earth would she want to behave like the men who had managed to do so little for her constituency?

Still, she dearly wanted the Center to succeed; for her approach to have credibility it ought to function within a major medical center, not at the periphery. She knew she was being watched, and she told her staff it was "hunker down time." Love would not change her method, but she could make sure that the Center worked as smoothly as possible.

The bigger question was how to buy an independent future. The Streisand auction viewing had yielded a meager $23,000, far below the six-figure dreams that had propelled her through February. She had stopped pretending that Streisand might come through as a major donor, and had so far failed to find a likely replacement. Individual donations added up to $60,000, not even enough to hire another nurse-practitioner. Revlon might in fact solve her immediate problems, but she worried that Slamon would then expect to play an even more active role.

She refused to fret in public, which would betray her nerves and weaken her position. So the anxiety imploded: she chewed her fingers incessantly, whenever her hands had nothing to do. Her weight sneaked up fifteen pounds, a tribute to chocolate, which she found irresistible, and comfort dinners that provided succor after a long day. At work Love was a model of caffeinated restraint—too many Diet Cokes and cups of coffee, perhaps, but lots of plain bagels and raw vegetables with yogurt dip. Once out of the office the pendulum swung the other way.

Moderation was out of the question. Love had always been

incautious about her own health, in defiance of the advice she handed out daily. The chain-smoking and daily birth-control pills had given way in later years to other, equally dramatic habits. She and Helen had decided they wanted a second child soon after Kate was born, and when Love got pregnant and miscarried she worried that at forty-one her time was running out. So she took Clomid, a fertility drug, until she got pregnant again, despite her concern that there might be an increase in ovarian cancer risk associated with fertility drugs.

She miscarried a second time and switched to Pergonal, which she took for a year, but she never again got pregnant. She switched her attention to the thirty extra pounds she had carried since Kate's birth, which she was able to lose only after resorting to a liquid diet program at UCLA. Love had no patience for smaller portions, which required a more subtle form of discipline. She preferred a radical approach—complete abstinence and a protein drink.

For the new fifteen pounds she decided on a booster program she invented herself, chocolate protein drink and as much air-popped popcorn as she could stomach. She also decided to take the five flights of stairs to and from her office instead of relying on the elevator. When she and Helen had first moved to the Palisades she had started her day at five in the morning with a half-hour of video-taped aerobics, but lately it was getting easier to think of reasons to roll over for another thirty minutes' sleep.

Love snickered to herself when she saw the medical students huddled in a knot at the end of the hallway. This was her annual opportunity to teach the second-year students how to do a proper breast exam, and the prospect made her laugh. There were a few women in the hall, but most of the white-coated students were men, whose only experience with the female breast was sexual—in a magazine, at the movies, on a date. They were about to spend a long afternoon learning a new way to palpate breasts, and the prospect clearly made them nervous. The hallway reeked of flop sweat.

"This place smells like a locker room," said Love, loud enough for the initiates to hear. She gathered together the five other doctors who would be instructing students and gave them one final piece of advice before dispatching each one to an examining room: she did not want the next generation of doctors to squeeze a woman's nipples during a breast exam. They would almost always get a discharge simply because they had stimulated the nipple, which meant that a panicked woman rushed to a specialist for no reason. Love had never thought that sporadic discharge was an indication of trouble. Persistent, spontaneous discharge on one side was cause for concern; otherwise there was no reason to scare people.

The students shuffled into the examining rooms, where an instructor and a volunteer awaited them. Love's model was Evelyn, a retired schoolteacher with a sprightly air, who liked the idea that she could help train the doctors of tomorrow. She sat primly on the examining table in her hospital gown while Love described proper examining room etiquette to five students.

Love opened Evelyn's gown and explained the visual exam. First she looked for gross differences in shape or size, though she was quick to explain that women's breasts rarely matched perfectly.

"I used to," said Evelyn.

Love smiled. She asked Evelyn to clench her arm muscles, because a tumor caused the skin to retract, "and it'll make a dent" where it attached to underlying muscle. She asked Evelyn to put her arms up above her head so that she could look for retraction underneath the breast—and to lean forward, because a tumor fought gravity and caused the skin to dimple.

Next she asked Evelyn to raise one arm, and she ran her fingers straight down from the woman's armpit to her ribs, looking for the "little blip" that meant a swollen lymph node. Only then was she ready to examine the breast itself.

Love preferred a lateral exam, fingers marching across the chest, to the more popular circular pattern that the students found in their textbooks, but which covered less terrain. She closed her eyes and narrated, as she ran her fingers across Evelyn's chest— "collarbone to rib cage, breastbone to the edge of the latissimus muscle. And use flat fingers. You're not playing the piano."

One young woman asked, "Do you always stand on the same side of the table?"

"One of the things that's important on a physical exam is to figure out how to do it in a way that's not crazy," Love replied.

"Changing sides of the bed is crazy. We teach complete physical exams by organ systems, but that's not the way to do it. When I did them, I thought about doing everything you need to do sitting up, and then everything laying down, so the patient isn't sitting up, then laying down, then sitting up, then laying down."

Suddenly Evelyn piped up, "Would it make any difference if they knew how old I was?"

"You could brag about it," said Love.

"I'm eighty-two," said Evelyn.

The group cooed appreciatively, and the first student, a woman, stepped forward to try to mimic what Love had done. Love stood right next to her, watching her every move, and as the student reached to feel for lymph nodes Love advised, "You need to have shorter fingernails."

She had suggestions for everyone—press harder, do not press so hard, put an arm at a woman's back to help her lay down, and again to help her rise, and always help her put her gown back on.

She also tutored them in compassion. The most comprehensive physical exam in the world was not enough, not if the patient was paralyzed with fear the whole time. A good doctor knew how to chat.

"Sometimes I say to the patient, 'Oh, you've got ribs, it's good to have ribs, you're supposed to,' " Love explained. "Because the patient's nervous. If you take a long time—or if you stop and feel something again—they've got themselves dead and buried before they sit up."

Once all the students had examined Evelyn, she sat up and said, "I'm going to tell my doctor next time to go across. I'll say, 'Dr. Love told me.' They won't believe I came here."

Love wrapped her arm around Evelyn's shoulder and said, "You ever find *anything*, you come to me. Don't let anyone else do anything to you. I'll take care of you. You've earned it."

When Love asked the students if they had any questions, the first young woman confessed that when she felt her own breasts they seemed terribly lumpy.

"I worry about it myself," she admitted in a small voice.

"But what you're looking for is a walnut—or a boulder—in a gravel road," Love said. "It feels different."

She apologized for the one flaw in the program, which was that none of the models had newly diagnosed breast cancer that had not yet been treated. The malignant lump remained a theoretical concept.

"I wish I had a cancer patient model," she said, "but the last thing a woman who's just been diagnosed with cancer wants is forty breast exams."

The best she had to offer was local psychologist and breast cancer survivor Ronnie Kaye, who had spoken to the entire group and the day before had been a volunteer like Evelyn, through forty breast exams. Young doctors also needed to learn how to look at a mastectomy scar without wincing.

Dr. Bernard Fisher's twenty-seven-year reign at the NSABP ended on March 28, 1994, with a National Cancer Institute order that he be removed from his position as principal investigator. Three days earlier the NSABP had notified the NCI of problems with data from a second Montreal hospital, this time one that had participated in the NSABP's tamoxifen prevention trial for high-risk women. Mammography dates for four patients appeared to have been altered, to make them eligible for the trial—and Fisher's team had known about the questionable data since September 1993. This new disclosure was all the NCI needed to turn indignation into disciplinary action. The NCI expected the University of Pittsburgh to comply immediately and name an interim replacement for Dr. Fisher, who quickly announced that he had requested an administrative leave of absence.

The NCI, which as the sponsor of the NSABP's clinical trials was under criticism for not having monitored Fisher's work as closely as it might have, also cut off enrollment in the group's studies, including the tamoxifen prevention trial for high-risk women. The prevention trial had eleven thousand women already enrolled but needed sixteen thousand, so the action guaranteed a delay in collecting data.

Immediately Love's phone began ringing with a new round of

interview requests. She stuck to her position: she would happily discuss the data, but she would not talk about Bernie Fisher. She revered him. The lesson of his life was not lost on her: he was a surgeon who spoke out against established therapies, pressed for radical change, and was about to become a victim of his own ego. Love felt that he had forgotten his obligation to his patients, a more damning indictment than some statistically insignificant data.

For his part, Fisher was caught between disbelief and rage, struggling to figure out the proper response to what seemed to him a completely misdirected attack. He considered what was happening a "contrived event, political inspiration," driven by activists and the media, neither of whom properly understood the world of clinical research. He believed that the furor over the falsified data, not the data itself, would eventually harm the women of America. It could make them wary of participating in clinical trials, or get in the way of the trials continuing. There had to be a way to explain that the data problems were statistically insignificant, that he considered himself his patients' greatest ally.

For the moment, though, he took refuge in silence and isolation. It seemed a safer place than the public arena, for a man who had spent his adult life in a kingdom of his own devise.

Newsweek reported on the NSABP scandal in its March 28 issue. It also alerted readers to the pending battle between two lingerie manufacturers—Gossard, which had just introduced its Super Uplift bra in the United States, and Playtex, whose long-awaited Wonderbra would arrive on U.S. shores in May. It was the perfect collision between medicine and fashion: the NSABP scandal made women wonder if they had been fools to try to save their breasts; the bra wars said that beautiful breasts were an essential.

Desire for the uplift bras had been mounting ever since January, when the rail-thin model Kate Moss told *Vanity Fair* magazine that a Wonderbra could provide even her with cleavage where none had existed before. Ample breasts—or the illusion of amplitude—were about to be the height of style. Cleavage was an imperative.

After a few seasons of a skinny aesthetic, the bra wars made for good copy, a voluptuous celebration of the female form. Gossard had started out selling the Wonderbra in Great Britain, thanks to a licensing agreement with a subsidiary of the Sara Lee Corporation. When the license expired in 1993 Sara Lee took it back and awarded it to Playtex. Undeterred, Gossard rushed into production with the Super Uplift, a padded bra made up of forty-six separate pieces, which hit the Manhattan Saks Fifth Avenue store weeks before the competition. Gossard's marketing director, Mark Pilkington, told *Newsweek* that he planned to "convert women who are 'functionalists' (a bra is a bra is a bra) to 'enjoyers' (a bra is a bra except on special occasions, when they want to take the plunge) to 'indulgers' (they want to take the plunge every day)."

Saks sold four hundred Super Uplift bras in a single day. The magazine cited several reasons for the sudden popularity of artificial cleavage: Madonna, whose infamous Jean-Paul Gaultier cone bra had focused everyone's attention back on the bosom; the popular Victoria's Secret catalogue, which offered sexy lingerie at reasonable prices; and women's new fear of breast implants, spawned by stories of a Pandora's box of physical symptoms connected to silicone leakage.

The bosom had returned, and anyone with twenty-three dollars could have a Wonderbra. *Newsweek* ran a photograph of Madonna wearing an uplift bra—eyes closed, a look of haughty serenity on her face, an eager member of the paparazzi in the background. A woman was supposed to have beautiful breasts—which was why Laura Wilcox insisted on reconstruction, why the plastic surgeon was so surprised by Jerilyn's resistance. Dee Wieman's Japanese radiologist had confessed bewilderment when she agonized over having a mastectomy. His wife would do it if she had to—but then, the Japanese did not idolize the breast the way Americans did.

Laura had tied her line to vanity. She was no longer pregnant, and her surgery was scheduled for May 24. It was all part of a calculated plan to be whole by the time her severance pay ran out at the end of the summer. She would recover, get back on the Hollywood circuit, get a new job, start a social life. In the autumn she would have her life back again.

She was thinking about how to network for a job when her

gynecologist at UCLA called to see if she could drive right over. The pathologist had found something abnormal in a tissue sample from the abortion. It was a possibly precancerous condition called a hydatidiform mole, a mass that fed on a pregnancy and could develop into a serious, sometimes fatal uterine cancer, gestational choriocarcinoma, if left untreated. It was a fluke coincidence, unrelated to her breast cancer, but for the moment it trumped that diagnosis. This was the kind of problem that required an immediate response.

When she got to UCLA she was breathless, flushed, a little high on drama and confusion. The doctor explained that Laura would have to have weekly blood tests to see if her levels of beta-HCG, the same hormone produced in a normal pregnancy, were still high. If they stayed high—or dropped and spiked up again the following week—she would have to have a course of chemotherapy immediately.

Her mastectomy and reconstruction might have to wait. This was far more of a threat than some DCIS. She went home numb, wondering how much more she was going to have to endure.

For Dee, looks had become a recreational luxury, something to occupy her when fear was taking a nap. She came back from Seattle terrified. The doctors at Hutchison had suggested she ought to have a double mastectomy before the transplant. Out of nowhere she told Gary they should take a week's trip to Italy before her next chemotherapy dose.

She talked about it happily for days, as though she could leave reality back home in a drawer. What a glorious time they would have. Springtime, rebirth, a romantic holiday as far as possible from the cold fact of treatment. They had just enough time to get there and back.

She told everyone she was going, and just as quickly she changed her mind. It was too far away. If anything went wrong she would not be able to get in touch with her doctors.

*   *   *

Having rejected Love's recommendation of radiation and a lymph node dissection, Barbara Rubin was determined to embrace her old life—which was, in turn, a celebration of her escape from the life that preceded it, marked by two divorces.

Her happy life, as she thought of it, was only about seven years old. That was when she had started buying flowers for herself and taking long walks with no destination in mind. For a long time she chose to be celibate, in the hope that enforced solitude would make her more self-sufficient. By the time she met her current companion she felt she could handle a relationship without drowning in it. So far she had been right.

There was a lot at stake. Barbara showed up for a follow-up appointment on April 4 in her standard exuberant attire, a burgundy blazer with a brocade vest sewn into it, burgundy stirrup tights, lizard-print sandals, and deep fuschia fingernails. Her long crystal and gold earrings dangled almost to her chin, and she wore two big gold hearts—one on her lapel and one on a long chain nestled between her breasts.

Only her haggard face gave her away. With a forced grin, she told Dr. Love about a persistent cough, which she feared was evidence of a lung metastasis.

Love said it sounded like a normal cough. "It could be anything," she said.

"I *hate* when you say that," replied Barbara, visibly relieved.

Love explained that mets were not subtle. If breast cancer invaded the lungs, bones, or liver, the physical symptoms were dramatic—great difficulty breathing, severe back pain that did not go away with over-the-counter pain medication, sudden weight loss and a deep fatigue.

"You know, it does get better, this hypochondriasis stuff," Love said. "It fades with time. You learn to be able to trust your body again—you don't regard everything as a possible betrayal."

She patted Barbara on the shoulder. "Call me if you have a pain that bothers you. Because a lot of these symptoms I can help you with. I can say, 'No, breast cancer never spreads to the big toe,' and then you'll feel better."

* * *

If Shirley was frightened, she refused to dignify it with conversation. Tracy, Mitch, and Kim kept a silent tally: Shirley was still smoking, not flying, not sleeping. The first mammogram since her surgery was scheduled for the end of April, and as it approached she seemed to sink into a trance. It was as though she had a sign around her neck that read DO NOT BRING IT UP UNLESS I DO. The anticipation was hard enough without getting into speculation about what might happen.

Dottie was quiet, too, frightened by the disorder that had so abruptly taken over her life. Nineteen positive nodes: so much for closure. She put all her energy into a new exercise regimen to combat the fibromyalgia, as though routine would keep trouble away. Someday the breast cancer might kill her. She tried not to think about it. She fingered her short white hair, thinner now from the chemotherapy but not gone altogether, and wondered how soon she might feel like putting on some red lipstick and a nice suit and having a Saturday dinner out with her husband.

Aside from Shirley Barber, who had only DCIS, Jerilyn Goodman had the best prognosis, a small tumor with good indicators and no lymph node involvement. But Jerilyn did not see it that way. Every detail of her life, everything she read about breast cancer, seemed part of a larger plan that undoubtedly culminated in her demise. Some days she could barely stand to make contact with the outside world. When she turned on the television at the end of a long work day and saw that CBS's *48 Hours* had a show called "Marked for Life" about genetics and disease risk, she turned it right off again.

Despite her instinctive distrust of groups—why on earth would she spill her guts to total strangers?—she continued to attend the weekly support group she had joined back in November 1993. It was for women with Stage 1 cancer, and had turned out to be a reassuring way to spend a Thursday night. They traded treatment stories with a certain sense of humor, safe in the knowledge that they were the ones who were supposed to survive. In the world of real breast cancer—not DCIS, but the kind that could move out and kill you—they were the lucky ones.

In March 1994 Cindy Gensler showed up for group for the first time and threw everyone, particularly Jerilyn, into a panic. Gensler was their worst nightmare—a thirty-eight-year-old nationally ranked bodybuilder who ate right, was in peak condition, had no family history, and had been diagnosed with a Stage 2 cancer and two positive lymph nodes. The wiseass redhead with less body fat than a bagel had been transformed, over the course of weeks, into a bony, bald chemo-cripple whose body ached so much that she could barely get out of a chair without help, let alone make it to the gym.

Three months had passed since Cindy finished her treatment. Now that she felt healthy she wanted to talk about what had happened to her, and the group facilitator thought she would be most comfortable in the Thursday night group, since its members were young, like her.

Comedy was the way Cindy coped. She made jokes about the Red Death, which was the nickname for Adriamycin, the drug she was given until the side effects overwhelmed her and the doctors put her on a milder one. She explained exactly how she positioned the plastic bucket between the seats of her BMW, so she could pull over and throw up without damaging the leather upholstery. Cindy Gensler talked about rashes and mouth infections and diarrhea and bone aches. She was living proof that life could get worse, and she wanted to be friends.

Jerilyn recoiled as though Cindy were contagious. Jerilyn had made what she considered a clean deal with fate—the sacrifice of her left breast in exchange for future health. No ambiguity, none of the uncertainty implied by extended treatment. She wanted to believe she was finished, which required as little contact as possible with women who might not be.

She had reduced her life to a comforting routine—the weekly visit to the acupuncturist, her Thursday night support group, quiet evenings at home in a spotless, spare little unit she rented in a house on the west side of the city. She had systematically eliminated almost all the fat from her diet and started swimming at the YMCA again. She even wore her Speedo tank suit without a prosthesis because it was more comfortable than her other suit, the one with a prosthesis stuffed into a pocket sewn inside. If anyone stared she chose not to notice, and considered it a personal victory.

It was a tidy life, but it depended for success on predictability. Jerilyn could not yet tolerate surprise, which she interpreted as threat.

So she became even more rigid with herself. A full carton of peanut butter granola bars sat ignored on top of her refrigerator. She had bought them a couple of weeks earlier during her low-fat phase—but now that she wanted a nonfat diet she refused to let herself eat them. She was sure that even ten percent fat was enough to cause a recurrence.

It was a severe regimen, but she liked it. All the reading and thinking and planning kept her away from her biggest fear, which was that nothing she did—the herbs, the nonfat diet, the vitamins, the exercise—would make any difference.

It was not an unreasonable concern. Love and her staff were trying to figure out what questions to include on a new patient form, and the first draft included questions about everything from sexual preference to pesticide exposure. The only problem was that women were probably not going to want to take the time required to fill it out.

Love considered the list with a rueful grin. Sometimes even she caved in, if just for a moment, wondering when the breakthrough was finally going to come, and from where. "You can collect all the data you want," she said, "and ten years from now it's going to be something we didn't ask about—like, 'Do you cut your fingernails once a week?' And we'll have this mountain of data that means nothing at all."

At four thirty in the morning on April 1 the car arrived to take Susan Love to ABC's Los Angeles studios for her satellite interview on *Good Morning America*. The other guests were Dr. Bruce Chabner, director of the Division of Cancer Treatment at the NCI, and Cindy Pearson, executive director of the National Women's Health Network and an outspoken critic of the tamoxifen prevention trial. Pearson wanted the trial shut down altogether because she felt that it exposed healthy women to an unacceptably high risk of uterine cancer, but Love vehemently disagreed. Shutting down the trial only meant that women would seek out tamoxifen on an individual basis, which meant no randomized control for the sake of comparison, no collection of data, no definitive answer. Love wanted the trial to continue so that researchers could figure out once and for all what the drug did, and did not do. Otherwise there could be more surprises farther down the road.

That afternoon she got a call from Dr. Ronald Herberman, director of the Pittsburgh Cancer Institute and a nineteen-year veteran of the NCI. Herberman had just been named as Bernie Fisher's temporary replacement, and one of his first acts was to form a new NSABP oversight committee. He wanted Love on the panel, which was going to meet in San Francisco in two weeks.

She said yes without hesitation, despite the complaints from Zinner and Slamon about how she spent her time. There was nothing she could do to save Bernie Fisher, but she worried that he would not be the only casualty. Harold Varmus, the new director of the NIH, might use this opportunity to remove Samuel Broder as the director of the NCI. Broder, whose wife had been diagnosed with breast cancer during the previous year, was fairly sympathetic to doing earmarked studies. Love worried that Varmus would try to replace Broder with someone who shared his commitment to basic science.

Not that she perceived Broder as a hero. But she talked to Visco on the phone and they agreed: better the evil they knew than the evil they didn't.

Breast cancer did not care how much of a big shot Susan Love was. On the way down the hall to see patients, she could not help but boast that she personally was going to save the NSABP. When she looked at the roster to see who was waiting for her, though, she was suddenly just another doctor slogging through the swamp.

Sometimes the discrepancy threw her and she lost her footing. One of her favorite patients was there with the kind of problem Glaspy had once joked about so bitterly—her breast cancer was incurable but not terminal, and she was suffering. She had a tumor on her chest that would not heal, but no metastatic disease. She might live for years. Local complications, like bleeding, or infection, might kill her before metastases did. Love wondered how long the poor woman was going to have to endure, in pain but denied the release of death.

It was Good Friday. When Love got off work she went to church to pray for a miracle. Medical science had nothing up its sleeve on this one.

16

PERSEVERANCE

T HE BILLBOARDS BOTHERED DENNY SLAMON. IT WAS IMPOSSIBLE TO drive through west Los Angeles without seeing that big, pale pink rose next to the words, WHEN YOU NEED THE FINEST, WE'RE HERE. At the bottom, in cursive script, THE JOYCE KEEFER EISEN-BERG BREAST CENTER, which was part of the John Wayne Comprehensive Cancer Center at St. John's Hospital. They had a dedicated center and an advertising campaign. All that Slamon had, after a year and a half, was the area's best-kept secret.

For all his criticisms of Susan Love, Slamon honestly thought that the multidisciplinary clinic was one of the best programs in the country for women who were diagnosed with breast cancer. If he pushed her as hard as he did, it was because he was so impressed with her work. He admired the way the multi forced a dialogue among doctors and made the patients feel that their needs came first. St. John's had the resources—a renowned surgeon in Armando Giuliano, a radiation oncologist, chemotherapy specialists, and all the rest. But they were private practice doctors who got together by choice, not mandate. Dr. Mel Silverstein, the surgeon founder of the Breast Center out in Van Nuys, had come up with the idea of putting all the specialists under one roof, back in 1979. It still was not the same as what the UCLA clinic team did, working together twice a week, all of them seeing a woman on a single afternoon and then discussing her case with the pathologist and radiologist until everyone reached a consensus. St. John's and Van Nuys offered comprehensive care. Slamon believed that UCLA offered synergy.

The problem was that nobody knew it. He had heard all sorts of frustrating stories. Women thought they could not get an appointment at the Breast Center without a referral. They thought all UCLA patients had to participate in research trials. Others were scared away by the word *clinic*. While the women who called about the multi got an appointment within a week, only some of those who came on Wednesdays actually got to see Susan; on Fridays she made her introductory speech and handled the conference, but let the other surgeons see the patients. The vast majority of women, the ones who wanted diagnostic appointments, had to wait as long as a month to see Susan.

Slamon agreed with Mike Zinner. The problem was not how long Love spent with her patients, but how often she was gone. He felt that her media presence hurt her credibility: whatever the reality, she looked like a director in name only, a marquee attraction who was rarely to be found on the premises, much less in an examining room. He imagined women watching Susan on television, and despite her reputation choosing another doctor who was likelier to be in town.

He faced a cyclical dilemma. If he got money from Revlon for a dedicated center he could demand that Love make a choice: advocate or doctor. If she would just give up all the politicking and devote herself to "moving the field," as he called it, Revlon might be likelier to underwrite the program.

Maintaining a diplomatic balance was almost impossible. When he questioned Susan she accused him of being paternalistic, but when he gave her her head on administrative issues she usually made what turned out to be a mistake. Denny had given up the idea of professional camaraderie; he would settle at this point for a profitable, efficient operation.

The Breast Center Steering Committee was made up of Love, Slamon, radiologist Dr. Larry Bassett; surgeons Dr. Dave McFadden and Dr. Bob Bennion; Mary Bading, the administrator for the Division of General Surgery; Tamara Sutton-Kasum, an administrator from the Department of Surgery who had filled in until Leslie Laudeman arrived, and Laudeman. On the afternoon of April 4 they gathered in the fifth-floor conference room to discuss the agenda Leslie had drawn up.

Did the Center's programs meet the patients' and physicians' needs?

Were staff members' talents and skills right for the tasks they performed?

What were the obstacles to, and opportunities for, continued program growth?

What was the best way to measure progress?

How could they meet financial and budget demands, and who were the potential donors?

"Does that sound about right?" asked Leslie.

"Pretty busy," complained Slamon.

"And then," Love said, in a nervous drawl, "in the afternoon . . ."

Slamon cut her off. There was no question in his mind: The two crucial issues were how to make the program grow and pay for itself. He cared about whether patients and doctors were satisfied—but first he wanted to make sure he had a viable program for them to talk about.

Love interrupted him before he could accuse her of disorganization. If Sherry Goldman was doing administrative work instead of making money billing patients, it was because they all had had to fill in the gap until Leslie arrived.

"Everyone had to pick up a piece of administration," said Love. "Now we're trying to pull all the pieces back into the right place."

"So you're satisfied," said Slamon. He made it a challenge. If Love said yes, he would expect everything to work perfectly from now on.

She eyed him warily. "It's not finished," she replied. "It's in process."

Slamon and Love went back and forth for two hours, interrupted by beepers, phone calls, and only occasionally by the other members of the committee. They agreed that the most important thing was to build up the multidisciplinary clinic, since it was, as Slamon observed, "the place where you get the most bang for your buck." What they argued about was how. Love reminded him that she did not yet have any advertising or promotional materials, despite the marketing department's promises. Slamon said they needed something more dependable to market. He wanted her there for weekend community outreach programs, for meetings with UCLA doctors who could provide referrals, for the women who had to wait a month to get on the schedule. The worst thing would be to market disarray.

The next morning there was a new notice on the Center's bulletin board: 350 multidisciplinary patients for March, the highest number since the clinic opened. Love walked down to see her patients in a jubilant mood. For all Slamon's worry, maybe she was not doing so badly after all.

O n April 6, after what she hoped would be a final physical exam, Susan Love announced the verdict to Dee Wieman.

"It didn't go from a grapefruit to a walnut. More like a grapefruit to a squashed grapefruit." The tumor had softened but not decreased in size, and Love wanted to be sure that Dee understood the probable consequence. Three times during the appointment Love repeated herself. It was unlikely that a lumpectomy would work, since the tumor had stubbornly refused to shrink. She was still willing to try it, but if the margins were dirty, if Love could not remove the entire tumor, Dee would have to have a mastectomy.

She was prepared to tolerate DCIS in the margins in a patient like Shirley, who had only a thirty percent chance of developing invasive cancer. An existing invasive cancer was another matter. All of the large mass in Dee's right breast had to come out.

"I'm not going to do something stupid," Love said. "If we try a lumpectomy and it doesn't look good to me, then I'm going to do what I have to do to save you. 'We tried. Tough.'"

"I'm clear on that with you," said Dee. "I understand that."

*   *   *

Dee had canceled a couple of appointments with the transplant team, so John Glaspy finally called and left a message on her machine: "You don't have to have the transplant. You just have to come in and talk about the transplant." When she finished with Love, Dee headed down to the first-floor oncology center, to hear what the research nurses had to say.

Linda Norton and Stephanie Chang were hell's ushers. As the research nurses who supervised the transplant program, it was their job to explain to each transplant candidate exactly what was going to happen—and then nudge her through the doorway despite that detailed description of what awaited her on the other side.

They were both small, circumspect women, disarmingly soft-spoken. They accompanied Dee into a low-ceilinged meeting room next to Dr. Glaspy's first-floor office and introduced her to the future—high-dose chemotherapy with autologous stem cell rescue, the more sophisticated descendant of a bone marrow transplant.

Once Dee was on the transplant schedule, her life would proceed in lockstep. First, an outpatient procedure, local anesthetic only, to install a two-channel catheter in her chest, into which her medications would flow, out of which the nurses would draw blood samples. Next, two procedures that were intended to save her life once the high-dose chemotherapy destroyed her body's bone marrow function. As insurance, a surgeon performed an inpatient bone marrow harvest from her pelvis, under general anesthetic, for a backup supply of marrow cells. Then seven days of injections of a synthetic growth factor hormone, Neupogen, supplied at no cost by Amgen Pharmaceuticals, whose future profits depended in part on the success of the procedure. Neupogen stimulated the growth of peripheral stem cells, bone marrow cells that spilled out of the marrow and into the bloodstream, where they were harvested through a blood-drawing process called pheresis.

John Glaspy said that stem cells were like "homing pigeons," that moved right back into marrow spaces and began to proliferate—far more efficient than the bone marrow cells, which could take from three weeks to thirty days to engraft. But the FDA had not yet approved the use of stem cells alone, so the marrow cells from Dee's pelvis were in cold storage, just in case they were required to bring her back from the near-dead.

Once the two harvests were complete it was time to check into the hospital, onto one of the two floors where transplant patients were treated.

Dee would arrive on a Thursday, and that night she would start getting intravenous fluids. One of the chemotherapy drugs could cause kidney damage, and another irritated the lining of the bladder. The fluids were meant to keep her kidneys working at peak levels, so that they could function through the onslaught to come.

The next morning a Foley catheter would be inserted into Dee's bladder so that she could urinate. Then the drugs started: cisplatin for seventy-two hours in continuous infusion, and Cytoxan once a day for three days.

"Enormous" doses, said Linda Norton, compared to what Dee was getting now. Ten times what she had already received.

The worst assault came on Monday morning—"BCNU Day," the nurses called it. Two hours of BCNU, or carmustine, a drug that made a woman act like she was falling down drunk, which meant an unpredictable response. She might get sleepy and sullen. She could feel disoriented, agitated, or angry. Loss of bowel control and vomiting were common. The one good thing was that women rarely remembered what happened to them that day. Dee would be sedated before she ever got the drug.

That was it. Over an average of five days, Dee could expect more vomiting and diarrhea, a fever, and a numbing fatigue. She would be put into isolation five to seven days after the infusion, as her white blood cell count started to drop, leaving her vulnerable to infection.

At that point Dee would get an infusion of her own healthy stem cells. She would start to feel better, and sometime in the third week she would be ready to go back home. She could expect to feel depressed—most women complained of feeling "cut loose" once that the dramatic treatment was over and they were on their own. And she had to watch for the one potentially fatal aftereffect— interstitial pneumonitis from the BCNU, easy to treat with antibiotics if found early, but a killer if Dee ignored the symptoms. She would have to be vigilant for a year.

Other than that, she would be finished. If it worked, her breast cancer would be gone. If not, she would develop metastatic disease and eventually die.

Norton and Chang did not pretend that a transplant was easy. They did tell Dee, over and over again, that many women had passed this way before and come out the other side.

She had only three questions. She had heard that the growth factor hormone might spike tumor growth as well as stem cell growth. Was it going to make the cancer worse?

Norton admitted that no one knew for sure—but if the chemotherapy was going to get rid of Dee's cancer, the assumption was it could handle a slightly larger enemy.

Dee also worried about what was going to happen to her, "bathroom habit-wise." Norton told her the truth: Some women lost control of their bowels completely, but the nurses on the floor were used to changing gowns and bedclothes; there was nothing to be embarrassed about.

Besides, she said with a pixie grin, Dee would not remember what had happened.

"I'm not worried about me remembering," replied Dee. "I'm worried about everyone else."

And she wondered what to do about her head. Gary still had not seen his wife without her wig on. Would the nurses be able to make sure it stayed on straight?

Norton suggested instead that she look for a cute cap or bonnet that tied under the chin. She knew from experience that Dee was only going to find that wig an irritation. She would be too busy staying alive to worry about her appearance.

But Dee lived by her looks; they might as well have told her not to worry about breathing. She had already decided on a tactical lie to protect herself.

"I have a rule," said Dee. "I'm going to tell everybody, protective isolation is from day one to day twenty-eight."

There was never any question about whether Dee would be able to have the transplant, since she and Gary had private insurance that covered the procedure. Women who could afford to pay lawyers to challenge a reluctant insurance company were also beginning to have success; *The New York Times* reported that nineteen of thirty-nine women who had been denied payments for treatment at Duke University had managed to get the insurers to change their mind when they threatened legal action.

They were the exceptions. There was not enough insurance money to enable most women to have a transplant, even if it became an accepted therapy, as long as the expense remained so high. As with any investment, it all came down to yield. Dr. Alan Garber, an internist and health economist at Stanford University, told *The New York Times,* "What if bone marrow transplants allow women to extend their life expectancy from one year to 13 months, but it costs $100,000? Are we prepared to say that because we know it works, we will pay for it, no matter what it costs?"

A generation brought up on medical indulgence—house calls when they were children, tests and treatments ordered by prosperous doctors and paid for by insurers—had run headlong into middle-age and medical rationing.

The twelve doctors who gathered in the radiology conference room on Wednesday afternoon were there to discuss the plight of metastatic patients, who in fact had more serious problems to face than whether they would be allowed to have a transplant. The question, as "cost-benefit ratio" became a standard for evaluation, was how to make sure that the metastatic patient was not abandoned.

The focus of the meeting, one of a series of "journal clubs" Love had initiated to help the multi team keep current with literature on research and policy issues, was metastatic patients and managed care—or, how to make sure that insurers continued to pay for standard treatments despite the fact that none of them could be shown to cure the disease. These patients might be terminal, but no one in the room was prepared to send them home to die as long as there were treatments that could slow their decline or make it less painful.

John Glaspy had begun to work with a national group, the University Hospital Consortium, to get the government to establish federal standards for managed care groups. He wanted guarantees that any woman whose disease had spread would receive at least two regimens of chemotherapy—in the name of stalling, if not stopping, the disease.

"There will be abuses," he said, "because there are abuses now. We have to look at what our competitors will be doing—if they're going to stop offering a lot of these chemotherapies."

Love found it a chilling idea. "You think people are going to come to UCLA because they say, 'I've had chemo, what else do you guys have?' "

"They already do," said Glaspy, with a shrug. Medicine was so in the dark on women with advanced disease. It was hard to know what was an opportunity and what was a joke, and he desperately wanted the chance to find out. He had heard about using diet to shift a patient's fatty acid levels, which might decrease cell proliferation, and he wanted to try that approach with metastatic patients.

"Right," said Love. "Those patients will try anything."

Another doctor quipped that the researchers at Houston's M.D. Anderson Hospital just threw darts at a board to decide which new rain forest plants to study.

"It's just as ethical as slinging 5-FU on the way to the funeral parlor," said Glaspy, referring to a frequently used chemotherapy drug.

"Shark cartilage. Wheat grass." Love understood why patients tried other treatments. She felt that chemotherapy, like its comrades surgery and radiation, had been oversold by doctors. A woman who did not get an instant response was likely to get angry and walk away. "They get disenchanted with chemo after two cycles that do nothing."

Glaspy considered a diagram on the board of the treatments currently in use for metastatic patients, none of which had yet shown any impact more than four years out. He was known for his compassionate attitude with patients, but with his colleagues he was blunt and often sullen—as though he had spent all his generosity helping women face the likely end of their lives. He was mightily offended at the meager resources he had.

"It's pretty pathetic," he said, gesturing toward the board, "that this is the state of the art for a disease that kills over forty thousand women a year."

No one replied.

"It's not for want of trying," he said. "A hundred thousand published trials each year."

"This is depressing," Love agreed, but she refused to give in to Glaspy's sadness. What made her irresistible to her patients—and to many of her colleagues, though they would admit it only grudgingly—was that she saved her sorrow for private moments. What the others saw was the public Susan Love, angry, impatient, eager for change. "It really shows me we have to look at this in a new way. We should be doing research on every patient in the Breast Center. Each one of them should be part of a study—especially with the metastatic patient, where we can't really help anybody."

If they could not save a life they could take knowledge from the effort. "At least we ought to be learning something."

Love was fed up at her inability to get Dee to make up her mind, depressed by the journal club—with its view of an ever more limited future—and concerned about Revlon.

The more she talked to Denny, the more she worried that the Revlon center was not the salvation she craved. She had taken him up to the sixth floor to show him an available empty space, lots of windows, full of light, but he had dismissed it as too small. He took her down to the basement to show her the excess space that radiation oncology did not need, and she worried that the Center was going to become part of a larger real estate agenda. Love's vision of a dedicated center had sunlight as an essential element; the women who came to the clinic were always wandering out to lean against the windows and stare at the sky. She thought that sending them down to the basement next to radiation oncology would only depress them. It was like purgatory.

It was time to get away. She looked forward to a conference she planned to attend in Bruges, Belgium, in mid-April. The British medical journal *Lancet* was sponsoring a three day meeting. The topic was "Toward a new paradigm for breast cancer." She was ready for that.

*   *   *

The beleaguered tamoxifen prevention trial was in jeopardy. The risk of uterine cancer was higher than originally thought. The data upon which the prevention trial was based, on the drug's effectiveness with breast cancer patients, was "polluted," as the NCI put it in a letter to clinical investigators, by questionable data from Dr. Roger Poisson. The NSABP's interim executive officer, Dr. Donald L. Trump, tried to reassure the investigators and their high-risk patients, in the hope of avoiding mass defections. Women who already had breast cancer might tolerate increased risk in return for a lowered chance of recurrence. High-risk women were a less dependable population.

The *Journal of the National Cancer Institute,* the most widely cited publication in the world, ran Dr. Fisher's defense of the tamoxifen trials on breast cancer patients in its April 6 issue—but it was not the anticipated re-analysis. The article, "Endometrial Cancer in Tamoxifen-Treated Breast Cancer Patients: Findings from the National Surgical Adjuvant Breast and Bowel Project B-14," still included disputed data from Poisson, a fact that Fisher and his co-authors had not mentioned in either their first draft or revision. The *Journal*'s editor made the discovery by chance—and added an editor's note on the first page of the article, alerting readers to the fact.

The NSABP team concluded, "Risk of endometrial cancer increases following tamoxifen therapy for invasive breast cancer; however, net benefit greatly outweighs risk." They argued that the uterine cancers did not seem to carry a worse prognosis than did uterine cancers among non-tamoxifen users.

The *Journal* also ran an editorial by three doctors from the National Cancer Institute's Cancer Therapy Evaluation Program, Division of Cancer Treatment. Under the headline TAMOXIFEN: TRIALS, TRIBULATIONS, AND TRADE-OFFS, Drs. Michael Friedman, Edward Trimble, and Jeffrey Abrams offered cautious praise for the structure of the NSABP's studies, while acknowledging new information on the risk of uterine cancer.

The authors agreed with the NSABP contributors that the increased risk "will probably have little impact on the risk/benefit ratio for patients in the adjuvant breast cancer treatment setting," but, they went on, "it could certainly affect the drug's use in cancer prevention."

They did not mean that the prevention trial should be halted. Quite the contrary: they endorsed a "broad research agenda" to refine tamoxifen therapy and so minimize the attendant risks.

The doctors stressed that women were not in an "either-or" situation. Now that the risks of tamoxifen were becoming clearer, researchers and doctors could look for ways to reduce the toxic effects of the drug "by endocrinologic or surgical intervention"— that is, by giving women another drug to block the pituitary hormones that made ovarian hormones work, or by suggesting a prophylactic hysterectomy.

"It would be no exaggeration to suggest that, globally, millions of women are directly interested in this research," they wrote. "We are not so naive to believe that cancer patients get 'something for nothing'—no patient does. However, we must continue to strive to diminish the toxic effects of our most effective therapies."

There was an assortment of other research reports, on April 6 and again on April 20, which primarily managed to prove how much more research needed to be done. It was as though some devil's hand kept stretching the distance between the researchers and their goal. A study of the relationship between premenopausal breast cancer and birth control pills found a "small excess breast cancer risk" among long-term users of oral contraceptives, not enough to recommend less time on the Pill, but enough to recommend long-term studies to look at risk as the population got older. A group of researchers in Milan, Italy, reported on their efforts to refine prognosis in node-negative patients by looking at a gene that seemed connected to slower cell proliferation, only to find that "such a relationship is relatively weak." The only way to determine its true significance was to watch it some more.

The list of things that might contribute to breast cancer risk seemed endless, and growing—organochlorines, DDT, dense breast tissue. The factors that determined whether a woman required and would respond to chemotherapy were also increasing. According to the NCI *Journal*, researchers needed to evaluate a "staggering array of candidates—one source counted fifty-eight."

The *Journal* article continued:

Thanks in part to earlier detection, nearly two-thirds of newly diagnosed breast cancer cases have no lymph node involvement, and an estimated 70% to 80% of these women can be cured without adjuvant therapy. Others will relapse despite drug therapy. The dilemma of whom to treat affects about 120,000 annually in the United States. Over and above the human cost, the potential annual cost of unnecessary or futile treatment—if all node-negative women were treated—has been estimated at $500 million.

The National Breast Cancer Coalition issued a position paper on April 6, headlined "Breast Cancer Advocate Involvement in the Research Process." Fran Visco continued to push for a more active role for consumers in the NIH grant process, along the lines of the Defense Department's Integration Panel. The NBCC release called for permanent NIH breast cancer study sections that included advocates—a long shot, but a nice way to remind the research establishment that the NSABP's high-handed behavior was not going to be tolerated by the patient community. If a woman was going to be a guinea pig, and maybe get the new treatment but maybe not, then she deserved something in return.

Dottie Mosk was the kind of patient who gave Sherry Goldman the willies. A clean mammogram, no palpable tumor, and here she was with a Stage 3 cancer. Nothing that anyone understood about breast cancer explained what had happened to Dottie.

She was resilient. Every morning she awoke at dawn for her daily exercise regimen, despite the fact that she was receiving chemotherapy and was scheduled to begin a seven-week course of radiation on April 26. She was in a wheelchair, but as Joe pushed her down the fifth-floor hallway to her follow-up appointment Dottie was the picture of stylish defiance—an oversize, buttercup-yellow cotton cardigan slung over her hospital gown, her chin jutting defiantly in the air, a cocky little straw hat with a flower on the brim to cover the tufts of white hair that chemotherapy had left her.

She always tried to schedule her appointments with Dr. Love, but that week Love's calendar was mired in conflicts and double bookings, so Dottie had been shifted to a Tuesday follow-up appointment with Sherry Goldman. The nurse-practitioner stood nearby as Dottie got up on the scale to be weighed, and when she got back in the wheelchair to have her temperature taken, Sherry stepped over to massage her back.

"Did you talk to Susan?" she said quietly. "She'll try to poke her head in. You may end up seeing both of us."

Once inside the examining room, Sherry looked at Dottie's mastectomy incision, which was still covered by a gauze pad.

"It's great, it's totally closed," she said. "If you pulled that scab off it might still be open a little, but when the scab falls off it'll be fine." She told Dottie she no longer had to wear the pad unless it made her feel safer.

To prove how well she was doing, Dottie showed Sherry the arm exercises she did—both arms fluttering gracefully above her head like some spindly ballerina. She was not going to become an invalid. Before the surgery she had been working with five-pound weights and driving a car. She could have lunch with a friend and spend forty-five minutes in a fitting room before her strength gave out. But fibromyalgia required daily exercise, and her cancer treatment had set her back. She traveled only as a passenger; no shopping, no social life.

Goldman suggested acupuncture, and Dottie gravely wondered how she was supposed to fit it in between all her other medical appointments.

"Later," said Sherry. They both smiled; the future was such a lovely idea.

There was nothing else to discuss, really. They were fretting about how tired Joe looked when suddenly the door swung open and Love burst in, her surgical mask hanging from one ear.

"Hi, beautiful," she said. "How are you today?"

Dottie and Joe beamed, and Dottie reached up to take Susan's hand.

"I'm *so* glad you're here," she said.

Susan looked at the scab on the incision, gently removed a small portion of it, and reported that there was still a tiny little open hole, but nothing to worry about.

"So how are you?" she asked.

"My fibromyalgia," said Dottie. "I wish that would go away."

Love raised her arms above Dottie's head like a faith healer. "Now what you have to do," she said, eyes closed, a blissful grin on her face, "is visualize that the fibromyalgia is seeping right out of this hole, and the radiation's going to just burn it all away."

"You look just like Kate right now," said Sherry.

"This is a good visualization," said Dottie. "When I do my relaxation exercises I'll think the fibromyalgia is leaving my body."

Love had another patient waiting for her upstairs in outpatient surgery, so she had to leave—but not before Dottie asked a special favor. She knew there was nothing medical that Love could do for her, but she wanted to come in, perhaps every other Wednesday after her radiation appointment, just to say hello.

Love could not resist. Dottie had stepped in over the past few weeks as a surrogate grandmother, asking to see family photographs, showing up just before Easter with two little straw hats for Kate. She was a lovely woman and she was stuck, and Love was not immune to her attentions. She told Dottie to go ahead and make the appointments.

17

LEVELS OF TRUTH

LOVE REVIEWED THE APRIL 13 MULTIDISCIPLINARY CLINIC ROSTER JUST before she left town for the first NSABP oversight committee meeting, which was being held in San Francisco. Only three patients. She could afford to miss the clinic and maybe even the conference, as long as she flew back in time for the five o'clock journal club. Slamon was going to make a presentation about his research. She would not insult him and miss that.

The goal of the oversight committee meeting was a simple one: to figure out how to make sure the NSABP survived as a large cooperative group dedicated to clinical trials. They needed an overall plan; as it stood now, according to Love, the NSABP was "very much an autocratic thing run by Bernie." A board of governors would help—but at the same time, the oversight committee had to protect the NSABP from turning into a paralyzed bureaucracy.

In the long run the committee would have to find a permanent replacement for Fisher—and define Fisher's new relationship to the NSABP. Member surgeons had been complaining loudly that Fisher was a saint, and ought to be saved, not pilloried. Love agreed with them, but saw no way that he could keep his job. Bernie Fisher had to be sacrificed to save the NSABP.

* * *

At three the following day the other doctors began to drift into the conference room, and Glaspy entertained a young oncologist and a radiologist with stories of his pugnacious behavior at a recent oncologists' meeting. The discussion at the conference had been about how to treat metastatic patients who either could not have a transplant or did not respond to it. The standard treatment was taxol, a drug derived from the Pacific yew tree in 1971 and now produced synthetically. If that did not work it was anybody's guess, and Glaspy was offended at the idea that some doctors behaved as though they had answers.

"I told them," he said with a satisfied laugh, "that after taxol anything else is a placebo. And there should be a balanced discussion about it, because you're not doing the patient any good."

The younger doctors nodded appreciatively. The radiologist recalled a speech he had heard recently. "The guy talked for an hour," he said. "It was, 'The hardest thing is knowing when to stop.' When we walked out of there it was like *Schindler's List*. Nobody said anything."

At that moment Love rushed into the room, all self-importance and smug pride. She had grabbed an early return flight just so she could attend the multi conference after all, and silence any detractors who might complain about her time conflicts. "I've been in San Francisco bailing out the NSABP," she bragged, tossing her purse and jacket on a chair and setting up her laptop computer.

Dave McFadden, a lanky, slow-spoken general surgeon who had been part of the multi team since its inception, slipped into his chair and regarded his colleague with amusement. McFadden was the one Zinner most often held up to Susan as an example of how a surgeon ought to behave: thirty hours a week in the operating room and so low a public profile as to be virtually anonymous outside of the medical center. McFadden was a Breast Center loyalist, despite the fact that he preferred gastrointestinal surgery, a discipline he found far more fascinating than performing mastectomies and lumpectomies. But he respected what Love was trying to do, and he liked what he called, in characteristic understatement, "her rather infectious enthusiasm." Despite his own scheduling conflicts—extensive surgeries that often ran overtime and VA patients who had been dispersed to other facilities—he managed to stay involved.

"Well," he drawled, with a wry grin, "*are* you going to bail out the NSABP?"

"Yeah," said Love. "We're trying. And the clinical people are certainly trying. But it's a mess. There's a lot to do. Bernie insisted on doing everything himself."

The three patients that day were casualties of bad medicine, bad insurance, and stale advice. The first woman was in her mid-fifties, already halfway through a neo-adjuvant chemotherapy regimen for a Stage 3 cancer, a five centimeter tumor with positive lymph nodes. She had three questions for the UCLA team: Given the side effects, was she going to make it through the full chemotherapy regimen? Could she have a transplant? Could she have a lumpectomy and radiation instead of a mastectomy? The chemotherapy, as difficult as it was for her, seemed to be working: on physical exam, doctors could no longer feel anything where the tumor had been.

The problem was that the slides from the original biopsy were no good. The UCLA pathologist could not make a definitive diagnosis from them, and Glaspy could not offer her a transplant without one.

"Here's the issue," he said. "She wants the BMT. Blue Shield insurance doesn't pay for a bone marrow transplant, so she's put down the cash with the hospital. But unless we get another tissue specimen from this pathologist, we've got to cut it short. We need tissue for a definitive diagnosis."

They were at sea. They had no tissue from which to make a formal diagnosis. They could try a new mammogram, ultrasound, and surgery—but if they could not find more malignant tissue, the woman could not have a transplant. It was a painful irony. The patient had responded well to standard chemotherapy, which meant that she might be one of the ones a transplant helped. But sloppy pathology slides precluded a diagnosis—and the chemicals had done their work so well they had eradicated evidence of disease.

Love recommended doing what she called a ghostectomy, in

which she removed a sample of tissue from the site where the tumor had been, or a mastectomy, in the hope of retrieving more malignant tissue. Sandy Barsky thought a core biopsy might get them enough samples, but Love disagreed.

"We ought to operate," she said. "And make sure we do it before she has much more chemotherapy."

"I hope they get more tissue back," said Glaspy.

"Pray," said McFadden.

The next woman was a victim of her managed care provider, which after almost a month still did not have her on a therapy regimen. She had a large tumor and eighteen of nineteen positive nodes. It was an unfortunately easy call. She needed a transplant—and she needed a recommendation from UCLA to that effect if she had any chance of getting the expenditure approved. Her HMO was not about to subsidize that kind of expensive, unproven treatment without a fight.

Glaspy wanted to move ahead quickly. He was more aggressive with Stage 3 patients, who did not yet exhibit metastatic disease, than with Stage 4 patients, whose breast cancer already had spread.

The last woman came to UCLA to see if the doctors there thought her own doctor was right. He had recommended a mastectomy and chemotherapy. McFadden chuckled.

"So they basically gave her the 'If you were my wife' speech," he said. The old guard still believed instinctively that removing more tissue improved a woman's chances, despite the data to the contrary. It was emotion masquerading as science, and McFadden was tired of it. He wanted to recommend a lumpectomy and radiation, and the others agreed.

Two days before the House Energy and Commerce Subcommittee on Oversight and Investigations began its April 13 hearings on the NSABP scandal, Dr. Bernard Fisher's lawyer asked the subcommittee to excuse his client from testifying. *The New York Times* reported that the seventy-five-year-old Fisher would not appear, "because of his age, and the distress and physical strain of testifying."

In his absence, the remaining witnesses tried to distance themselves from the scandal. The *Times*'s Dr. Lawrence Altman would report on April 14 that the first day of testimony had been marked by apologies, promises of better behavior in the future, and condemnations of Dr. Fisher's "arrogant and cavalier attitude." National Cancer Institute director Dr. Samuel Broder implied that Dr. Bernard Fisher's heroic status in the research community had temporarily clouded his own judgment, and kept him from pressing Poisson for a timely reanalysis of the lumpectomy data. He had no explanation for Fisher's delay in reporting the uterine cancer deaths of four of the women who had taken tamoxifen.

"We clearly understand the principle that we cannot allow a grantee's formidable reputation, history of prior accomplishments, or service in science to stand in the way of prompt, corrective action and oversight," said Broder. "We cannot, and will not ever again, defer or appear to defer to the timetable of a grantee in reporting fraud and fabrication to the public."

The NCI was about to begin a series of unannounced audits at sites around the country to make sure that no one else involved in the NSABP breast cancer trials had falsified results.

Broder's boss, NIH director Dr. Harold Varmus, was securely wrapped inside the cloak of time. The initial discovery and most of the subsequent delays had taken place before he took the NIH job, so he could credibly promise to improve the way the NIH responded to accusations of fraud and kept the public informed. He had already requested an inquiry into Imperial Chemical Industries' 1988 offer, four years before the tamoxifen prevention trial got under way, of $600,000 to endow a chair at the University of Pittsburgh in Dr. Fisher's name—a rather hefty compliment to a man whose research findings would help determine the profitability of I.C.I.'s then-subsidiary, Zeneca Pharmaceuticals.

Zeneca officials did not attend the hearing, but the committee chairman, Michigan's Representative John Dingell, cited a July 1993 memo of a telephone conversation between Zeneca senior director of clinical and medical affairs, Dr. Paul Plourde, and Dr. Fisher. Plourde had called Fisher to discuss Zeneca's intention to alter its Nolvadex label to reflect data on the increased risk of endometrial cancer. Fisher approved of the idea, but commented on "the potential negative publicity" that could result. It might hurt the European prevention trial, which would in turn affect the trial in the United States. They ought to prepare in advance for the possibility.

Fisher was "relieved," according to the memo, that Zeneca did not intend to discontinue providing the medication to the National Cancer Institute.

The activists, for their part, behaved as though Fisher were already part of the ignominious past. Fran Visco intended to step over the rubble of the last few weeks to claim the activists' rightful seat at the table, implying that consumer participation was the one thing that would keep the process honest. Her colleague, Women's Health Network executive director Cynthia Pearson, was more strident. She repeated the demand she had made when she appeared on *Good Morning America* with Susan Love—that the government shut down the breast cancer prevention trial because it exposed healthy women to an unacceptable risk of a new disease.

One by one they made their case to the committee, except for Zeneca and Fisher. He had remained silent for a month, through the furor of the initial disclosure and the professional humiliations that followed. When he turned down interview requests he told reporters that he intended to wait and make a formal statement at the hearing.

Instead, he retreated. He did not plan to present a reanalysis of the lumpectomy data at upcoming scientific conferences, though the April 6 NCI *Journal* had reported that he would; he intended instead to publish later in the year in the *New England Journal of Medicine,* which had published the original lumpectomy studies. The new analysis, which excluded the tainted data, was supposed to show the same results, that lumpectomy and radiation were as effective as mastectomy, but until it was available to the public it was all too easy to take his reluctance as an admission of trouble.

Doctors who admired him, like Love and Glaspy, believed he had kept the falsified data a secret to protect women from unnecessary anxiety, but if so, his good intentions had backfired. The promise that the study's conclusions held up even without the Ca-

nadian data was cold comfort. Fisher's decision made women feel
that they were no more important to the scientists who studied
them than a cageful of lab rats.

With Dr. Fisher removed from the stage, the most vulnerable
player in the NSABP drama was Dr. Samuel Broder, who had been
director of the National Cancer Institute since 1988. Love had said
from the beginning that Varmus might use the NSABP as a wedge
to force Broder out, and now her fears seemed to be coming true.
The rumor among doctors was that Broder would be replaced to
show the NIH's good intentions.

Love continued to be diplomatic in her support of both Fisher
and Broder, and wrote to the NCI director to reaffirm the importance of the NSABP trials. She told interviewers again and again
that personalities and poor judgment were not the important issue.
What mattered was that the data from both American and European studies supported the conclusion of the NSABP lumpectomy
trial. Fisher had been wrong to keep the falsified data a secret—and
the NCI had allowed him to do so for too long—but one sacrificial
lamb was enough.

When she got back to her office after the multi, she found a fax
from Broder at the top of her stack of mail.

"Thank you very much for your kind note," he wrote, "and all
your words of support. We at the National Cancer Institute want
you to know how much we are in your debt for bringing some
sense of order to the events surrounding the NSABP trials and the
tamoxifen prevention study.

"I watched your interview on *Good Morning America*. The
clarity and precision of your statement reminded me of how during
a storm, a skillful and firm hand at the wheel of a ship can save the
day. You are quite correct that there are no substantial scientific
doubts regarding the value of breast-conserving surgery. Moreover,
if we do not learn whether tamoxifen can have a role in preventing
breast cancer with the current trial, we will never know the answer
at all and women will be left to fate, and fate alone."

He was preaching to the converted. The critics continued their
attack: two members of the Senate's ad-hoc breast cancer coalition
had announced plans to hold their own hearings, and Congress-

man Dingell planned a second House subcommittee hearing in mid-June.

The next piece of mail made Love catch her breath. It was the pathology report from Laura's abortion—but Love had not known about Laura's abortion until this moment, nor about the hyda-tidiform mole. It was impossible to keep up with patients' lives between appointments, and the double sadness contained on that single page stopped her cold.

"Abnormal cells," she whispered. "A mole. Pregnant, but there wasn't a kid in there. I didn't know she had the abortion." She slumped in her chair, the folder full of mail splayed open on her lap, and stared vacantly out the window.

She had to call Dee's oncologist at St. John's, Dr. Boasberg, to schedule a fourth cycle of chemotherapy. She also wanted him to know that Glaspy was willing to do the transplant first followed by the surgery, because that seemed to make Dee comfortable.

Boasberg replied that the doctors in Seattle and at Los Ange-les's City of Hope hospital had insisted on a bilateral mastectomy before the transplant, and Love confessed that at this point she simply wanted Dee to do something. It hardly mattered what, as long as she got started. Besides, with so many positive nodes there was a reasonable argument for treating the systemic disease first.

But she wanted Boasberg to understand that she did not buy Dee's theory about the transplant shrinking the tumor down to lumpectomy size. She repeated what she had told Dee: since stan-dard chemotherapy had failed to affect the size of the tumor, there would likely be enough tumor left even after the high-dose drugs to require a mastectomy.

When they were finished talking Boasberg walked back into the examining room—where Dee had been waiting while he took the call.

He repeated what Love had said.

Despite all of Love's warnings, particularly at their last meet-ing, Dee was stunned. "Why do you think she told me we'd try lumpectomy?" she asked.

Boasberg shrugged uncomfortably. He decided to tell her his own feelings on the subject.

"I think you should have the bilateral mastectomy," he said. "I think you should consider it." That would get rid of everything—the large invasive cancer, the smaller tumor, the DCIS. She would have to wait about a year to have reconstructive surgery, until she recovered fully from the transplant, but he thought she would be happier with the results than if she had plastic surgery on one side only. Her breasts were too large to reconstruct. If she had a single mastectomy the surgeon would have to reduce the size of her other breast before he could attempt to build a new one. It was not going to be a simple one-step procedure.

She left his office reeling. Both St. John's and UCLA were talking about more aggressive surgery, and those were the two places where she had felt safe. She had promised Gary that she would have a lumpectomy first. She had given her word. She had told the doctors: We have to ease Gary into this slowly.

Giuliano had replied that it was her life, not her husband's, and a lumpectomy was not going to save it. Gary called him a butcher, and wanted to have nothing more to do with St. John's. When he heard that City of Hope recommended a bilateral mastectomy he started referring to it as City of Death. Dr. Love had been their one hope, and now that was gone.

Love's plan to back gradually into the truth had failed. Dee always heard the hopeful part of the message and chose to ignore the rest.

This was the scenario Dee had feared the most. For all her yearning, information was not power. When it came to breast cancer, information was too often just that—a pile of facts that led nowhere.

She felt betrayed.

The future of breast cancer was quite literally outlined on Denny Slamon's face. He had begun his lecture to the Wednesday afternoon journal club in proper professorial stance, just to the side of the screen where he projected his research slides. But the more he talked, the more enthusiastic he became, until he was standing right in front of the screen. Statistics and cell lines played across his forehead, cheeks, and chin: he was enveloped by the work that had consumed him for twelve years.

This was a departure from the standard journal club agenda, a "requested talk," according to Love, who introduced Slamon. The doctors and students who worked at the Center heard a lot about Slamon's research, including discussions about whether individual patients might qualify for his clinical trial, but most of them did not really understand it.

Gene research like Slamon's HER-2/neu work was the bridge between Bernie Fisher's systemic regimen and the new age of genetics, in which doctors hoped to identify and manipulate damaged genes or their products before they led to disease, or to treat disease by targeting mutated genes and leaving the rest of the body alone. That future was probably farther away than anyone wanted to admit; Slamon liked to say that researchers had all seven thousand pieces of the breast cancer puzzle—the only problem was that they were all blue and all the same shape. In the meantime, he hoped at least to enhance systemic treatment for women with a particularly aggressive type of breast cancer.

Normally, there was a single copy of the HER-2/neu gene in every cell in the body, but it was expressed only in cells in the kidneys and the respiratory and gastrointestinal tracts of men and women, and in the breasts and ovaries of women, where it helped to regulate cell growth. Most breast cancer tissue samples contained that single copy of HER-2/neu—but about twenty-five to thirty percent contained extra copies of the gene. There was nothing abnormal about the genes themselves, only the number of copies, as many as twenty instead of one. The protein produced by HER-2/neu told the cell to grow faster; the alteration made too many copies of the gene, which meant too much protein, and uncontrolled malignant growth.

"When we started to look at those women whose tumor had this alteration, they had shorter disease-free survival—more prone to relapsing—and a shorter overall survival," said Slamon.

The lab work was frightening. To see exactly what an altered HER-2/neu gene would do, Slamon's team worked with cell lines, established groups of cells that were grown under laboratory conditions. Introduce extra copies of the HER-2/neu oncogene into a human breast cancer cell line that had a normal copy of HER-2/neu, and it took over. Slamon pointed to the cell line projected on the screen. "In every instance the cells behave more aggressively," he said. "Most important, their ability to form tumors in experimental animals goes up significantly. . . . The most recent data—we're just starting to get the data in—is that looking at metastatic potential, there is a significant increase when you introduce this alteration. They will travel and form metastatic sites, and those sites will grow much more quickly when these genes are introduced."

But HER-2/neu could not cause breast cancer single-handedly. When Slamon put the gene into normal cells, those cells did not become malignant. HER-2/neu had an accomplice, or perhaps several of them—other genetic alterations that in combination with the gene would lead to breast cancer.

If he could develop a therapy to deactivate the gene, Slamon could conceivably alter the course of the disease for women who historically had not responded well to treatment. He began to work with synthetic monoclonal antibodies, to find one that would block the protein produced by the HER-2/neu oncogene—antibodies developed at UCLA as well as antibodies from other research laboratories and from three major pharmaceutical companies: Berlex, Amgen, and Genentech. The Genentech antibody acted like the brake Slamon had been looking for. After four years the effort that a colleague had dismissed as a "fishing expedition" had yielded results.

The problem so far was that the antibody worked on human tumors in laboratory mice only as long as it was administered. There was no lasting effect to the treatment: Once it was stopped, the tumor began to grow again. The next step, Slamon explained, was to "convert this cytostatic effect into a cytocidal effect that would kill the tumor cells."

He had found a clue to that step lurking in an Israeli study of antibodies used against a relative of HER-2/neu. The Israeli researchers were looking for what Slamon called "a smart bomb" to deliver the antibody more effectively. What got Slamon's interest were the controls the researchers had used for reference points.

Potential hid in the oddest places—not always in the central experiment a scientist conducted, but in the ancillary work he did in an attempt to structure a responsible, durable study.

Slamon was distracted by one of the study's controls, in which a patient received the antibody and the chemotherapeutic drug cisplatin, delivered separately. He wondered if the same regimen might extend the antibody's ability to suppress HER-2/neu, perhaps even after a woman finished her treatment. One of Slamon's researchers immediately tried a similar regimen in the laboratory, producing "some beautiful studies," Slamon said, "in a very short period of time."

They got a "significant decrease" in tumor growth, first in cell lines grown in petri dishes, then in transgenic mice—animals who had been implanted with malignant cells, guaranteeing that they would develop breast cancer. It worked in the laboratory. It was time to see if it worked on human subjects.

Slamon began his Phase 1 clinical trial, designed to determine toxicity levels, late in 1991. It gave him great hope: after eighteen months of what he called "rigorous" testing done with the help of Genentech, there was no evidence of toxicity in the patients who received it, and only five to ten percent of those women experienced slight, intermittent fevers. Over the summer of 1993 he began his Phase 2 trial, in which the antibody's efficacy was tested—another eighteen-month to two-year gamble. If it caused a fifty percent or greater reduction in the size of a measurable tumor, it was a success. Anything less than that was a failure.

If it worked, Slamon would be able to start a Phase 3 trial comparing the HER-2/neu antibody to accepted therapies for women with metastatic disease.

A handful of subsequent studies by other researchers had failed to show a prognostic link, and it had sometimes looked as though the clarity of Slamon's results might not hold up. But now, eight years after the discovery of the alteration, there were over forty studies assessing the relationship between HER-2/neu and prognosis, and only seven failed to show an association. When two of those studies were combined and reanalyzed, the link between HER-2/neu and a bad prognosis did appear. Only five studies conflicted. Slamon was convinced he was right. The presence of HER-2/neu in larger than normal amounts was a predictor of aggressive disease.

Journal presentations usually precipitated noisy debate, but the eighteen people in the room had few questions for Slamon. Most of them were clinicians, and as breast cancer research entered the genetic era the gap widened between the research laboratory and the examining room. Other than the women enrolled in his study, Slamon saw patients only two months out of the year—having made a rule that all the doctors in his department would spend that much time on the clinical service, he felt obliged to obey it himself. His empathic skills had atrophied over time; he had to remind himself of how to act with patients. In the same way, the clinicians who had asked him to speak could do little but absorb the material he presented. They did not know enough about the topic to ask informed questions.

When he talked about the trials, though, once science entered the clinic, they knew what mattered. Did the treatment work, and for how long?

Slamon chuckled. "As is always the case with these exciting new trials," he admitted, "the first patient is your best." She had failed to respond to chemotherapy or to tamoxifen and radiation, and by the time she joined Slamon's study she had pulmonary lesions. After receiving the HER-2/neu antibody the lesions, and any evidence of nodal disease, were gone.

"She's still in remission," he said proudly, "a year and three months posttherapy." The combination of cisplatin and the antibody did seem to produce the desired synergy.

The next two patients did not do as well. One only responded to the HER-2/neu antibody for seven months before her metastatic disease began to progress. The next woman received treatment for almost a year, but she had to give it up because she could no longer tolerate the cisplatin doses. Slamon would never know how she might have responded if she had been able to see it through.

At this point, he was still limited to working with what he called "the hardest patients," the ones with advanced metastatic disease. What he hoped for, in the coming Phase 3 trial, was the

chance to treat women who had just had their first metastatic oc-
currence. The more he knew, the more he wanted to know. Would
the antibody work better earlier? In combination with a different
chemotherapy agent? In different sequence?

The dosage that killed tumor cells did not seem to affect normal cells—unlike standard chemotherapy, which attacked the body
indiscriminately. If Slamon could find an effective way to deliver
the antibody without using traditional drugs, he might be able to
save lives without simultaneously damaging them in other ways.

His long-range hope was to help the unusual cases—the women
with early cancer and good prognostic indicators who died from
what should have been manageable disease. "It may be that HER-
2/neu is a trump card over other prognostic factors," said Slamon.
"You can have ER-PR negative, low nuclear grade, diploid—but if
it's a HER-2/neu expressor you'll crash and burn." Women
hoarded their positive indicators as though they were precious jewels, proudly displaying them as evidence of their security, but
Slamon had seen too many of them show up as his surprise guests,
all because of HER-2/neu.

Love was uncharacteristically silent during Slamon's presentation. On her way into the room she had heard a disturbing rumor—that Mike Zinner was going to Boston to run the Department of Surgery at Brigham and Women's Hospital. He had
mentioned the offer a couple of weeks ago and Love, who knew
too well the hospital politics in Boston, had tried to joke him out of
it. Going to the Brigham and Women's Hospital was like "going to
Guadalajara," she said. No one would notice Zinner there. UCLA
was a much more high-profile post.

She thought she had convinced him, but clearly she had not. He
had chosen not to take her advice; he was deserting her; and he had
not even bothered to make sure she heard the news directly from
him. Love was disappointed. For all the tension between them over
Love's role at the Center, she had thought until now that Zinner
considered her his partner in the effort.

After the meeting one of the other surgeons confirmed what she
had heard: Zinner had announced that very afternoon that he was
leaving. Love made sure that everyone in earshot heard her initial

reaction, which was that Zinner's departure was tough for the Department of Surgery but would have no impact on the Breast Center. But she accepted Slamon's invitation to grab dinner on the way home. She was prepared to let him reassure her that the Breast Center was not in any immediate danger—and even to listen to his litany of suggestions about how to make sure it remained safe.

18

THE TRANSPLANTERS

I T WAS ONLY HUMAN NATURE TO YEARN FOR AN ANSWER THAT WAS too good to be true. Glaspy saw it all the time on both sides—women who came to him certain that high-dose chemotherapy and a transplant would leave them cancer-free, doctors who maintained a simple optimism despite mortality statistics that refused to yield. He bought into it himself, to a limited extent. If a woman qualified for a transplant, who was he to deny her?

"Everyone deserves a swing at the plate," was the way he put it. He was not God. He could not look at a woman and tell if she was going to respond to high-dose chemotherapy—or if she might be one of the freak exceptions who lived some good years with metastatic disease no matter what the doctors did.

What frustrated Glaspy was his realization that transplants would not generalize. They might work for certain patients, though no one yet knew how to identify those women in advance, but they clearly did not work for everyone. The standard regimen, what he called "lunch-pail chemotherapy," had reached the same dead end. Despite everyone's initial hopes, lunch-pail chemo would not generalize. Some women got better without it and some got worse despite it, and there was no way to tell who was who.

For all the decades of hope invested in them, standard and high-dose chemotherapy were not the answer. Still, Glaspy was obligated to continue on this road, if for no other reason than to confirm that it was the wrong way. He reminded himself that history was full of doctors and scientists who made a great contribution to medical research by posting a sign that told others to turn back. Negative results were a contribution—not the kind that won prizes, but a contribution nonetheless.

He had come to think that he was working the wrong end of the disease, stepping in too late, when the odds were against him. The future probably lay in prevention, but that would belong to other doctors, younger ones with entire careers before them.

It would take that long. When Glaspy surveyed the terrain he came up with a cold conclusion. "It's possible for human beings to play chess with nature and win," he said, "but you don't play chess with nature without a really thorough understanding of the playing board, or you're going to get burned." The environment was a wilderness, as far as breast cancer prevention was concerned, despite all the headlines about various diets or vitamins.

He believed that breast cancer was an "oncogene disease, a failure of normal on/off switches" in the body, and with his trademark black humor he liked to tell people, "The real question is how come we're not all dead of cancer when we're two. The regulating switches work so well. Every time you nick yourself a switch gets turned on to make new cells—but not cancer." The body did a very good job of maintaining a healthy balance until something—a faulty gene, or an environmental insult—caused a switch to break. Perhaps the key to prevention required a change in perspective. Researchers needed to figure out what made the body's switches work so well in the first place, and then devise a way to supply more of it.

The best he could hope for in the meantime was anecdotal success. "I think I'll be able to go to my grave pretty much convinced that there are a few people who lived because we did these things," Glaspy said. "I won't know who they are, because of the ones who do real well, you don't know which ones would have done so without the treatment. But I'll feel I prevented some pain. Prevented some tragedies."

*   *   *

The tantalizing promise of Glaspy's field, medical oncology—slightly shopworn, but still appealing—was that researchers simply had not yet stumbled on the magic combination of drugs. Perhaps chemotherapy did work; perhaps the limitations of drug therapy were the doctors', not the drugs'. There was a dizzying array of variables to consider: dosage, combined effect, sequence of drugs, even the time between treatments and the speed at which a given drug was administered. As weary as the combatants had become, they could not rest.

There were four cooperative oncology groups in the United States, whose member doctors and researchers conducted clinical trials at participating hospitals around the country: the Southwest Oncology Group (SWOG), the East Coast Oncology Group (ECOG), Bernie Fisher's National Surgical Adjuvant Breast and Bowel Project (NSABP), and the Cancer and Leukemia Group B (CALGB). On the weekend of April 16 to 18, the members of SWOG gathered at the Hyatt Regency Hotel near the San Francisco Airport for three days of presentations and discussion about new studies that needed to be done.

The breast cancer working group that Susan Love attended was run by Dr. Silvana Martino, the chair of SWOG's Breast Committee. A small, dark-haired woman with a fierce, impatient manner, Martino was quick to put the forty people in the room on notice. She still hoped for an answer on the easy side of a transplant for patients with recurring disease.

"It's my hope that before the end of my days I'll see some recurring patients cured," she said, "and not with a stem cell transplant. That's what I'd like. And I think I want to charge this group: That's what I want you to bring me."

They could not, not yet. After two presentations about dose toxicity in new chemotherapy combinations, the meeting was turned over to the doctors who called themselves "the transplanters." It was an important distinction. They did not treat breast cancer patients unless those patients required a transplant. They were not part of the community. The transplanters were like hired guns who rode into town because the local folk had failed to roust the villains.

Immediately the meeting turned into an acrimonious exchange

between the two sides. The transplanters complained that doctors did not refer patients to them, and the doctors replied that too many of their clinical trials were single-arm studies that would not provide conclusive data. The transplanters agreed that a random-ized study, which allowed researchers to compare two treatments using like populations, was preferable—but if a woman insisted on a transplant there was no way to force her into a study where she might land in a control group.

The doctors admitted the problem, but they blamed the trans-planters for the increased demand as well. Transplants were creep-ing down the ladder. There was talk of administering transplants to women with between four and nine positive nodes. The treatment was about to become standardized, not because it worked, but be-cause patients wanted it. The doctors chastised the transplanters. Supply and demand was not the proper way to treat disease.

Still, the challenge for SWOG was to determine how to effec-tively conduct transplant research; they could not sit this one out. If the group backed off it would jeopardize both its professional status and its ability to get money for the studies it wanted to initiate. "If we don't have the ability to get patients in these trials we're not going to be taken seriously," Martino said. "It's numbers that talk."

She was determined to collect enough data to retire the question once and for all. "To me, one of the worst things that can happen in this decade would be if we said, 'You can't have breast cancer with-out a transplant,' " she said. "It may turn out to be true, but I want research so I know it. I don't just want to *think* it might be so."

One of the transplanters insisted that with enough subjects re-searchers would have the answer in six years—and the data would prove that transplants did work. Her pronouncement was met with a collective groan. Most of the doctors in the room were not so sure.

There was the desire for knowledge, and then there was the desire to be the one who defined knowledge. When the next trans-planter got up to present his pilot study, a young man in the front row interrupted in protest. He knew of about forty studies on high-dose chemotherapy and transplants. The only reason for that many studies, he felt, was professional ego.

"Everyone's competing to further their own careers," he said, "and the women of this country are paying. Lots of them don't even have this treatment available to them."

He figured there were two possible truths: the transplant worked, in which case the researchers should combine efforts to prove it as quickly as possible; or the transplant was no good, in which case they were harming the women who received them. The shared goal had to be to limit experimental stem cell transplants to a smaller number of clinical trials until they resolved the issue. Private doctors should not be doing transplants and billing insurance companies until the medical community arrived at a consensus.

His complaint came too late. Outside the auditorium a company had set up a poster advertising the future of transplants: an on-site service that could treat patients on an outpatient basis and drastically reduce hospital time and the threat of infection.

The lobby was crammed with pharmaceutical company displays, souvenirs, and sponsored snacks: coffee service from Glaxo Pharmaceuticals; bite-size chocolate bars from Wellcome Oncology, a division of Burroughs Wellcome; literature booths from Zeneca Pharmaceuticals and U.S. Bioscience, all of them waiting to find out which therapy—and which manufacturer—was going to hit the jackpot.

Love, who had flown in just in time for the breast committee meeting, zigzagged between them with her suitcase. Dozens of doctors were crowded into the lobby, but all she wanted was to get up to her room and out of her good suit. She refused to expend any more energy on the topic of transplants. High-dose chemotherapy was the logical extension of Bernie Fisher's systemic approach, but Love did not think it was going to work. This was not a paradigm shift like Fisher's early work, or what she hoped to hear the following week in Belgium. Transplants were a refinement of the existing paradigm, and that was not enough.

* * *

She was much more interested in the women's health committee, chaired by Dr. Kathy Albain, an oncologist at Chicago's Loyola University Medical Center. Advocates were at the conference for the first time—Amy Langer from the National Alliance of Breast Cancer Organizations, Ellen Stovall of the National Coalition for Cancer Survivorship, and a representative of the Chicago-based Y-Me hotline. The agenda was full of consumer issues.

While the government, the NCI, and the NSABP debated the consequences of giving tamoxifen to high-risk women, the SWOG women's committee wanted to talk about how to prevent or predict the endometrial cancer everyone was so worried about. They could monitor trial participants more carefully, conducting endometrial biopsies for participants in two SWOG trials, one studying women with node-negative cancer, the other postmenopausal women with node-positive disease—or they could try a more aggressive intervention. The drug Provera might arrest premalignant uterine abnormalities, but the notion of adding yet another medication to the mix made the doctors in the room uncomfortable.

"I'm *very* nervous about diving in with yet another drug we know nothing about," said Love. The only argument in favor of the approach was that women who were scared by all the news about tamoxifen were going to their own doctors, being treated in what one doctor called a "hodgepodge way." If SWOG had a policy about Provera, at least the data would be better.

"I'd rather randomize them for a hysterectomy," said Love. "Do a hysterectomy instead of Provera."

Albain and Martino gasped so loudly that Love instantly recanted.

"Okay," she said, "maybe I'm a surgeon." Still, she resisted the suggestion that another drug was the answer. Provera was a progesterone sometimes used in addition to estrogen in hormone replacement therapy after menopause, and no one knew enough about its side effects. If a woman took it long enough to change the lining of her uterus, it could change breast tissue as well. Love reminded the others about DES, diethylstilbestrol, the drug that was widely used in the 1940s and 1950s to prevent miscarriage—and, a generation later, caused increased cervical cancer in the daughters of the women who took it. Provera presented a similar problem. None of them knew what the long-term consequences would be.

Kathy Albain suggested a complex schedule of endometrial biopsies and short courses of Provera, with a recommendation that women be taken out of tamoxifen studies if they showed abnormal pathology that did not respond to the drug, but Love still resisted. At the end of an hour they were stuck.

They finally agreed to settle for careful monitoring, and hold off on more drugs for the time being. The increased risk of uterine cancer was real, but too small to expose the entire population of a study to yet another drug.

As people left the room they broke up in pairs or small groups, eager to continue the conversation or make dinner plans. Love did not join them. She always looked forward to the time off she had at medical conferences. She could work for the rest of the afternoon, take a walk by the water, order room service, and get to sleep at a decent hour. She had no interest in the socializing that went on at SWOG conferences. She liked solitude, which she got too little of these days.

19

THE REBUILT BODY

LAURA PRANCED AROUND THE PLASTIC SURGERY EXAMINING ROOM LIKE A high-strung racehorse, too excited to sit down, too nervous to hold still. The pregnancy was behind her, and the second week's blood test showed that her levels of beta-HCG had dropped. One more week like that and she officially would be safe—no need to have chemotherapy or postpone her surgery. The doctor who discovered the abnormal uterine cells had explained that she undoubtedly would have miscarried, which absolved her of any guilt over the abortion. She was seized by the desire to have her mastectomy and reconstruction and get on with her life.

On April 18 she showed up at Dr. William Shaw's office straight from a power lunch, in tailored olive green pants and a cropped jacket over a coffee-color lace T-shirt. She was full of confidence. She had seven people coming over for dinner, several of whom were in the industry, and she had a friend's script to sell. The guy who had got her pregnant was coming into town and wanted to see her, and a producer she liked was being flirtatious. She did not want a man in her life right now, not until the surgery was behind her, but the attention made her feel good.

She took off her jacket and top to reveal a dark green silk bra edged in black lace. Without thinking, she reached back to unhook it—and when it came undone the half dozen cotton balls that Laura daily stuffed under her right breast, to make it look larger, fell softly to the carpeted floor. Laughing, she reached down to retrieve them and tucked them into her pile of clothes. She shrugged into her hospital gown and waited for the man who would make her body right.

Before he came to UCLA, Dr. William Shaw had spent twelve years putting lives back together as the director of the replantation service at New York's Bellevue Hospital. An expert at micro-surgery, Shaw could undo reality, sew a severed limb back on and make it work again. He could make a person whole. He allowed that his years at Bellevue gave him a "little different sense of confi-dence, in terms of what could be reattached," than most plastic surgeons.

A quiet, introspective man, he was always interested in new procedures—an unusual predilection, since surgeons were known for their resistance to change. He had read in 1976 about a plastic surgeon in Japan who used buttock tissue to reconstruct a breast—removed it completely and used microsurgery to reattach it to a new vein and artery pulled down from the armpit. Shaw was in-trigued. In 1978 he tried what he believed was the first buttock flap surgery in the United States—called a "free flap" because the tissue was severed from the body. It was successful, but Shaw found it a "very tedious operation," and expected to use it primarily as conso-lation surgery for women who had what he called "implant fail-ures."

The silicone implant, introduced in 1963, had revolutionized reconstructive surgery. For sixty years women had sought a way to conceal the effects of a mastectomy, but until the implant, satisfying that desire required a rigorous round of surgeries. During the first half of the twentieth century surgeons developed the waltzing tube flap, an arduous set of six operations in which a piece of abdominal tissue was gradually moved up through the body, one end of it always attached to its original blood supply. The process took from six months to a year, the woman misshapen the entire time, and the results were hardly aesthetically pleasing.

Other surgeons attempted to use the tissue of a woman's healthy breast by splitting it and moving one section of tissue over to the side where she had had a mastectomy. But this, too, was a difficult procedure, with questionable results. For the most part women settled for prostheses and endured what Shaw called "the aesthetic and emotional devastation" of the radical mastectomy—a concave chest and skin so thin that a woman could see through it to her ribs below. Shaw began his general surgery residency in 1968, and he had never been able to forget that mutilating procedure.

"It was scary," he said, "and ugly, and you look at it and feel a little queasy."

Under those circumstances, the implant was, he said, "like magic." A few surgeons continued to work on reconstruction using a patient's own tissue, but even Shaw considered it an inferior alternative to the implant.

Still, many doctors preferred using tissue. It gave the plastic surgeon greater aesthetic control, and the result looked more like what Shaw called "a normal breast." In 1980 an Atlanta, Georgia, doctor described the "tunnel tram-flap" procedure, an alternative to the free flap that did not require microsurgery. It was a sophisticated descendant of the waltzing flap: in a single procedure, the surgeon took tissue from the abdomen and tunneled it through the woman's body up to her chest, still attached to its original blood supply. The tram-flap was easier than Shaw's free flap, though more painful for the patient, and it soon became the accepted model for reconstructive surgery with a woman's own tissue, with implants still the most popular choice.

In 1985 Shaw saw a patient who convinced him that this was not the proper order of things. After listening to his standard speech about implants and reconstruction, the woman announced that she did not want an implant, though that was supposed to be her first choice. She preferred that he build a breast out of her own tissue.

Her response stunned him at first—but when he thought about it, it made all the sense in the world. His implant patients often had complaints: the implants felt hard, or sat unnaturally high, and never had the look or feel of a real breast. His flap patients seemed on the whole to be a much happier group. It was inherently a more natural reconstruction. Perhaps women should have a choice.

When he thought about what kind of reconstruction they ought to have, the answer was clear. The tram-flap might be easier, but there were more problems with it. In his judgment, it was not a very hardy flap. The blood supply that kept the tissue alive had a long way to travel, so surgeons had to be careful about screening patients. A woman with potential circulation problems—a smoker, or someone who was overweight—did not qualify.

The free flap that Shaw performed was more reliable and more versatile, if more challenging for the surgeon because of the microsurgery. He decided that it ought to be the primary operation, and an equal option to the implant.

But the tram-flap was in widespread use, and having mastered one approach, doctors were reluctant to adopt a new procedure. Shaw started performing the free flap on a regular basis in 1986, and eight years later he was still one of only a handful of plastic surgeons in the country who did so.

Now he was in demand, as the controversy over the safety of silicone implants suddenly made Shaw's alternative look more and more preferable. Although Laura had chosen implants for cosmetic reasons, she looked forward to getting rid of them. She would not have to worry about leakage, or hardening, or the laundry list of physical complaints that women attributed to their implants, and the manufacturers denied. Though there was only anecdotal evidence to support the claims, and a frustrating lack of scientific data linking the implants to various ailments, the stories had snowballed until it no longer mattered if there was a real connection. Women believed that there was.

In 1988 the FDA had given implant manufacturers three years to prove the safety of their product, but their research was as shaky as the evidence from the other side. The FDA withheld approval; silicone implants could be used only for breast cancer patients, as part of a clinical study. By the end of 1993 there were more than three thousand lawsuits over implants manufactured by Dow Corning—and in March 1994 the company and three other manufacturers agreed to a $4.2 billion settlement over thirty years.

Women were terrified of implants—and many breast cancer patients were angry at the implication that they were expendable. They turned instead to Bill Shaw, who came to UCLA to head the Division of Plastic Surgery and a new microsurgery unit in 1989 and began to perform simultaneous reconstructions.

Laura would wake up with her new breast already in place. She would not be able to feel it; medicine knew how to reconnect the blood supply but had not yet conquered the network of nerves that supplied feeling. It was Shaw's next goal—to create a sensate breast. He liked to think that anything was possible.

Dr. Shaw studied Laura as though she were a piece of sculpture—looked at the proportion of shoulder to hip, of breast to belly. Reconstruction was never a simple matter. He had to take into account the age and appearance of each patient, as well as her expectations. Laura was relatively young, in good physical shape, and as far as he knew, still interested in having a child someday. He had to consider all of these things when he made a recommendation.

He asked her to stand up and remove her slacks, so she stood, unzipped her pants, and let them and her silk bikinis fall to her ankles. He sat on a low stool in front of her, reached up, and squeezed her left breast, the one that still had the implant in it.

With the same mute detachment he reached down to feel how much fat she had in her abdomen. Not much. He reached over to squeeze her hip and her buttocks, looking for enough tissue to approximate her healthy breast. His expression never changed.

"Okay, now," he muttered, without looking up. "You would like the size to be about the same as what you are now?"

Laura looked down at her scarred right breast. "Do you mean this one . . . ?

Shaw gestured toward the left side, where the implant was still in place.

"No, we can go much smaller than that," she said, flustered. After two bouts with breast cancer, even residual breast cancer, Laura no longer cared about having large breasts. "I don't mind a small breast on me. I've been around the block with my breasts. As long as they look okay, I don't care. I don't need to go big."

"Okay. And let's see, you might get pregnant again in the future."

"I don't know," said Laura. "I'm not sure about it."

Shaw leaned back on his stool. "What I try to do is kind of look at the problem of reconstruction in totally different ways—separately—and then put things together," he said. "It's what I call a hillside architecture project. You're given an assignment to look at a particular reconstruction. First you need to understand the geology, the mechanical aspect. The ideal way of approaching it is to have a clear understanding of the material you're working with.

"You define the structural, architectural possibilities. Next you put into context the particular patient, her functional requirements or priorities. Then we go over preferences in terms of where the scars might be."

He spoke quickly, and more to himself than to his patient. There were drawings of classic Greek columns on the walls of Shaw's examining room. Each time out he aspired to come as close as possible to an ideal form, within the practical limitations he faced.

That included finance. When Shaw had completed his initial exam he paged through Laura's folder looking for information about her insurance. Simultaneous reconstruction required the services of Shaw, one or two other plastic surgeons, and two plastic surgery nurses—as well as the breast surgeon's team, the anesthesiologist, and the operating room staff. If Laura's file had not contained a preapproval letter from Aetna, which had provided the health insurance at her last job, she would have had to pay his $14,000 fee out-of-pocket—or forgo the procedure.

Since she had sufficient coverage, they could draw up a plan. Shaw laughed quietly. "In some ways," he said, "surgery is just like doing houses. The sky's the limit. You can keep building, but the reality is that you don't want to spend your whole life doing one house—not the patient and not the architect."

He wanted to have what he called a "realistic" conversation about what Laura could expect. If he removed the implant from her left breast and built a right breast to match it, they would be about half the current size of the left breast—larger than the right one, which had been excised twice for cancer. The advantage was that he could take tissue from her abdomen, buttocks, or hip. If he left the implant in he would have to take tissue from her buttock, for she did not have enough fat anywhere else.

Laura liked having the choice. He could remove the left implant. The only issue was what to use for her new right breast.

Older women usually preferred the abdomen. "It's saggy," explained Shaw, "so it's definitely a plus to use the abdomen."

"Because of the tummy tuck," said Laura.

"Because you gain something there," Shaw agreed. But a younger woman might be better off not using the abdomen. If Laura did get pregnant again she would lose the cosmetic advantage, and there was a slight increased chance of a hernia. Just in case, Shaw recommended that he remove the necessary tissue from her buttock, or the side of the hip.

She was not ready to commit. She told Shaw that she had been "nickle and diming my brain cells to death for weeks," trying to figure out where the scars would be the least obvious. Yes, most people chose the abdomen, and Love had told her it was a slightly easier procedure. But Laura had other considerations—not the least of which was the way she would look naked, from the front, to a man. Maybe hiding a big scar in the back would be better. She wouldn't have to look at it every morning in the shower, and neither would a guy.

Laura had more questions before she made a choice. She did not understand how Shaw could make a breast to match her left one without first removing the implant. The one thing that worried her even more than the scars was the possibility of being lopsided, and the fact that most women's breasts were uneven was of no consolation. Part of the allure of reconstruction was that it carried the promise of improvement. It was, after all, plastic surgery. Laura would not settle for looking like a healthy version of herself. She wanted something better.

She asked Shaw if he could remove the implant on the day of surgery to give him a proper model to copy.

"No, I think we have a pretty good idea. I can look at your left breast and say, Well, I think this is going to be half the size. Maybe wrong by ten percent. It sounds okay to do both at once, but it's kind of chaotic."

Laura began to jabber nervously. She knew that the implant surgeon in 1988 had tried different models to see which gave the best appearance. She knew they had raised her up to a sitting position to check the way she looked. For reconstruction she would be on her back the whole time. How could Shaw possibly build a breast that looked right when she moved, when all he saw was a supine figure still wearing a bag of silicone?

He smiled reassuringly. After over six hundred reconstructions, his imagination was quite sophisticated.

"You see," Shaw said, in an attempt to calm her down, "I'm looking at you now. I'm seeing your left breast as if it were fifty percent of its size now. I'm looking at your right breast as if there's nothing."

He could build a new breast that was ten to fifteen percent larger than Laura's left breast without the implant. He designed the excess on purpose. Ninety percent of patients required a second surgery to refine the shape. If the new breast was slightly oversize, it was only because Dr. Shaw planned it that way.

Laura could not envision the scars on her hip or buttock, so Shaw took out his purple marking pen and began to draw the incision lines on her skin. This way she could go home, look in the mirror, even try on some clothes or a bathing suit to see if the lines would show.

He drew three elliptical shapes—one at the top of her hip angling slightly toward the buttock, another about three inches lower, where a bikini would rest, and a third at the base of her buttock. On each he made a cross-hatched line where the scar would be—and then they discussed the consequences.

A small bikini bathing suit would be "tough," Shaw allowed, with either of the first two options, "but a regular two-piece would be fine." The higher hip incision was more trouble with clothes but better for shape; with the middle incision Laura might find her hip oddly flattened, and the buttock incision definitely would make her uneven.

He pushed and prodded her body so that she could see what he was talking about. Shaw preferred the highest incision—and if Laura was unhappy with the way she looked when he was finished, he could always perform some liposuction or do a small tuck on the other side, so that both hips were the same.

She sighed. "I've got scars here," she said, pointing to her breast, "and scars here," she said, pointing to the laparoscopy scars on her abdomen. "I'm single. I'd like to think of myself dating

again someday in my life, and the idea of all these things here"—
she gestured at the front of her body—"I don't think I can handle it.
Can I handle something back here, where I'm going to be
crooked?"

"I think so, yeah," said Shaw. "You're going to have a scar
somewhere, and my personal experience is that for younger
women, scars in the hip and buttock tend to go a little bit better."

"Okay," said Laura, suddenly confident again. "Then I feel
very good about choosing this area. At first I said, 'I have breast
cancer, I can't worry about aesthetics.' Well, yes, I can. It's important to worry about aesthetics."

"Cancer or no cancer," said Shaw, "it's the same."

"Thank you for saying that."

"Unless you can put it back together in a reasonable shape," he
said, "the patient is going to have a hard time."

He got to his feet to leave. He would see Laura once more
before the operation to review her decisions and refine the drawings.

20

NO FUTURE PAIN

EVERYONE HAD TO LEARN TO COPE, ONE WAY OR ANOTHER. THE AP-pointments with Susan Love were anchors, but there were lots of days in between, enough time for a woman to lose her way. All the survival statistics dealt with physical recovery; doctors measured time by external markers. True recovery required a healed heart as well, something that not even Love could provide her patients.

Jerilyn saw evidence of her distress everywhere. Piles of paper covered her usually tidy apartment. The mess had been growing since December, and she felt defeated by it. Her desk was covered. She had not been able to eat at the dining room table for four months.

One day she simply could not stand it anymore. She sat on the floor in front of a big box and sorted all her papers, into the box or into the garbage. At her next acupuncture appointment she asked Dr. Zhou what to do about the tension in her neck, shoulders, and lower back, which refused to yield to Dr. Zhou's steel needles, a chiropractor's hands, or swimming laps. The acupuncturist gave Jerilyn the phone number of Adi Herman, whom she described as a healer, and Jerilyn called him from Zhou's office to make an appointment.

She had one question. Did he do shiatsu or Swedish massage?

"I do body work," was all he would say. He could see her that afternoon.

Jerilyn had some time to kill, so she drove home to pick up her mail. There was a birthday card from her ex-lover, whom she had not seen since a disastrous visit two weeks after her surgery, when the woman had flown out to tell Jerilyn she had fallen in love with someone else. It was a glib little note, as breezy and impersonal as if it had been sent by a business associate. If she needed external proof of her loneliness, she had it.

Adi Herman's office was in a red brick building on a quiet street at the edge of the Santa Monica business district. He asked Jerilyn a few questions about her health and then ushered her into a treatment room, where he had her lie down on a table. A short wiry man with close-cropped dark brown hair and deep brown eyes, Adi had a palpable distrust of words. He looked to the body for clues about a person's health—for evidence of stalled energy, old emotional insults, the physical residue of psychic pain. When he found it he set about untying the knots.

Jerilyn was mystified. This was hardly traditional massage. After about forty-five minutes she suddenly lost sensation in her arms and legs—she doubted she could move them. Her face felt contorted in some kind of palsy. Then she began to feel something moving along her arms and legs, almost like an electrical current. They were pulsing on their own, and there was nothing she could do to stop it.

At first she was thrilled; the journalist in her was fascinated. But when Adi told her he was going to go out and get a drink of water, she panicked.

"Don't leave me alone," she said. "I don't know what's happening."

"Just let go," he said.

Aha, she said to herself. He wants me to cry. I am not going to cry.

"Just let go," he said again.

Jerilyn said to herself, Fuck, what am I holding back for? I don't know this guy.

"I don't care anymore," she said aloud. "I just don't care." She began to cry. It felt as though her arms and legs were crying. If she ever told her friends back in Wisconsin about this they would think she had gone totally off the deep end. "The California Zulu state," they would say, shaking their heads.

She truly did not care. She cried and cried, and after a while Adi stepped over and stroked the bottoms of her feet.

"Tell me what's going on," said Jerilyn, "because my hands are still numb and I'm frightened."

Adi calmly replied that he had released all the oxygen in all the cells in her body. What she usually felt was all the emotions she held in check. That was why she had problems with her lower back.

"You're holding in a lot," he told her.

Out of nowhere she recalled a trip her family had taken to Los Angeles when she was thirteen. Her mother had taken her and her younger sister to see *The Sound of Music,* and when the lights came up Jerilyn was in tears.

"Oh, look," her mother had said. "Hard-hearted Hannah is crying."

Jerilyn was on her way to a place where Barbara Rubin had resided for years, a universe made up of body work and breath therapy, of trance states and reflexology. Alternative therapy could get expensive, since it was not usually covered by medical insurance—not unless a healer had the savvy to hook up with a medical doctor whose name appeared on the bills. So Barbara turned to barter to get what she wanted, her therapy services in return for weekly breathing sessions.

For forty-five minutes once a week she concentrated on breath in, breath out, healing breath directed to her breast, big breaths to relax her body. The feeling of bliss did not always come immediately—"Surrender is hard," Rubin told her breath worker—but it did come eventually.

It was enough to get her through the week and keep fear at a reasonable distance. It was even enough, sometimes, to make her feel brave. She and her young boyfriend went to a barbecue where everyone was happily devouring big juicy hamburgers—and Rubin broke her discipline and had one.

She was feeling fairly invincible. "When in Rome," she told her beau, "do what the Romans do."

Every day Dee tallied the toll her treatment had taken so far. The hair on her head was gone, but that was just the most obvious indignity. Chemotherapy had robbed her of her pubic hair, of the pale fuzz on her upper lip, of the hair under her arms and on her legs. Her eyebrows and eyelashes had fallen off. Even the thin hairs at her jaw line, which she attributed to too many years on birth control pills, had disappeared.

And this was just the standard dose. With the transplant she might experience hallucinations and hearing loss. She remembered what the women at the support group had said about their fingernails and toenails coming off. Dee felt she had no choice—without the transplant her chances of survival were almost nonexistent—but she was paralyzed, unable to move ahead with her treatment.

One night she turned the television on to keep her company and stumbled on an interview with the songwriter Henry Mancini. Mancini, who had inoperable cancer, was telling an interviewer that he would like to live long enough to see the millennium, and Dee thought how nice another six years would be.

It sounded like success. Six years. Time for her toddler grandson to grow old enough to remember her. Time for someone to come up with a miracle cure. She went to UCLA's April 22 transplant support group looking for a little hope.

It was hard to find. The topic that evening was "What happens if a bone marrow transplant fails." Almost forty women and a half dozen husbands showed up for the lecture, and what they heard was daunting. Dr. Melani Shaum, an oncologist and UCLA professor, laid out the options.

Taxol was the drug of choice for women who still showed signs of malignancy after a transplant, the last decent outpost before the treatments John Glaspy derisively referred to as "placebos." But Shaum reminded her audience that taxol was a toxic drug, a chemotherapeutic agent; it was not gentler because it was originally derived from tree bark. It could cause hair loss, low white blood cell counts, numbness of the hands and feet, muscle aches, and in some patients a potentially fatal allergic reaction.

She got a rueful laugh from the crowd. These women were used to death threats. Taxol had undeniable appeal: over fifty percent of women with metastatic disease responded to taxol, even some who were resistant to the dread Adriamycin, the drug that had devastated Cindy Gensler. There was no cumulative dosage lid, like there was for Adriamycin—women could take taxol as long as it did any good.

The only problem was its lifespan. So far taxol's benefits seemed to run out at four years.

Navelbine was a new drug taken from the periwinkle plant, awaiting FDA approval. The clinical trial data looked promising, because there was no hair loss or nausea associated with the medication. It would be the first new drug approved specifically for breast cancer treatment in seventeen years.

"Is *this* curative?" asked one of the women. Everyone was waiting for the drug that stopped cancer—not one that diminished its impact or slowed its progress, but a drug that wiped it out.

"This is not considered curative," said Dr. Shaum. "This is a palliative drug with results that run anywhere from a few months to three or four years." Another drug to make the descent less painful; relief but not release. Everyone in the room looked disappointed.

The University of Southern California had a new vaccine study for women with breast cancer. A preliminary Canadian study of thirteen metastatic patients had shown that the vaccine extended survival for seven of them, to an average of twenty-two months so far, compared to typical survival of eleven months. But the requirements for admission to the USC study were strict: three or fewer bone metastases, no chemotherapy or radiation for six to eight weeks before starting the program, and no large tumor burden. Only forty-five women would be accepted.

One of the husbands interrupted Dr. Shaum. Women with advanced disease often found themselves unable to meet the rigorous requirements of clinical trials, despite their willingness to try an unproven treatment. This man had begun to wonder. Were the guidelines "to make sure the guinea pigs are homogeneous," he asked, "or to guarantee positive results?"

"A little of both," admitted Shaum. "It's always hard to publish negative results."

She mentioned Slamon's HER-2/neu study at UCLA, with his injectable antibody, but Shaum interpreted the literature differently than Slamon did. She was not so sure that HER-2/neu was a powerful prognostic indicator.

Doctors in Long Beach were looking at RU-486, a pill that had gained notoriety for inducing abortion but seemed also to hold promise for preventing breast cancer.

One woman asked, "What else do you see on the horizon?"

"I see some very encouraging research."

"How soon?" demanded another patient.

"I'm sorry to say, not in this decade," replied the oncologist. "Maybe 2000. 2005. Some way to turn off the oncogene. And I think the treatments will be very nontoxic. We'll look back on this era and see it was like giving arsenic for syphilis."

On the weekends Dottie often woke up and began to cry, and Joe would turn to her and ask what was the matter. She did not snap at him—she was too reserved a woman to lose control like that—but sometimes she had an angry thought: Don't you *know* what's the matter?

They had read the literature together. Once breast cancer moved into the lymph nodes there could be millions of microscopic cancer cells traveling throughout the body. With nineteen positive nodes, there was little doubt that such cells had got loose in Dottie's body. The only question was whether the combination of chemotherapy, radiation, and her own immune system could keep them from forming metastases.

She tried not to dwell on it, but on the day of her first radiation appointment, the one where the radiologist took measurements and tattooed the spot where they would aim the radiation, she found herself falling apart. Though she was usually rather restrained with strangers, Dottie started telling the radiologist the whole sad story of her son's death. Dottie had a photograph of him on the table in the master bedroom, and she confessed that she talked to him from time to time. As she told the radiologist about the boy she began to cry.

"I just never do this," she said apologetically. "This is something I just don't do. I've been so upbeat. Nothing has been bothering me." But she continued to weep, and to wake up sad on the weekends.

She did not care about a cure. Dottie had no interest in living to be as old as her eighty-seven-year-old mother; the fibromyalgia made ripe old age a cruel joke. But she desperately wanted five more years, because she had made a promise she wanted to keep.

Dottie's daughter was divorced, with two children. Her sixteen-year-old granddaughter was living with Dottie and Joe that year, and her grandson, who was nine, had already asked for a turn once his sister went away to college. Dottie and Joe doted on their two grandchildren—Joe took them on a trip each summer, Europe or Hawaii, and Dottie was always happy to have them in the house. She was aware of just how little she could do with her grandson, given her physical limitations, so she was determined to have him live at the house.

She told everyone involved in her care: she had promised the boy. It was up to them to make sure she came through.

Shirley and Tracy had plenty to keep them busy in the coming months—the high school carnival, Mitch's junior prom, Kim's graduation from junior high, a Memorial Day family camping trip. But life was not quite back to normal. The pain in Shirley's right breast kept her from going back to work, and sex was as much a matter of tactical planning as it was physical pleasure. Dr. Love said the discomfort could last for up to a year after radiation treatment, so as far as Shirley was concerned she was in nuclear purgatory. She and Tracy had learned a measure of patience, after twenty years together and the year-long bout with infection, but she yearned for the day when she could hug her husband without thinking about it first.

She fought the urge to dwell on her upcoming doctor's appointment. When friends worried about Shirley's health she always brought them up short. She would not allow herself to suffer future pain. The next mammogram would show what it showed, no matter how much she yearned for the calcifications to disappear. She was not going to let it bother her now.

The trick was to enjoy the time before that day, just in case it turned out to be the happiest life was going to get.

Shirley liked to cook, but she had always hated feeling responsible for what she called "maintenance meals," the dependably nutritious three squares a day. As her appointment got closer, though, routine became a pleasure, and she assembled the occasional oversize dinner, designed to yield leftovers for three or four days, just to keep busy. She thought about signing up for a required day of emergency retraining, so she could get back to work in May.

The kids' defenses were not as highly developed. Shirley kept a watchful eye on Mitch, who tended to internalize his worries. Two nights before her appointment she took Kim out for a cup of coffee, because her daughter had been following her around like a scared puppy all evening.

"This isn't surgery," Shirley reminded her.

"I know, but I'm worried," said Kim. "Suppose it's bad."

"Okay. Suppose it's bad. What's the worst thing that can happen?"

"You have to have a mastectomy," whispered Kim.

"Okay," said Shirley. "So I'll have a mastectomy. What's the worst thing that can happen then?"

"You die with breast cancer," said her daughter.

"Okay, so fine, I die with breast cancer," said Shirley. "So what's the worst thing that happens then?"

"You're not around to see your grandkids."

"Oh, okay." If that was the worst thing Kim could imagine, Shirley had an answer. "If I didn't have breast cancer I still might not be around."

That hardly helped. They agreed to be apprehensive until the appointment on Friday—and Shirley promised to drive by school on her way home from the doctor to let Kim and Mitch know what had happened.

Tracy did his best to match his wife's cool discipline, but some nights it was too hard. He looked at Shirley and the kids and could not understand for a moment why she should have to endure this nagging fear. She was such a decent person, and she had known such unhappiness as a child. This new worry was an affront, and he hated the fact that there was no real way to comfort her. He could offer distraction but no solution. On a fundamental level, Tracy felt that he could not take care of his wife. When he got too blue he got out of her way, drove over to a nearby bar and had a couple of beers. No future pain.

On April 27 the Breast Center got its first piece of bitter proof that even the most aggressive treatment did not work. Three months earlier a young woman with positive nodes but no distant disease had undergone a transplant. Now she had metastases. When Sherry Goldman heard the news from one of the oncologists she had to lean against the wall for support. This was the first recurrence Sherry had heard of in a woman who did not have metastatic disease before her transplant—and so soon. Three months was nothing. The patient was still recovering from the procedure.

That same afternoon the Breast Center staff was confronted with a new class of casualties—the young children of young women whose diagnosis was due to improved methods of detection. Twenty years ago these women might not have been diagnosed so quickly, and their kids would have been teenagers by the time they got the news. But there were three women in their early thirties in the General Surgery waiting room, each with small kids.

Psychologist David Wellisch found it harder and harder to talk to such patients. His heart ached for the children. Before the clinic began he pulled his two young trainees into a room to advise them on how to proceed.

"What we want is for the mother not to get depressed," he said. "The three-year-old asks her mother, 'When will your ow-ee go away? Does your ow-ee hurt?' She can tell the child it is healing— but our greater concern is that she not get depressed."

One resident had already met one of the patients, whom she feared was dangerously upset. Six weeks ago the woman's gynecologist had told her that the lump she felt could not possibly be cancer. In fact, she had eleven positive lymph nodes and was sched-

NO FUTURE PAIN   265

uled for a transplant. She could not eat and had to take Halcion to get to sleep.

Wellisch shook his head in disgust. "This is getting a little old," he said. "They shouldn't be saying 'It can't possibly be cancer' anymore to women in their thirties."

"I think they say it," replied the resident, "because they don't *want* it to be cancer."

During the third week of April, Love went to the *Lancet*'s conference on breast cancer in Bruges, Belgium, and came back revitalized, confirmed in her belief that the best way to treat breast cancer was to walk away from all the old accepted notions about the disease.

She brought back a copy of a 1993 *Lancet* article entitled "Breast Cancer 2000 B.C. to 2000 A.D.—Time for a Paradigm Shift?" by Michael Baum, a surgical oncologist and director of clinical research at the Royal Marsden Hospital in London, who had organized the conference. It was all she wanted to talk about. Baum, like Susan, believed that the modern approach to breast cancer treatment, based on surgery and systemic therapy, had only "limited success." He believed that research would show more aggressive systemic therapy to be of little value. The answer lay somewhere else.

The possibilities were truly fabulous. Love boiled down what she had heard to an accessible formula: Instead of trying so hard to kill cancer cells, doctors ought to be working to figure out how to tame them. Alter the environment and they would not be able to find a comfortable breeding ground.

It was a radical notion, and she felt she was just the one to popularize it. People had kept coming up to her in Bruges to tell her that—to entreat her to use her celebrity to gain attention for the approach. Love had been complaining loudly for years about "slash, burn, and poison." If she could articulate an alternate direction, research dollars and scientists might be ready to follow her lead. She could enhance her own position within the academic community. All that was required was the discipline to follow through—much less fun than the joy of discovery, and not something she was good at. Still, she let everyone at the Center know that she was working on an idea. Perhaps if she told enough people, it would come true.

21

HEARTS AND MINDS

FOR THE FIRST TIME IN HER LIFE SHIRLEY BARBER HAD WRITTEN DOWN A doctor's appointment on the wrong date in her calendar, and when Dr. Love's office called on Thursday, April 28, to find out why she was late, she panicked. She thought the mammogram was scheduled for Friday, the twenty-ninth, the day when Tracy planned to come with her, the day the kids expected to see her at school. Shirley had anticipated a cozy Thursday night watching sitcoms, all of them curled up together on the bed, but here it was Thursday morning and the facilitator wanted to know if she could drive up right away.

An hour later she was signing in at the reception desk of the Iris Cantor Center for Breast Imaging in the basement of the Medical Center, her nerves on edge. First she had to explain to the technician that she had different problems in each breast. The technician had to mark every one of her surgical scars with a little strip of tape that looked to her like miniature rosary beads, so that no one who read the film would mistake a scar for something else. She had to take two standard views of each breast and a magnification view of the right breast.

Shirley stood in front of the mammography machine as the technician positioned her breast between two clear plastic plates, and for once the wisecracks deserted her. A tear ran down her cheek. When the technician was finished Shirley quietly got dressed and headed up to the fifth floor to see Susan Love, like a comic who had suddenly forgotten the next chunk of her routine.

Fate let Shirley down again. In the six months since her last mammogram a new crop of calcifications had appeared. Love was unconcerned. These were large, unlike the ones that had led to Shirley's cancer diagnosis, and were almost certainly the type that signified what Love called "the normal wear and tear" of breast tissue. Everyone who participated in the tamoxifen study would have a mammogram in late June, which was only two months away. They could take another look then.

She sent Shirley home with orders not to worry. These could be residual calcifications from the radiation treatment. There was no reason to be upset.

Shirley managed to pretend that she felt fine for most of the ride back to Irvine, but by the time she pulled into the driveway she was agitated. She immediately took out Love's book and read the section on calcifications. Shirley knew that radiation killed cells. Dead cells could calcify. So the radiation had given her more calcifications. It made perfect sense.

On the other hand, she wanted to run around the house and scream. Was she two months away from a mastectomy? Was she going to be this worried forever? For a moment she could not decide which was worse—losing her breast or losing her peace of mind. A mastectomy might not be such a bad trade-off if it meant she could stop wondering about the future.

She decided to clean the house, with a vengeance. If she could not have a normal mammogram, she could have the most pristine kitchen counters in Orange County. When an unsuspecting Mitch and Kim got home from school she drafted them as well. By the time Tracy got home from work the place was spotless, his wife was pulling at a cigarette, and the kids were disgruntled.

She tried all night to calm herself down. Dead cells, calcification, dead cells, calcification. There was a clear causal link. There was nothing to worry about.

The voice of emotion replied, "If I can't get a clean mammogram after going through radiation, what does it take?"

* * *

Susan Love walked out of her office late that afternoon and collided with the delicious consequence of having a wealthy donor—the official opening ceremony for the Rhonda Fleming Mann Center for Women with Cancer, the psychosocial center whose newly decorated suite of offices was just down the hall from the Breast Center's makeshift digs.

Elegant women in pastel afternoon suits and impeccably tailored men nibbled hors d'oeuvres and accepted drinks from black-tie waiters. There were sprays of fresh flowers everywhere, and a gay ribbon stretched across the doorway. Chancellor Charles E. Young himself was here to welcome the crowd and congratulate the actress and her husband, who had fully underwritten the center's operation. Young handed a huge pair of scissors to Ted Mann, who cut the ribbon to great applause, and then everyone went back to eating arugula and cream cheese on walnut bread.

Center director Dr. Ann Coscarelli ushered appreciative guests in to take a look at the center, which included a resource library, a conference room with video equipment, a private kitchen, and comfy staff offices. Even the chairs were perfect—reclining easy chairs into which the most shell-shocked of patients could collapse.

This was the way new programs were supposed to be born. Rhonda Fleming had nursed her sister through terminal cancer, and in the process came to realize how little emotional help was available to patients and their loved ones. She pledged her financial support to UCLA, which enabled the university to take a year to plan and develop a program that offered comprehensive psychosocial services to women with cancer. Coscarelli and her staff had never been hungry like the Breast Center, never bothered about numbers and profits. To Susan it seemed they had the best possible arrangement: financial autonomy and the university's resources; a medical boutique protected from the normal exigencies of the small business. The Breast Center, in contrast, had been born of ambition, and ever since had been involved in an irksome game of economic catch-up.

Love stood off to one side with Shannon and Christi, two

of the Breast Center facilitators, staring at the sumptuous spread and wondering where she was going to get the funding she needed.

A photographer for the Manns approached Love to ask her to pose with them, and she amiably slung her arm around Ted Mann's shoulder as though they were old buddies. When he thanked her for coming she could not resist bragging, just a little. She might not have funding, but she wanted everyone within earshot to know that she was working harder than anyone else.

After work she had to take the red-eye to Atlanta to chair a selection committee for the first Walt Disney–American Cancer Society Research Professor for Breast Cancer, an endowment for a doctor anywhere in the country who specialized in breast cancer care or research. Friday night she would fly home to plan Kate's Saturday birthday party, after which she would take another red-eye to Washington for an all-day NBCC board meeting on Sunday. There were more NBCC meetings on Monday morning, and at noon the artist who was doing the line drawings for Love's revised book would show up at her hotel. An NBCC reception at the French Embassy followed that night, a congressional breakfast Tuesday morning, and then a meeting with Samuel Broder at the National Cancer Institute. She would get out in time to head back to the airport for the Tuesday evening flight home.

Mann was suitably impressed.

"Somebody has to do it," Love said, beaming, and strode down the hall to where her patients were waiting.

The notion that the heart could help to heal the body—that comprehensive care for the breast cancer patient required emotional as well as physical therapy—was a popular one, promoted since the 1980s by an assortment of self-help titles. The most startling research in the field, however, came from a reserved, self-effacing man whose work was motivated in great part by a desire to refute what he saw as a "blame the victim" mentality. Stanford University's Dr. David Spiegel did not believe that a woman could make herself sick, but he found that she might be able to improve her outlook—and that, in turn, could affect how long she lived.

Spiegel was the psychiatrist son of two psychiatrists, a composed, erudite man who considered becoming a philosophy professor before he decided to go into the family business. His father had used hypnosis with combat soldiers in World War II; the younger Spiegel found himself drawn as well to the way the mind and body interacted. He went to medical school at Harvard University, where he distinguished himself early on for advising a young asthmatic to use self-hypnosis to short-circuit an attack. It worked. The woman and her family were effusively grateful; the hospital administration, equally outraged. Spiegel emerged thinking that anything that got such a dramatic response—from both the patient and the other doctors—must be worth looking at.

As a young professor at Stanford in the late 1970s, Spiegel worked with group therapy expert Irvin Yalom, who took a different tack than traditional therapists. Instead of analyzing the past, Yalom wanted to talk about the future, because he believed that a person's anticipations defined how he felt in the present. To test the theory, Yalom gathered together a group of women who were more aware than most of their mortality, women with metastatic breast cancer.

Spiegel and Yalom recruited eighty-six women and randomly assigned them to one of two groups. One participated in an experimental support group, while the other received standard care. When the study was over, the two doctors had the results they expected: the support group had helped women feel better.

That was a simple enough notion. What troubled Spiegel was that in the 1980s popular writers of self-help books took it too far. If therapy helped the mind, perhaps more work would help the body. And the troubling reverse: If people did not work on their feelings they might quite literally make themselves sick. Spiegel was uncomfortable with the idea that the mind could heal or harm the body, as popularized by Dr. Bernie Siegel in his 1986 book *Love, Medicine and Miracles*. It sounded like anyone who was sick was an accomplice in his own disease. Siegel, a Yale University professor of surgery, had been quoted as saying, "I try to heal lives by teaching peace of mind," and liked patients to consider what "benefits" they derived from their disease, a point of view many of his colleagues found appalling.

Spiegel realized that he had a perfect opportunity to refute the concept that people made themselves sick. All he had to do was contact the women who had participated in the Stanford study. He would find out who had died and when, and publish a paper that quashed all this talk of self-healing. The support group might have made the last months of those women's lives happier, but it could not have had a real impact on the disease.

Except that it did. Spiegel was stunned to learn that the women who attended the support group lived, on average, twice as long as the ones who did not—thirty-six months instead of eighteen.

The results of Spiegel's follow-up study were published in 1989 in the *Lancet,* and in his book *Living Beyond Limits,* in 1993. While he did not become a bestselling fixture on the talk show circuit, like some of the authors he criticized, he was something of a hero within the medical community. His point was a more subtle one: the mind did not cause disease, but a woman who was at peace with her mortality might just avoid it, at least a little while longer.

Or maybe he had just got lucky the first time. The women who lived longer might have done so anyway, without intervention; doctors were always telling stories of the one patient they had who confounded everyone and lived for years with metastatic disease. In 1993 Spiegel mounted a new study of breast cancer patients and the impact of group therapy. He intended to recruit more than one hundred women, to see if he could duplicate his 1989 results.

In the meantime his services were much in demand. Members of Spiegel's staff visited the Rhonda Fleming Mann Center, as they did other psychosocial programs around the country, to tutor group leaders in the fine art of effective listening.

The women in Jerilyn Goodman's support group had only their breast cancer in common. Jerilyn was forty-four, single, gay. Joyce was a full-time mom in her early thirties. Susan was a prim, divorced fifty-year-old, and Nina, a wealthy, fashionably dressed

Frenchwoman. They had managed to make room in their midst for Cindy Gensler, despite her Stage 2 diagnosis, because she brought a new element to the group—a wicked sense of humor. Cindy taught them how to stop swapping prognostic indicators and have a good time.

The group leader, Mann Center social worker Carol Fred, had to keep the evening from deteriorating into a litany of manic one-liners. Humor was a release, but there were issues to discuss. With her half-glasses, short hair, and elegantly tailored clothes, the soft-spoken Fred was the grown-up in the room, responsible for not letting the kids get too wacky. They regarded her, in turn, as the outsider, the disciplinarian who both irritated and reassured them.

They gathered in a small meeting room an hour after the grand opening of the Mann Center, but Jerilyn was in no mood to celebrate. She showed up last, plunked herself into the only available chair, and looked around with a dour gaze, as though daring the others to cheer her up.

"Anybody see *The New York Times* obituaries today?" she asked.

"Who died?" said Gensler.

"Forty-one. Breast cancer."

"Do you *always* read the obits?" asked Joyce. "Did you before the breast cancer?"

"Yes," said Jerilyn. "And I thought, I wonder what her S-phase is."

Carol Fred knew what Jerilyn was really thinking. " 'How much is she like me?' "

Jerilyn would not be roused. "I just have this weird feeling I'm not going to live past forty-seven," said Jerilyn. "It's my birthday today. Maybe that's it."

As if by magic, Nina produced a bottle of champagne and a half dozen plastic glasses. "Another excuse to have champagne," she said gaily.

"We'll make you feel better," said Joyce.

"Or you won't," cracked Gensler, "but you won't care."

They toasted Jerilyn's birthday, and another forty-four years.

"When you die at eighty-eight," said Carol, "you'll know you were cured of breast cancer."

Joyce said that over the weekend she had told her husband the names of the songs she wanted sung at her funeral, to the consternation of his eighty-eight-year-old grandmother, who happened to overhear.

She clapped Jerilyn on the back and laughed. "I wanted to say to her, 'Wise up, sweetheart.' "

"See?" said Jerilyn, to herself as much as to anyone else. "I'm not the only one who has these thoughts. I just wonder—is this the beginning of the next forty-four years, or just as it gets interesting it's going to end?"

Carol gently wondered if Jerilyn saw putting her life in order as the last step before death.

"I don't want to die," Jerilyn protested. "But I don't have great dreams for the future."

The conversation rolled like the tide, the jokes building until they all felt too silly, then subsiding into a little bit of serious talk, until the comedy started again. They talked about all the dumb things their friends and family said, and how dependent they were on favorite doctors. They wondered if they were likelier than most to die of other cancers, and gossiped about the rumor that vitamin E would lower the chance of recurrence.

Carol observed that they were bouncing their fears off each other, but that was all they wanted to do. There was an implicit pact among the members of the Thursday night group: honesty was good, humor was better, and heavier issues were to be meted out in small doses.

"One of the biggest issues in coming to terms with this," Carol said, "is the uncertain future."

"It was always uncertain," Jerilyn said. "It just didn't loom."

Carol persisted. The other problem, for these women, was that their cancer had come at such a young age.

"They all ask how young I am," complained Joyce. "Like I need to be reminded one more time, guys."

Cindy said that her pals at the gym had concluded she must have the breast cancer gene to get it so young, as though that were somehow a comfort.

They wondered if they ever would get to be old—and since there was no way to tell, they wondered how to live in the meantime. Should they do all the things they had never done—take off to Europe, quit that dead-end job? Or should they behave like everyone else, go to work in the morning, save money for the future? Healthy people deceived themselves, but the women in this room had irrefutable proof that the body could betray you at any moment, without warning.

So they debated and marked time. The five-year cure statistic might not hold up, but there was one thing that was true—each year out the chance of recurrence declined. Sixty percent of all recurrences happened in the first three years. If they got past that marker, the odds would shift in their favor. Maybe by then there would be a new treatment. That was what survival was really all about—hanging on long enough to find something that worked.

Laura's route to inner peace was daily meditation, but toward the end of April the world conspired to overwhelm her. Prudence demanded that she move her May 24 surgery back a few weeks, even though she expected a call that very afternoon telling her that the third blood test was normal and she was out of danger. If she did need treatment she would have to delay the surgery, because chemotherapy weakened a patient's immune system and left her more vulnerable to infection. Better to change the date now, before Love's and Shaw's schedules filled up.

She called the Breast Center to find a new date. "My severance pay is about to run out," she said, in her best Hollywood deal-making manner. "You want your doctor to get her fee? Let's get this organized."

Rescheduling was a nightmare. It turned out that her insurance company had mistakenly provided preauthorization for the second, follow-up surgery to correct the size of her reconstructed breast and construct a nipple—and not the initial, more expensive free flap procedure. UCLA had to start that communication over again, and in the meantime Shaw's office wanted a $2,600 cash deposit.

Laura was feeling sorry for herself in the first place, for having to change the date, but as the day wore on she began to feel that everyone was against her. The nurses in Shaw's office, who had seemed so accommodating when she first came in, now struck her as cold and unsympathetic. One of them tried to explain why she would have to wait: Since she had had a wide excision to get rid of her invasive cancer, she was less of a priority. There were others ahead of her in line.

"The insurance companies don't give a damn about anybody if they don't have cancer," said the nurse. "You'll be lucky to have your surgery by the end of the year."

Laura had to fight not to burst into tears. One of her unspoken terrors was that the pathologist would find more cancer in her right breast, or that Shaw would discover a tumor lurking behind the implant in the left. In a tremulous voice she asked the woman, "How do you know I don't have cancer?"

At five o'clock that same day Laura got the call she had been waiting for from her gynecological oncologist. The third blood test was emphatically not fine. Laura's hormone levels had shot up again dramatically. He wanted her to start her chemotherapy early the next week.

Six to eight weeks of treatment, followed by a three-week recovery period before she could undergo major surgery. Frantically Laura started to work the phone. She called Shaw's office back and left a message that she had interesting new information—she thought bitterly that if they wanted a patient with cancer, maybe now she could oblige. She called Susan Love's office and asked that Dr. Love call Dr. Shaw. She called the insurance company, terrified that she would lose another month to insurance certification.

An hour later she had her deal. Shaw's office called to say that she could have her surgery on July 19, which was the earliest date possible given her chemotherapy schedule. The insurance company would precertify the surgery and guarantee one hundred percent payment, so she did not have to spend $2,600 of her dwindling severance pay.

The future was secure. Now all she had to face was weekly injections and the probable side effects.

Deepak Chopra, the forty-seven-year-old endocrinologist and bestselling author of *Ageless Body, Timeless Mind* and a dozen other titles on spirituality and health, had been a friend of Laura's for eight years. Chopra, who ran the San Diego–based Sharp Center for Mind-Body Medicine, was a Hollywood industry favorite, full of suggestions for how to get just about everything anyone could want—affluence, the perfect weight, a good night's sleep, endless energy, and good digestion. Laura, who felt at the moment that she had very little of what she wanted, recited her litany of woe to him.

"You really have cancer karma," Chopra said. He did not mean that she deserved what was happening to her, or that she was somehow responsible for it. Laura understood: he was telling her that life was trying to teach her a lesson.

She could tick off the things she needed to learn—patience, tolerance, forgiveness, a more loving nature, less concern with the way she looked. She had confessed to Love at her last appointment that she was ready for therapy, but there was no way she could afford a private therapist. Group therapy was too public. If you were at the top in Hollywood you could talk about your triumph over breast cancer, like Lucie Salhany, who ran Fox Television, or Margaret Loesch, who was in charge of that company's children's network. Laura lacked their high-profile autonomy. She could not afford to give a prospective employer an excuse to choose someone else.

Still, she had to do something. Love urged her to talk to Carol Fred about the kinds of groups the Rhonda Fleming Mann Center had to offer. Carol got her the names of two women who had already had simultaneous reconstruction—and explained that the only ongoing group at the moment was the one for women with early stage cancer, which Jerilyn belonged to.

Laura mistook the explanation for an invitation, and the next Thursday called Carol to say she wanted to come to that evening's session.

Carol was taken aback. It was a cohesive group, and she feared that Laura's presence would rattle the others. Besides, this was Laura's second round; she had different problems. She suggested that Laura find a private therapist; some organizations offered inexpensive counseling.

Laura got furious. "I know you're a professional, but you're wrong," she said. "I need a group *now*."

Carol Fred gently suggested that a group for women with early stage cancer was perhaps not the most appropriate place for Laura, but what Laura heard was, "You're too sick to join." It made her feel as though she had the plague.

There was a point every day where she felt she was going to lose her wits. Laura reminded herself that she had no choice but to cope. She had no family to support her, no savings to fall back on. She had to keep moving forward.

She had talked to Chopra about the irony of her life—that after living on her looks for years she was being systematically relieved of everything she had preened over, her thick, healthy hair, her flawless pale skin, her surgically enhanced breasts, her dependably trim figure. But enough was enough. She had gained six pounds since the abortion. She was sick of the cotton balls she was using to make up for the missing implant. Laura decided she might break down and buy a prosthesis after all, to get through the summer.

On April 20 the University of Pittsburgh had filed a reorganization plan with the National Cancer Institute, the result of the oversight committee's efforts. Dr. Bernard Fisher was given the newly created role of scientific director—an attempt to move him out of a central, controlling role while acknowledging his ongoing contribution to the field. He would have to wait for the NCI's reply to find out if he had a future, or if the events of the last month had forced him into an early, unwanted retirement.

The answer came with harsh speed. In a letter dated Monday, May 2, the NCI sternly rejected the NSABP oversight committee's attempt at a compromise peace. There was no room for Fisher as the scientific director of the group he had brought to prominence—and to prove its resolve, the NCI threatened to cut off funding to the University of Pittsburgh unless he was removed from the program.

Dr. Herberman, the interim chair of the NSABP and the man who had invited Love to join the oversight committee, told *The New York Times* he was "surprised and disappointed" by the NCI letter, since clearly the proposed reorganization did not put Fisher in a central role. But the terms of the NCI letter made compliance an imperative. The university had a choice: dump Fisher or lose $16 million in annual funding.

22

STUBBORN LUCK

SOMETIMES THERE WAS SIMPLY TOO MUCH TO DO, AND THE WELL-OILED machine that was Susan Love—surgeon, program director, advocate, mother, teacher, author—broke down. She arrived in Atlanta to chair the Walt Disney–American Cancer Society selection committee meeting with two right shoes, a casualty of thinking about something else when she was packing, so she wore a business suit, pantyhose, and her Birkenstock sandals.

Harmon Eyre, the American Cancer Society's deputy executive vice president for Medical Affairs and Research, shanghaied her after the meeting and offered to drive her back to the airport so that he would have a chance to lobby her to change her position on mammograms for women under fifty. He wanted her to embrace the existing ACS guidelines recommending screening mammography for women between the ages of forty and fifty. There was no definitive study to suggest that mammograms for women under fifty were completely useless. Why confuse them?

Love replied that she was not in the habit of making recommendations just because a particular approach had not yet been proven unnecessary. She wanted to see convincing data that mammograms before fifty made a difference, and so far she saw no research to support that position. The ACS might as well change its recommendation. Women were not children. They could handle a little confusion.

Late Saturday night, after Kate's sixth birthday party, she was back on a plane for Washington, and when she arrived at dawn on Sunday morning she headed for the ladies' room to change out of her sweats and into her business clothes. She pulled out the pair of pumps she had been careful to pack—only to realize that this time she had failed to bring stockings.

The long weekend had been a mess of missing clothing, a laptop that refused to function, and too many meetings, but Love showed up at the Breast Center on Wednesday morning, May 4, ready to go. She told everyone what she had done, almost as though she were evaluating a patient's symptoms, wondering if two right shoes and no stockings were emblematic of anything more troubling than a temporary lapse in concentration.

Leslie Laudeman waited with a rumor: the word was that Revlon had decided to fund the expanded women's health center. Ronald Perelman was coming to town for the first annual Revlon Women's Health Luncheon and 5K Run/Walk on May 6 and 7. There would probably be a meeting to discuss plans the evening of May 5.

Love greeted the news with unexpected crankiness. "Do I have to wear makeup?" she said. She did not like surprises, and her first reaction was to wonder why no one had called her personally to tell her what was going on. Slamon should have been in touch, unless he intended to make decisions without soliciting her opinion.

"Want to bet they've already approved the plans?" she complained. "The ones they told us they wouldn't hold us to?" At Slamon's request Love had talked to an architect about how they might fit out the basement suite of rooms, even though she still held out hope of finding daylight space.

"I bet," said Leslie sympathetically.

"But that's life in the big city," said Love. "I'd rather have my own donor who I was in charge of, but that didn't work. I couldn't find one. I can't say anything about this because I didn't bring them in. I just don't get to speak up."

Dr. Linnea Chap was an oncology fellow and one of Love's hand-picked recruits, a thin young woman with efficient short blond hair and an incipient crease between her eyebrows. She caught up with Dr. Love right before the May 4 multi with bad news. The woman who had a recurrence only three months after her bone marrow transplant was dead. They both knew that women died despite the procedure—and some, because of it—but this was the first patient in their care who had died.

When they reviewed the multi patients who were waiting for them it became clear that the bad news was just beginning. Chap was assigned to three patients. One had already had leukemia. One had had ovarian cancer. One was twenty-seven weeks pregnant.

Love glanced at her. She wanted women on her staff whenever possible, and she thought the young oncologist was a bright, dedicated soul. The trick was to keep her from feeling overwhelmed.

"I tried," said Love, with a droll look, "to give you the interesting ones."

Abbas Ardehali was Love's surgical resident, and it was his job to take medical histories from the patients before Love saw them. His first case was a forty-six-year-old woman who for five years had been involved in a fertility program at a local hospital. In May of 1993 she had felt a mass, but the radiologist could not see it on a mammogram, and a surgeon who performed exploratory surgery could not find anything.

Ann Donaldson finally got pregnant in November of that year, and was due on July 31—but she had felt the lump again in early April. This time a surgical biopsy revealed infiltrating lobular cancer, a tumor over two centimeters in diameter with dirty margins. She needed either a re-excision to try for clean margins, or a mastectomy, if they were dirty a second time, and a lymph node dissection.

She was twelve weeks from her due date. She and her husband were expecting a girl.

"First pregnancy?" asked Love.

"She's been pregnant several times," replied Ardehali, "but never carried for this long." He hesitated. "She has a feeling the lump's been there."

"She's probably right," said Love.

Ardehali winced. Everything about him bespoke a desire for order—his impeccable shirt and tie, his low, soothing voice, a precise, reserved manner. This patient offended him. It was too much sadness, even in this arena.

"She's gone through so much to get pregnant," he said, as though there were a ceiling on distress.

Love knew what that felt like. She had gone through her own bout of middle-aged baby lust, and at least she already had a child. Ann Donaldson had finally succeeded in getting pregnant, only to be blindsided by such bad news. They could save the baby and try to help Ann, but she would never, ever have the chance to be just a happy new mom. That unadulterated pleasure was out of her reach.

"Okay," Love said brusquely. She could not allow herself to be swept away by her feelings. "She can deliver at thirty-two weeks, deliver early. We can wait. The bad thing would be if she were at twelve to fourteen weeks."

"She's been on very heavy-duty hormone treatment for fertility."

Love gave a tired nod.

"And birth control pills on and off."

Love took a moment to collect herself before she went into the examining room.

"Hi," she said, with her usual breezy smile. Ann and Rick Donaldson stood plastered against the wall of the room like kids on the centrifugal-force ride at the carnival. They could no longer feel the floor beneath them. They were too dizzy to walk over to the chairs.

"How are you?" asked Love.

"I'm fine," said Ann, and then she smiled. Ann owned her

own small public relations firm, and everything about her bespoke the charming diplomacy of her field: a gracious smile, understated clothing, a congenitally sweet manner. Suddenly she remembered that she did not have to perform, not in this room.

"Habit," she said, with a tiny laugh. "No. I'm not fine."

Love wanted the couple to understand that they had done nothing wrong. Lobular was a sneaky cancer to diagnose, hard to detect, able to appear and disappear. "But the pregnancy didn't bring it on," she said, emphatically. "Forget it. That's bullshit."

Ann managed a wan smile. "That's what I decided," she whispered.

Love also reassured her that her prognosis was as good as if she were not pregnant. Studies showed the same likelihood of progression, stage for stage, whether a woman was pregnant or not.

As Love did the physical exam Ann quietly told her the history of her attempts to get pregnant—the four surgeries, the fertility drugs, the hormone injections her husband gave her twice each day. She had "maximum doses" and still did not respond. She had gotten pregnant with a donor egg.

At that news Dr. Love brightened considerably. She patted Ann on the shoulder and helped her to sit up.

"Well, then, if it's a donor egg it's not your genes," she said, relieved to find even the smallest cause for optimism. "So you don't have to worry about your daughter and breast cancer."

At three thirty Love got back to her office long enough to glance at the mail. Connie had placed the most important letter on top—the one from the FDA granting her conditional approval for the first phase of her ductoscope study, which was essential to her DOD grant application. She had to answer some procedural questions, a bother but not an obstacle. There was one query she could not answer, about "the potential for distant tumor seeding by cells in distant areas of nonmalignant ducts"—the chance that inserting the device might itself spread the cancer—but at this point it did not matter, since the only women she was allowed to study were ones who were scheduled for a mastectomy.

She read the letter quickly and kicked the partition in front of Connie's desk. "Hot damn," she said. "On our way. Call Denny's office and tell them—and then let's call Hawaii and say, send us the scope. Move and groove."

She strode into the conference and announced the news. Radiologist Michael Racenstein had some advice. "You better pick and choose your patients carefully," he cautioned. There were always two goals for preliminary research: learn what you want to learn, but select patients who would yield enticing results and ensure support for the next phase. Nobody would want to fund the continuation of what looked like a dead end.

"Hey, at least I got it," said Love, who was not interested in talking about limits. "Damn. This makes my day. Finally, something good in my life."

Racenstein shot her a harsh look.

"I think," he said, slowly, "that your life's pretty good."

Love was chagrined. "You're right," she said. "I have a great relationship, a great kid, a decent enough job, and I work too hard."

"Hey," he replied. "I look around at the women we see. I think you're pretty well off."

Luck stubbornly refused to break in Ann Donaldson's direction. At the multi conference pathologist Sandy Barsky slipped one of her slides into his microscope and predicted that Love would find positive nodes when she operated. He could already see evidence of lymphatic invasion. Love exhaled loudly, and the entire room fell silent.

David Wellisch was concerned about the patient's emotional state. For all her effervescence, Wellisch found her very depressed. She woke up every night after only three hours sleep and often could not go back to sleep at all. She could not concentrate on her business. She confessed to him that she blamed herself for the cancer—despite everything Love had said, she was convinced that the fertility drugs had done it. She had no idea how she would manage to bond with the baby.

The doctors considered their options. They could try an immediate re-excision because of the dirty margins, along with a lymph node dissection, but the general anesthesia might kick Ann into premature labor, and she had twelve weeks to go. They could wait until she delivered naturally. They could wait just a little longer but not to full-term, and induce labor at thirty-two weeks. Glaspy, who was eager to start chemotherapy but preferred not to do so while a woman was pregnant, liked that option and encouraged Love to present it to Ann and her husband.

They agreed that Susan would recommend a re-excision and lymph node dissection under general anesthesia as soon as possible after the birth of the baby—which she would suggest they induce in three to four weeks. She would tell them that Ann would need chemotherapy so they could start to get used to the idea.

Ann could have a few more weeks to pretend that all she had to do in the world was await the child she so yearned for, but no more.

Michael Zinner chastised himself for what he called dime-story psychiatry, but he had come to believe that people ordered their lives to achieve their definition of satisfaction. He was fulfilled building programs and working within the academic community; Susan Love seemed happiest dealing with patients, an almost unassailable position, except that her definition of patient care included political advocacy and the kind of follow-up care that he thought ought to be delegated.

He had told her time and again: the president of General Motors does not fix hubcaps. She was not supposed to be speaking at ladies' luncheons and seeing follow-up patients. She was supposed to build a program and establish relationships within UCLA, to ensure the stability of that program.

He wrote her a blunt letter on May 3, a farewell communique in which he asked her once more to consider what she was and was not doing. He said it was time to start minding the store.

It was not what Love needed to hear, sandwiched between her shoeless weekend and the upcoming conversations with Revlon. She reviewed her calendar and had Connie prepare a rebuttal, a list of her activities over the past two years. It was designed to prove two things—that a lot of what she did outside of UCLA benefitted the program, and that her political activities were at a national level. She proudly pointed out that she had in fact cut back her local speaking engagements.

The V.I.P. Lounge of the Beverly Hilton Hotel was a public relations dream. Friday, May 6, was the first annual Revlon Women's Health Luncheon, and the lounge was crowded with celebrities: Revlon models Lauren Hutton and Veronica Webb, television newswoman Maria Shriver and her mother, Eunice, and actor Pierce Brosnan, all of whom the photographers recognized immediately; and Dr. Love, Dr. Slamon, and Revlon's Ronald Perelman, whom they did not. Lilly Tartikoff moved coolly through the crowd, herding the proper individuals together for group photographs.

Perelman had not had time to meet with Slamon and Love the night before, nor had he announced any formal decision about increasing his investment. But thanks to Tartikoff, photographers from the *Los Angeles Times, People* magazine, and *Allure* captured the image of an incipient partnership: Slamon, Love, Tartikoff, Hutton, and Webb with their arms around each other—medicine and cosmetics, the future.

No one pretended that private money replaced government funds, but it protected medicine from two harsh economic truths— the government did not have the funds to keep up with medical research, and the practice of medicine was not as lucrative as it until quite recently had been. Slamon and Love had already begun to spar about how to divide the new money, since Love wanted more money to underwrite clinical operations than Slamon thought she ought to have. Revlon was supposed to help compensate for the gap between income and upkeep—not subsidize bad business. He insisted that the bulk of the money go to new programs and research.

They smiled while the flashbulbs popped, though, and hoped that the weekend's activities would help to cement the Revlon deal. The success of Slamon's research program had had an unintended effect, which was that other institutions had approached Perelman for funds—most notably Memorial Sloan-Kettering, which was talking about a $3 million to $10 million program, a women's center to complement the Evelyn Lauder Center, one that would provide cancer screening and services for high-risk ovarian and breast cancer patients.

Slamon was hardly in a position to push Perelman for an answer. He could only hope that events like this luncheon would strengthen Perelman's commitment to UCLA. He had warned Susan twice not to talk about anything but breast cancer at the afternoon's panel. No matter what the other experts said—no matter how wrong she thought they were—she was to stick to her topic and not start any arguments.

The baby boomers' collective medical history was one of easy solutions. Medicine had always had an answer. There were vaccines to stave off childhood illnesses, pills to keep from getting pregnant, medications to get pregnant, more pills to ease the transition of menopause. That generation wanted—expected—tools to prevent or eradicate the major illnesses that threatened them.

Seven hundred women, most of them in their late thirties and forties, paid seventy-five dollars to attend the Revlon luncheon and hear a panel of doctors discuss the major issues in women's health—breast and ovarian cancer, osteoporosis, and heart disease. The panel, moderated by Maria Shriver, provided a range of expertise—Dr. Love on breast cancer; Dr. Beth Karlan, director of gynecologic oncology research at Cedars-Sinai Medical Center and a UCLA assistant professor, on ovarian cancer; Dr. Susan Johnson, from the University of Iowa, on menopause; Dr. Michael Kleerekoper, a professor of medicine at Wayne State University, on osteoporosis; and Dr. Linda Demer, chief of UCLA's division of cardiology, on the risk of heart disease after menopause. After a brief statement from each one, four women walked into the audience with microphones, and women quickly raised their hands to ask questions.

Were birth control pills a good idea?

Dr. Karlan liked them as a preventive for ovarian cancer—if

taken for five to ten years they reduced the risk of the disease from 1 in 70 to 1 in 350.

Love did not take up the challenge. She had previously publicly disagreed with Dr. Karlan on the issue, but she was not going to debate the first question.

A few moments later Dr. Kleerekoper fielded a question about calcium's benefits against osteoporosis. He dismissed it: calcium helped only if a woman took it when she was young.

For older women the choice was clear. "There is nothing better than estrogen."

Maria Shriver turned to Susan.

"You want to comment on that, Dr. Love?"

"No."

She maintained her self-control until they came back around to the topic a second time. Kleerekoper said that women over fifty were as likely to die of osteoporosis as breast cancer, a claim Love disagreed with. Women, he insisted again, needed estrogen.

Love raised her hand. This was Western medicine at its worst: *Got a problem? Take a pill.* She did not want to see the next generation inherit such a limited solution.

"The biggest thing we could do to prevent osteoporosis, heart disease, and breast cancer is to promote grammar school and high school athletics for girls."

She got a big round of applause, and then a woman who had breast cancer raised her hand to ask why she had got it.

"We don't have a clue," said Love, "because until recently there wasn't enough funding for breast cancer. So we all need to get angry and obnoxious and loud."

Denny Slamon walked with Love to the parking lot, full of adrenaline and unmet expectations. He worried that the luncheon had done his cause more harm than good. Women wanted answers. All his panel had provided was conflict. Hormones were good or bad, depending on which disease you wanted to fight. Birth control pills, the same. If his hand-picked experts could not agree, weren't women going to come away more frustrated than ever? Ronald Perelman wanted to be associated with optimism, not random fear.

Love told Slamon the same thing she had told the American Cancer Society's Harmon Eyre. Women could handle confusion. That was where change came from.

23

CLINICAL TRIALS AND KITCHEN MEDICINE

DAY AFTER DAY LOVE FACED WOMEN TOO CONCERNED WITH THEIR own survival to think about political change. She had to figure out who could handle conflicting truths and who merely needed an escort past the perils of treatment. Shirley Barber could juggle five options without panicking; Laura, and so many women like her, just wanted to come out the other end.

Love tried to get them to see beyond their own predicament. "Come the revolution," she always began, and then listed the improvements she expected once society came to its senses. Come the revolution, Clinton's health care reform would pass and the thirty-seven million Americans who lacked health insurance would have coverage. Come the revolution, research would provide data that led to answers. Come the revolution, managed care would live up to its promise and provide reasonably priced, quality health care.

Love thought there was great potential for a partnership between HMOs and specialists. For months she had been after UCLA's Managed Care Programs staff to shop a breast care package to the large HMOs. Private practice physicians and those with university affiliations were scrambling to create groups and market their specialized services to HMOs, who could use those treatment packages to distinguish themselves from the competition. The managed care provider who could boast of a comprehensive breast program designed and delivered by Dr. Susan Love and the UCLA Breast Center would have a real edge in the marketplace.

The contract department staff was receptive to the idea, but they needed Love to refine it. If she devised standard practice guidelines to describe the care that each category of patient ought to receive, they would have something to sell. And they needed her to create a fee structure—necessarily less than a private doctor might charge but high enough to guarantee profits. They could not market good intentions and idealism.

The idea languished, a casualty on one side of Love's schedule, and on the other by the often confusing demands of managed care. Should UCLA compute its services on a reduced fee basis to make the package look more attractive? Or should the university pursue a capitation payment structure, where the managed care provider paid a flat monthly fee per patient—a system that rewarded doctors who kept expenses down. Love held weekly meetings with the Breast Center staff to try to thrash out the guidelines, but it was slow going. They had to distinguish private practice excess from necessary treatment, and at the same time make sure they left nothing out. In exasperation Love wondered why she had to work so hard to convince people of her position—that it was possible simultaneously to cut spending and provide quality care.

Come the revolution, everyone would have access to decent health care. Otherwise the dread scenario of bad managed care would prevail: a two-tiered universe where most people got minimal care and the rest, the wealthy minority with discretionary cash, got something better, as unfair as the system it replaced.

Susan Love had no idea that Dee Wieman had felt betrayed by her comment to Dr. Boasberg about the likelihood of a mastectomy. Dee's behavior, when she came in for her May 11 appointment, was not unusual. The only difference was her willingness, for the first time, to admit that the drugs might not be working.

"In my heart, I don't think it's smaller," Dee confessed. As the words came out of her mouth, her eyes overflowed with tears.

"Okay," said Love. "It's not gone. It may be smaller, it may not be."

Dee rummaged in her purse for a tissue and tried to repair her face. "I'm only emotional because I haven't slept," she said.

"You're allowed to be emotional," Love replied.

"But I'm *not*," insisted Dee. "I'm really very calm—even though I'm going off the cliff."

"What is it that's making you feel like you're going off a cliff?"

"Oh, just because it's the next thing." Each new effort scared Dee—not only the literal threat of a more aggressive treatment, but because it meant a door was closed. The next therapy was proof that the last one had failed.

Love saw her resignation as an opportunity. If Dee had accepted the fact that she had to move on, perhaps she would agree to schedule the surgery first, a smaller step than the transplant.

Methodically they paced through Dee's history—another look at the mammograms, another physical exam, another discussion of the side effects of chemotherapy. This time Love did not argue, nor did she elaborate. She acknowledged each one of Dee's complaints and pressed forward, determined to get a signature on a surgery consent form.

Halfway through the appointment she sat down on a footstool, inches away from Dee.

"Our choices," Love said, "are to do surgery now—let's say, do a lumpectomy, see what happens. Follow that with a transplant, and if the lumpectomy isn't clear we could do a mastectomy at the end. If it is clear we'll just do radiation at the end."

"It's probably not going to be clear," Dee muttered, staring at her hands. "I shouldn't prejudge my condition, but . . ."

"I think it's fifty-fifty," said Love.

Love reminded her that Dr. Glaspy preferred surgery first, before the transplant, so that the drugs had a smaller enemy to fight.

All Dee had to do was say "yes" to that first step. They could handle the consequences of it later.

"What about what's already been sent out?" began Dee. "We're sure it's been sending out its little babies."

Love cut her off. "Yeah, but that's why you've been taking it— the poison—to kill those babies."

"My concern was, because the tumor wasn't responding dramatically, maybe the rest of it wasn't either. Maybe it's kind of resistant."

"That's possible," said Love. "But the other thing we know is that tumors don't respond as well as microscopic cells."

"Okay."

"That's one of the reasons they like to debulk the tumor, because the chemo works better on microscopic cells."

Dee seized that tiny particle of optimism and brightened considerably. She allowed herself to forget about what Love had said to her oncologist, swayed by the seductive promise of a minor procedure she just knew would work. Language was a crucial part of Dee's arsenal; she stored up every positive comment, however slight, memorized it, quoted it—and in this case, gave in to it.

"I like that idea," she said, suddenly compliant. "That's the plan I think would be a good plan."

Love moved ahead quickly. She reviewed Dee's chemotherapy schedule and her blood counts, and decided that she would be ready for surgery in about two weeks. Two more weeks after that she could start the transplant, no matter what the surgical pathology report showed.

It sounded fine to Dee, especially since she still believed that the transplant would rid her of every last vestige of cancer.

Susan grabbed a surgical consent form before Dee could change her mind, slid a Kleenex box under it so Dee could sign without even getting out of her chair, and went out to check the surgery schedule. She came back a moment later, triumphant. For once the gods of coincidence had conspired in her favor. Dee could have her surgery on May 24, in the space vacated by Laura Wilcox.

* * *

Once Dee was gone Love collapsed in a chair in the doctors' consultation room. It had been an exhausting half hour, but she had what she wanted. Dee Wieman was on the surgery schedule for a lumpectomy.

"The whole thing is a dance," she said to Christi, the facilitator who handled the surgery schedule, "of knowing when the right moment is to do things. Real estate is a dance; everything is. You have to be ready, both medically and emotionally, before you can make the deal."

For all the economic problems it presented, the Breast Center was popular with patients, who appreciated the individual attention as well as the ease with which they were able to see all the doctors they needed. Dr. Alison Estabrook, a breast surgeon at Manhattan's Columbia Presbyterian Medical center, had been given the happy task of designing a new program there, and in early May she embarked on a trip to look at various models. She visited the University of Southern California and St. John's, and planned to look at the Breast Center in the San Fernando Valley. On the afternoon of May 11 she and her colleague, Dr. Freya Schnabel, met with Dr. Love in the physicians' consultation room. Lunch was a shared tub of popcorn; the accompanying sermon was about why the multidisciplinary approach was better than all the rest.

Estabrook listened attentively to Love's explanation of how the multidisciplinary clinic worked, only to confess that she had doubts about it. She had found that older patients in particular were used to the confidentiality of the individual appointment. She worried that they would be overwhelmed by the five-hour schedule—and intimidated at the notion of having to sit in a waiting room with a bunch of other patients.

Love disagreed vigorously.

"They're all informed in advance," she said, dismissively, "so there's no surprise." She was willing to admit that the program was far from perfect. Her team of doctors continued to complain about the number of patients they saw for free, patients who never came back to them for treatment—and if the surgical residents happened to be delayed in operating rooms when the clinic started, the surgeons themselves had to take medical histories, a terribly impractical waste of their expensive time. The clinic often ran an hour or two late, a casualty both of Love's disregard for time and last-minute staff defections.

Still, she believed that multi patients got better care than they otherwise would, and she was prepared to ask women to sacrifice their privacy in return for access. Besides, Love believed that privacy was just a second cousin to secrecy, which was part of the problem in the first place—women ashamed to speak up, to complain or ask questions. There was a dependable momentum to the clinic, and she liked it. At first no one looked at anyone else—but by the time the nurses herded the patients into examining rooms there were a few shy glances, a nervous smile here and there. By the break some patients were ready to start up conversations.

They were no longer quite so cut off. Where some patients saw privilege—the tasteful waiting room, the string of appointments with specialists all over town, the false comfort of anonymity—Susan Love saw isolation. She brought the doctors together to provide what she considered the best treatment; she brought the women together so that they would understand that they were not pariahs. They had lots of company.

Estabrook's primary concern was her high-risk patients, the ones who did not yet require any kind of medical treatment. The future of the tamoxifen prevention study was still in doubt, until the government finished reviewing the NSABP data. Beyond that, there was nothing concrete to offer a woman with increased risk. Worse, Estabrook had heard that finding the exact location of BRCA-1 on the seventeenth chromosome was turning out to be much harder than anyone had anticipated.

"Nobody's saying anything about it," she told Love. "I think they can't find it. I heard they don't know where to look."

Love reflexively defended her friend Mary-Claire King. "Nobody's talking," she said with a blithe smile. "When people stop talking that means they're close."

"Mary-Claire's having trouble," insisted Estabrook. "I heard she said she can't find it. She's running out of families and she can't find it."

Love was noncommittal. "Well," she said grumpily, "I've never believed in prophylactic mastectomy anyhow."

Estabrook gently disagreed. She had seen young women who had had preventive mastectomies. They were so grateful for the chance to do anything to improve their odds; their peace of mind had to count for something.

"But *did* we do anything for them?" Love shot back. "God knows." She had come across one study that disturbed her, of rats that had some of their twelve breasts surgically removed. Researchers removed either three, six, nine, or all twelve of their breasts and then gave them a carcinogen—and the rats in each group got the same number of breast cancers. In a similar study mice were given prophylactic mastectomies without the introduction of a carcinogen. Again, the incidence of breast cancer was the same in mice who had had their breasts surgically removed as in those who had not.

Love allowed that the procedure might slightly reduce risk, but she insisted that common sense in this case was wrong: removing ninety-five percent of the breast tissue did not reduce a woman's risk proportionally. Denny swore that she had misinterpreted the results, and that the procedure did in fact reduce risk, if not eliminate it, but Love complained that this was yet another treatment being sold before it was proven. She worried that it would become even more popular once there was a gene, and a test to detect it.

She performed the procedure rarely, and with great reluctance. One patient came to her after another doctor had performed a bilateral mastectomy to prevent breast cancer—and Love found breast cancer in the scar tissue from her incision. That woman was one of the angriest patients Love had ever met.

Estabrook knew about the rat study, and wished that there were more data on women who chose to have the procedure. But they had the surgery done privately, not as part of a randomized control study, so there was no way to make a definitive judgment. Love recounted her single attempt to get data from a plastic surgeon who did a lot of prophylactic mastectomies. She told him she would be happy to be proven wrong, if only she could see his data. He never got back to her.

Estabrook sniffed derisively. "Plastic surgeons."

At five that afternoon the multi team assembled for a particularly exasperating journal club. The topic—hormone replacement therapy for postmenopausal women—was a mystery about to collide with a marketing blitz. Love saw a major sales pitch on the horizon, as pharmaceutical companies tried to convince baby boomers that hormones were the only way to protect quality of life—but she was still waiting for data that showed it was safe to take hormones for an extended period of time. Hormones were already in widespread use, despite the lack of information about their long-term consequences, and she worried about what would happen to breast cancer rates once younger women, who represented a bulge in the population, began to take them.

The eight-month-old Women's Health Initiative, which had started up in September, promised to track 27,500 women in a randomized trial of estrogen replacement therapy and a placebo, and would collect additional data in an observational study of 100,000 women. Love's only concern was that as soon as researchers found a single endpoint the study would be shut down. What good did it do to show that hormones diminished the risk of heart attack at sixty-five, if no one waited to see what it did to breast cancer risk at seventy?

She also wished that more women would think about the difference in risk. She told her patients again and again that they could make lifestyle changes to protect themselves against heart disease and osteoporosis. There were no proven preventives against breast cancer.

Love had assigned the topic of hormone replacement therapy to medical student Brooke Herndon, who apologetically informed the dozen doctors in the room, "The data is really confusing."

She reviewed the studies she had found, including one Love had been telling everyone about, which showed an increased risk of breast cancer among hormone users in their late sixties—while heart disease and osteoporosis posed a greater threat to women in their seventies and eighties. But there was no definitive science. The only conclusion Herndon could make was that the drug's allure outstripped any rational analysis. Herndon had been to England recently and brought back a copy of *Chic* magazine with a cover photograph of actress and author Joan Collins. The headline read, ETERNALLY YOUNG ON ERT AND EXERCISE.

On the same day, May 11, 1994, a Senate panel convened its hearing on whether the $68 million tamoxifen prevention trial ought to continue. The prevention study, like the other clinical trials conducted by the NSABP, was still under suspension, two months after the *Chicago Tribune* first reported the discovery of fraudulent data.

Federal health officials recommended to the panel that the prevention trial be reopened. There was no reason to wait. Dr. Fisher was no longer in charge at the NSABP. The National Cancer Institute promised an improved audit procedure. Consent forms had been revised to apprise participants of all the potential risks.

Amy Langer, herself a survivor and the executive director of the National Alliance of Breast Cancer Organizations, was the voice of practicality. No woman wanted to be at the mercy of irresponsible science, she told the Senate panel—but the only way to retire the controversy was to continue the study. Otherwise it could take longer to find an answer, which meant more women at risk. She told *The Washington Post* that "women would conduct their own private trials in kitchens and offices," if the NSABP trials were halted.

A week later Dr. Bernard Fisher made his first public appearance since his forced departure from the NSABP, speaking at a Dallas, Texas, meeting of the American Society of Clinical Oncology. Fisher was the immediate past president of the group, which responded enthusiastically to his presence with several standing ovations.

He spent almost an hour presenting reanalyzed data, which, he said, reached "monotonously similar" conclusions to the original analysis, with its falsified data. According to *The New*

York Times's Lawrence Altman, "Dr. Fisher did not apologize, admit to any errors, or explain what the National Cancer Institute has said was his team's failure to follow its own guidelines in conducting the studies." Officials of the society prevented reporters who were there from getting close enough to Fisher to ask questions.

The next day the *New England Journal of Medicine* ran an editorial complaining that none of the principals in the NSABP scandal had "fulfilled their responsibilities." The journal, which had first learned of the falsified data not from the medical research community but in a phone call from *Chicago Tribune* reporter John Crewdson, wanted to establish a new chain of accountability.

The journal had just received the long-awaited reanalysis from Fisher, but that did not keep the authors of the editorial from adding their voices to the critics' chorus: "There is no excuse," they wrote, "for the four-year delay between the first indication of misconduct in 1990 and the publication of a reanalysis, which we hope will take place in 1994."

The immediate issue was the lumpectomy data; the long-term question was how to balance the government's desire to maintain confidentiality during an investigation with the public's right to know. It turned out that the ORI had, in fact, published news of the falsified data, almost a year before the *Tribune* ran its story—in the April 1993 ORI newsletter, and in the June issues of the NIH *Guide for Grants and Contracts* and the *Federal Register*. The public had been informed, at least that segment of the public that read government publications front to back.

The journal hardly considered those notifications sufficient. The public, and the medical community, had a right to know without having to play detective. "When Mr. Crewdson phoned," said the editorial, "we were as surprised as anyone else who is not a regular and careful reader of government documents."

The article called for new procedures. The NCI and ORI had already agreed to notify journal editors immediately, once an investigation had been completed, but that was not enough. "We believe that journal editors who may have published seriously flawed or fraudulent work should be considered among those with a 'need to know' during the formal investigation," the journal editorial suggested. Disclosure was essential to the future of clinical research. Without it, "the public may become disillusioned with clinical research and indiscriminately skeptical of its results. Such seems to be the unfortunate outcome in this instance."

24

NAVIGATING SORROW

W HEN THERE WAS NO ROAD MAP, WOMEN TURNED THEIR HUS- bands into doctors, their friends into specialists, their feelings into decisions. There was no clear path for a middle-aged pregnant woman with breast cancer—just a series of heartbreak detours that might never lead back to the main road. Ann Donaldson could only do what her doctor, and her heart, and her husband and friends thought was best.

Love had suggested induced labor in three or four weeks, fol- lowed by a lumpectomy and lymph node dissection, and Ann wanted to cooperate, but in the end she could not wait. She had to know how sick she was before the baby was born. If the anesthesia sent her into premature labor, it would be only a couple of weeks earlier than Love's plan. On Thursday, May 12, she and her hus- band Mark came in for a preoperative appointment. Love had wedged her into an early morning surgery slot for the following Monday.

Ann was uncharacteristically quiet. "I always felt smug about my health because of my family history," she said, afraid to look either Love or her husband in the eye. "I never felt victimized until now."

She reluctantly confessed her fear that there were, in fact, posi- tive nodes. She swore she could feel them, though Rick had run his fingers firmly down her armpit, as he had seen Love do, and said she was wrong. He could not feel a thing, and he did not want to feel a thing.

Love examined her a second time and reiterated her position: she did not feel anything either. But she did want Ann to be prepared for standard chemotherapy, whatever the nodes looked like, because her tumor was over two centimeters. She drew her standard diagram of ten circles and explained the percentages—of ten women with negative nodes, seven would get better without chemotherapy, two would die regardless, and one would improve because of it.

Ann managed the smallest grin. "I'm a businesswoman," she said, "and if I saw these odds I wouldn't invest." If seventy percent were supposed to get better anyway, why would she want to take the drugs?

"But you don't have a choice," said Love. Even if the nodes turned out to be negative, the size of the tumor made chemotherapy an imperative, not a choice.

Tears welled up in Ann's eyes. Rick leaned over and rubbed the little bandage that marked the place on the inside of his wife's elbow where blood had been drawn. He tugged at the sleeve of her T-shirt, his fingers searching for some way to comfort her.

Ann wondered if she ought to have a mastectomy instead of a lumpectomy. They had been to three other doctors before they came to UCLA, all of whom advised her not to waste time with anything less.

"That's old school," said Love. "Either there are microscopic cells or not." Having the lumpectomy first was not going to put Ann in any more danger.

There was no point in talking any further about the surgery, and they knew it. What really mattered were the lymph nodes. Love told Ann and her husband that she wanted to stop doing node dissections in the next few years if someone discovered a more reliable prognostic indicator. Nodes were a faulty way of predicting the likelihood of metastatic disease—twenty to thirty percent of women with negative nodes had disease that spread, and thirty percent of those with positive nodes did not. She hoped for another type of marker, perhaps something in the tumor itself that better predicted the cancer's future.

For now, Ann's fate lay in the hands of the anonymous pathologist who would look at her lymph nodes and deliver a report to Dr. Love about thirty-six hours after surgery. Until then they might as well talk about baby names as anything else.

On May 16, Susan Love performed a lumpectomy on Ann Donaldson. When she was finished she stepped back from the operating table to prepare for the lymph node dissection. The OR nurse broke out a new set of instruments and helped Love change her surgical gloves and gown. Theoretically, an invasive cancer could survive and spread to a new location. Researchers gave breast cancer to lab mice and rats by injection all the time, and the cancer survived that transmission. Love had seen recurrences in scars—and even one case where a cancer recurred at the site where a surgical drain had been placed. Maybe it tracked along the drain. Or maybe it dripped off a tainted instrument or glove, took hold and grew.

Fear accompanied her every time she operated. Nobody knew that surgery roused dormant abnormal cells in a woman having a biopsy, but nobody was sure that it did not. With a cancer patient there was always the ugly chance that a single incautious gesture could inadvertently help the cancer on its way. Doctors even had a name for cancer cells that were spread to a new site off the end of an instrument or glove. They called them "drop mets."

Love always excised an old scar when she operated, just in case it was a breeding ground for breast cancer. She told people that if breast cancer was contagious she was in big trouble: Love frequently nicked herself while performing surgery, cut through her double gloves and into her skin with a dirty knife. It was only half a joke. She could not catch someone else's disease, but she respected cancer cells.

Love got the pathology report on Ann's re-excision and lymph node dissection on Tuesday, May 17, but she did not call her patient. Dirty margins at all the edges of a piece of tissue the size of a golf ball, and five positive lymph nodes. There was still cancer left in Ann's breast, and a good chance of micrometastasis. Love's first thought when she heard the news was that Ann would be dead in five years. Fewer than half the women with more than five positive nodes survived that long.

Immediately she chastised herself. She could be wrong. There were always patients who did not live up to the statistics. But she did not feel wrong. She was glad she had told a small fib and instructed Ann to expect the results on Wednesday. If they had been good she would have picked up the phone right away. This way she had an extra day to figure out how to tell a woman who was about to have a baby that she had to have chemotherapy, probably a mastectomy, and a transplant, just for insurance, because of the size of the tumor.

She told no one at the clinic. When she got home she confided in Helen, who had no good advice to offer her. Helen said that giving Ann Donaldson the news was like dropping napalm on a Vietnamese village. Life would never be the same again.

"Hi, how ya doing? But feeling okay? Good." It was Wednesday at noon, and Love was on the telephone in the doctors' consultation room in the General Surgery suite. She had only a half hour until multi began, and it would be dinnertime before she took a breath. It was time to talk to Ann.

"Now, I've got mixed news," she began. "Not great, but not awful—in the middle. The cancer's all through the tissue, which means ultimately you may have to have a mastectomy. But I don't think I cut through any cancer, and I don't think there's a lot of cancer left in you." She believed she had "shelled out" the tumor, as she put it, scooped it out with just a rim of dirty margin remaining. She did not think there was a large segment of malignant tissue left behind.

"Now, there were five nodes that were positive for cancer. It certainly doesn't mean you're doomed, but it also doesn't mean you've got a touch of cancer. Ten is bad, zero is best, so this is halfway. But chances are you're going to be around. You have to look at the numbers. And that's what we want to sit down and talk about—and discuss how to proceed with the chemotherapy.

"I don't think we need to do anything to the breast right now," she went on, "though ultimately we may. This shifts your attention to 'Are there microscopic cells elsewhere in the body?' And that's where chemo comes in."

She took off her glasses, rubbed her eyes, and propped her feet up on the side table, waiting while Ann digested the news.

"What would I do?" Love said. "Chemo, three to four cycles, one now and three after the baby. And if it were me I would consider a stem cell transplant. *After* that, I'd consider another lumpectomy and radiation, or a mastectomy, but that's tagged on at the end. What's important is the cells that might escape into your body."

Ann wanted to know how many nodes had been taken out altogether.

"I don't remember," said Love. "I think it's eleven, but the fraction doesn't matter. It's the number of positive ones. Over ten we always suggest a transplant, but this was a big cancer."

That was not what Ann wanted to hear, and her despair ate away at Love's usual resolve. She backed into the same kind of anecdotal defense that her patients so often used. What Ann needed was a morsel of hope—as did her doctor, for once.

"I've had women do fine," said Love. "I have one with seventeen nodes, alive ten years later. In her forties, like you."

Ann was afraid to believe her.

"You are not doomed," said Love. "I know it's really scary—but we can get there." She invited Ann and her husband to come in to see Love and an oncologist late in the afternoon, after the multi, or the following day, whenever they were ready to talk.

"We'll be around," she said. "But I still do think there's hope for you. Do you hear me? I know. But guess what? We don't have any choice, except to take one step at a time. It would be nice to fast forward through this year, but we can't. Okay? You okay? Okay. We'll see you. Bye."

She walked out of the room with a tight, fake smile plastered on her face, her eyes downcast. She punched a clenched fist into the air, took a deep breath, and strode into an examining room to look at a patient's mammograms.

Right before the multi she heard the news that had been circulating through the Breast Center offices all morning, and her frustration turned to bitterness. The word was that the Defense Department had notified the successful grant applicants by phone—so Susan, who had heard nothing about her three applications, assumed that she had failed to qualify for funds. Denny supposedly had won big with an $800,000 grant for a statewide tissue bank. Love, without whom there might not have been a DOD program, had been left out.

She grumbled about a system that required so much effort and rewarded so few. "People spend all this time writing grants," she said to Connie, "and only five to ten percent of those judged worthy of being funded actually get the money." So much for desire and discipline. She had played by all the rules, jumped through the FDA's hoops on the ductoscope, applied for the grants, and at the moment had nothing to show for it except a brochure for a piece of equipment she still could not use.

Her last multi patient that day brought a friend along, a retired general surgeon in his seventies. After the appointment he wandered out into the hallway and approached Dr. Love. He had taught at SUNY's Brooklyn campus, where Love went to medical school. He had done "some breast work," he said. His wife had died of bilateral breast cancer, and he was trying to get his daughter to come to the high-risk program at UCLA.

He remembered what breast surgery was like in the 1950s, radical mastectomies and skepticism about anyone who suggested a less extreme procedure. To this day he doubted the wisdom of such extensive operations.

"You know something?" he said. "I think extensive surgery just stirs things up."

Love warmed to the subject, happy to find someone who agreed with her. "I think you may have a point. One thing I'd like to do— if I *ever* had the time and money—is to try not taking out the tumor. Go in with a probe, freeze it, and leave it there. Maybe there would be an immune system response to the dead cells. Because I think the scar and healing process is similar to the action of metastases. All those leaky capillaries." She already knew what she wanted to do—take mice with breast cancer, freeze the tumor, and let it sit. All she had to figure out was how to image the tumor, or when to remove it, to make sure it was dead. That, and find enough hours in the day to talk to the cryosurgeons and find funding.

She stared past the man at the empty hallway. She could see Ann and Rick sitting in the last examining room, waiting for the oncologist.

"I'm not sure," she said to the retired surgeon, "that we're doing much good at all."

At the end of the afternoon Love lingered at the clinic's reception desk with Leslie Laudeman and Lisa, one of the facilitators. She had spent the day thinking about Ann. Love often said that patients blamed the messenger for the message—lots of them went to a doctor for a second opinion and stayed there for treatment, not because the news was better, but because it was easier to take the second time around. Sometimes doctors had the same problem. Faced with a patient whose sadness defied solution, they berated themselves for being the one who made her feel that way.

Love confessed her dismay to her two staffers.

"I didn't *give* her the cancer," she said, as though wishing for confirmation. "But it feels that way, because I had to tell her."

On Thursday, May 19, UCLA hosted the American Cancer Society's "Look Good, Feel Better" program, a day-long workshop in cooperation with St. John's Hospital, designed to teach patients how to handle the physical fallout of cancer treatment. The place settings included a lavender-rimmed plastic makeup mirror, an assortment of makeup samples, a plastic caddy holding Q-Tips and cotton pads, and an array of scarves. A film crew from the cable television station CNBC had set up at the far end of the room for a segment on the program.

The introductory speaker was an impossibly beautiful woman, a professional model with porcelain skin and long, sculpted waves of auburn hair. She wore a fitted black pantsuit with ivory cording at the cuffs and down the front of the jacket. As the ten women who had signed up for the workshop filed in and took their seats—their faces wan, their eyebrows and eyelashes a memory, their bald heads covered by wigs or scarves—they gazed sidelong at her as though she were a cruel joke. Why was this woman here, this person whom even a healthy woman would envy?

She explained immediately: she was a breast cancer survivor. She told them about getting into the shower one day during chemotherapy and watching her hair come out in tufts as she washed it. After her first month of chemo she went back to work; she handed out photographs of herself in an assortment of wigs. And she had since had a baby, a boy. She was here not to reproach, but to encourage—vibrant proof that the treatment did end, and life got back to normal.

Ann Donaldson walked tentatively down the hallway with her husband—small steps, her arms wrapped in front of her as though she were afraid she might break. She was there to see Susan again, but suddenly she was surrounded by staffers from both UCLA and St. John's, where she had gone before coming to Dr. Love. They thought she might be cheered up if she sat in on the program. Her eyes widened in fear and her lower lip began to tremble.

"I don't think I'm going to make it," she whispered.

Love came up behind her and said loudly that she thought it was too soon for Ann to worry about how she looked. But her husband offered to sit with her, and two people from the Rhonda Fleming Mann Center encouraged her to sit on the sidelines, so she could leave without disrupting the program—or stay without having to become an active participant.

Hesitantly she moved toward the door. At that moment Ann Donaldson believed she was dying, and the people who surrounded her were the only ones who might be able to save her. Her own feelings did not matter. She had to get over her desire to dart into a side room somewhere and cry. They could save her, and they wanted her to walk into the conference room.

So she did. She took a chair, her husband at her side. A half hour later Rick was in the hallway, pacing back and forth outside the door while his wife listened to the lecture on skin care. Ann managed a wistful little smile. These other women were coping. Perhaps she could too.

Outside, a woman from the St. John's psychosocial program approached Rick about getting Ann into a support group there.

One of the UCLA staffers overheard, stepped over to the woman's other side, and quietly informed her that her behavior was inappropriate.

"They don't have to *go* anywhere," said the UCLA staffer. "They can walk right into the Rhonda Fleming Mann, right here."

The woman from St. John's was indignant. She was not trying to steal a patient. She knew the Donaldsons from St. John's.

"Our paths have crossed," she said. "I'm just giving him my card." She turned away from her competitor, pressed a business card into Rick's hand, and offered to come to the Donaldsons' home to work with them.

Ten minutes later, once the woman from St. John's was inside the conference room, the UCLA staffer approached Rick and introduced herself.

"You can get everything you need right here," she said. "That's what I was trying to explain."

She sat and chatted with Rick for a while—and then she quietly stepped into the conference room and took the seat next to Ann.

25

ONE STEP FORWARD, TWO STEPS BACK

"OH, HOT *SHIT*!" SUSAN LOVE BIT HER FINGERNAIL NERVOUSLY while Connie recounted her conversation with the woman from the Defense Department.

"She was very careful," said Connie, while Love struggled to contain her excitement. "She asked about the ductoscope. I said, 'It's as big as a hair.' She said, 'But we may have trouble on human subjects protection.' I said, 'No, we've been fine with ours.' "

"So then she said, 'Then there shouldn't be any problem.' "

They both stared at each other for a moment. Love was going to get a Defense Department grant after all, it seemed; her name had merely been farther down on the list than Denny's. The ductoscope grant was the smallest of the three that Love had submitted, but it was better than nothing at all. Far better: Love had refused to admit how badly she wanted to win a grant until now.

"Hot damn," said Love. "That's great. We got it."

"Now, she said it's not official," warned Connie. "She's just the contracting lady, but—"

"It's great," said Love. "I mean, I would rather have had the bigger grant, but this is great." Susan had applied both to the DOD and to UCLA's Jonsson Comprehensive Cancer Center.

Now she had the satisfying task of telling UCLA she no longer
needed the money.

At four o'clock Dr. Armando Giuliano called, and he and Susan had what she considered a reasonable conversation about the
patients who kept switching back and forth between them. There
was one woman who had left UCLA and was busily badmouthing
Love to everyone at St. John's. There was Ann Donaldson, who
had seen Giuliano before coming to Love. And there was Dee,
who seemed determined to have both of them.

But Susan had won the first round with Dee. "We're going to
do a lumpectomy," Love told Giuliano. "We may have to do a
mastectomy eventually, but I think with her it's easier to do the
two surgeries."

They talked a bit more about Dee's problems making up her
mind, and for the first time Love felt at ease. Giuliano admitted
that he had performed two surgeries on a few patients to ease
them through the process. It was a comfortable exchange.

She went home feeling better than she had in weeks. It looked
like she was going to get a DOD grant—not a big one, but a grant
nonetheless. Dr. Giuliano had treated her with respect—and his
opinion carried outsized weight with her, because he had been the
preeminent breast surgeon at UCLA before she arrived. She had
research money and the esteem of an admired colleague. It was a
new level of professional acceptance. Susan Love's patients adored
her, but the medical and academic communities had been slow to
come around.

She liked to think that this was all evidence that it was possible
to foment revolution from within. She had not done anything to
curry favor, and yet she had got the results she wanted. When she
got home she told Helen that she and Dr. Giuliano were on their
way to a better relationship.

The next afternoon Dee Wieman showed up at UCLA unexpectedly and told a facilitator she needed to speak with Dr. Love
for just a moment. She knew Love was busy, but she would wait
as long as she had to. Dee had important news. Dr. Giuliano had

performed a lumpectomy on her on Thursday, May 19—just hours before his telephone conversation with Love.

She sat down on a bench in the hallway to compose a note.

> *Dear Dr. Love,*
>
> *I came today (without an appointment—I'm sorry) to let you know that I had the surgery w/Dr. Giuliano yesterday. I intended to try to see you on Tuesday but they told me you weren't available. I needed to tell you in person.*
>
> *It seemed the right thing for me when he shocked me by telling me he would do it. I hope I haven't offended you. I still hope I can see you. You have been the single most important person to me in the handling of this disease, and I hope you will continue to see me. This has no reflection on my feelings about your surgical abilities. I have just had a strange connection to him and when he surprised me by agreeing to the surgery I felt it was right. It was a difficult decision.*
>
> *I love you and respect you greatly as a physician and a person.*
>
> *I'll call next week and hope you'll continue to see me.*
>
> *Warm regards, Dee Wieman*

She stood up and gently tugged at the bandage that covered her breast. Tears ran down her face. Dee had gone in for what she swore would be her final appointment with Dr. Giuliano, intending to tell him that she had a surgery date at UCLA. When Giuliano said that he would perform the lumpectomy after all, she was caught off guard. How could she offend him and say that she would prefer to have Love perform the procedure?

He was standing right in front of her waiting for a reply—and all that Dee could think was that she somehow owed him the chance to take care of her. He had taken her wishes into account and changed his mind. He could perform the surgery on the nineteenth, while she would have to wait until the twenty-fourth at UCLA. And the cosmetic results of the biopsies he had done were wonderful. Walking out on him under these circumstances was unthinkable.

Surely Susan would understand.

Dee's best friend, Suzy, had slept over the night before, so that they could be on the road at four thirty in the morning for the drive up to Century City Hospital, where Giuliano had operating privileges while St. John's main hospital building underwent earthquake repairs. Gary was not going with them, but he got up early, and even made the bed while they got dressed.

"I hope you're fine," he said to Dee when she was ready to leave. "I want nothing but the best for you." He was fighting tears. He asked Suzy to call him as soon as the surgery was over.

By mid-morning Dee was out of the surgery, awake and raring to go. She and Suzy invited Dee's father, stepmother, and aunt, who had come to the hospital, to come back to Dee's for drinks— and an hour later, although she was not hungry herself, Dee was puttering in the kitchen, putting together hors d'oeuvres. Gary was not yet home.

When he did show up an hour and a half later, Dee could not resist baiting him.

"What's the deal?" Gary asked, confused by the merriment.

"Oh, they didn't do the surgery," lied Dee, with a languid smile.

She held up most of the afternoon, until someone pointed out that her eyes looked bleary and insisted that she go to bed. She fell asleep easily. Dee had finally made a choice, always a difficult process for her, and she felt secure that she had made the right one.

As she stood in the hallway on Friday afternoon, waiting for Dr. Love, Dee worried that she had made a mistake. "I can't not see her again," she thought. "I'm a person with her, not a patient. But Wednesday, for the first time, I felt like a person with him."

Love was genuinely confused when she finally emerged and saw Dee. Was she going to back out of next Tuesday's surgery? She ushered Dee into an examining room and slumped onto the footstool, while Dee quietly took a chair.

"I had surgery," whispered Dee, handing over the letter.

Love looked at her sharply. She had spoken to Giuliano late the day before, and if Dee had had surgery today she would not be sitting here. Something was very wrong.

"What time?" she asked.

Dee thought that was an odd question. "Eight in the morning, yesterday."

A tight grin, no teeth. "I was talking to Dr. Giuliano at four about another patient," said Love, "and I mentioned doing a lumpectomy on you next week. He said nothing."

Dee chattered on about how this was a personal victory for her, but Love had trouble concentrating.

Dee said that she still wanted to come to Love for whatever treatment she needed next.

Love turned her down. This had to be the end of their relationship. "If he's going to do the surgery, then he ought to take care of you," she said.

"But I don't *feel* like he takes care of me," said Dee.

"You can't have it both ways," said Susan. "For me to take care of you, I had to have been there for the surgery."

She got up and walked out of the room, and Dee began to weep. Her voice wafted into the hallway. "That wasn't the answer I wanted to hear. If I'd known that I would have changed my decision."

She wandered down the hall to cancel her surgery and her follow-up appointment.

"My husband's going to be so angry at me," she told the facilitator.

Love was reeling. She stormed into the Breast Center offices, where the facilitator who helped Dee was busily erasing her name from Tuesday's surgery schedule.

"Are you angry?" she asked Love.

Love was, in fact, furious—not at Dee, whose departure she regarded with a mixture of irritation and relief, but at Giuliano for not telling her about the surgery. She was angry at herself for being naive. So much for mutual respect.

Leslie Laudeman came out of her office when she heard the commotion. Laudeman was extremely concerned about what she heard—not because of the personal slight to Love, but because to her this was not civilized professional behavior. She advised Love to call Giuliano immediately and confront him with what he had done, but Love sheepishly admitted that both of them had taken patients from each other before; neither one had called the other to acknowledge it. A woman did have the right to choose her own doctor.

Laudeman insisted that this was different. They had been on the phone together, talking about Dee. He owed Love the courtesy of telling her what he had done. "I think you ought to tell him," she said.

"Well, we don't call him every time we get a patient from them," Love persisted. For all her outspokenness, she did not like confrontation. She preferred to operate inside a cocoon of loyal, like-minded colleagues.

"But if you were already talking to him you would mention it," said Laudeman.

"I'm a chicken," said Love.

Laudeman was not going to let her off the hook. "Maybe write him a letter," she urged. "Put it in the context of, 'I saw Dee today, and I'm referring her care back to you.' And then say, 'I would have preferred that I find out about her surgery from you.' Just to let him know that it's not okay with you."

Love did not want to do it, so she changed the subject. "What upsets me, too, is now there's a surgery slot open on Tuesday."

"It's going to be hard to fill," admitted Leslie. "We don't have time to do pre-op for someone else." Every surgical patient had to meet with the anesthesiologist and the surgeon and have a blood workup—but with the weekend in the way there was no chance to process another patient before Tuesday morning.

"And she's on the list for the bone marrow transplant," said Love, her voice rising irritably. "She acts like there are no consequences to her actions, and there are."

Sherry Goldman walked up and Love began her litany of complaints over again, trying, in the retelling, to find a way to defend herself from the double slight.

"I think it's a whole Mommy/Daddy thing," she said to Sherry. "You know, Mommy's always the one who's going to forgive you. Well, guess what. This Mommy says, 'Forget it.' "

She stomped into her office and immediately began dictating a letter to Dr. Giuliano. Just as abruptly, she got up and went to the staff lounge to make some popcorn. When she returned she had come up with new targets to siphon off some of her rage: Denny Slamon needed to get someone to help him run oncology; Bill Shaw had to get other plastic surgeons doing free flaps; and she was going to talk to Zinner about both of them. She was throwing her weight around, reminding herself, and anyone else within earshot, that she was an important figure.

Then her beeper went off. Giuliano was calling. She returned the page and talked amiably to him about another patient who had just defected from UCLA, the troublesome one who complained so much about the way Love treated her.

Susan took a breath, and in a tone more appropriate to discussing the weather, said, "I just want you to know, Dee Wieman came in today. . . . She told me, Yeah, and then she said, 'But I'll still want you to take care of me.' But I said no."

Giuliano told her the grave news he had received from pathology: there was cancer in Dee's nipple and in all the tissue samples Giuliano had taken, in addition to the lumpectomy tissue. She had cancer in all four quadrants of the breast.

Love thought to herself, You keep her. Neither of them said anything about the previous afternoon's phone call. Love felt that it was up to Giuliano to bring it up. Giuliano, who considered himself more strict than most on the issue of patient/doctor confidentiality, did not do so. Unless a patient gave him explicit permission to discuss her case with other doctors, he talked about her only to the colleagues he knew to be actively involved in her care. The day before he had not known if Dee intended to see Love again, so he told her nothing. Now that Dee had returned to Dr. Love, he seemed comfortable divulging the pathology results, and did not explain his earlier silence.

Leslie was waiting outside to hear what had happened. Love confessed, "I thought about it and thought about it, and I just couldn't do it. I'm too well-socialized as a woman. I just couldn't do it. I mean, I told him Dee was here—so he knew that I knew."

She shook her head at her own cowardice.

"I want to keep the communications open," she told Leslie. "I really believe in the high road, but I couldn't talk to him about the phone call. I chickened out."

It was too familiar a slight for her to handle easily. Love remembered what it had been like when she first started seeing patients. Women came to her for information and went to a male surgeon for the operation Love recommended. Fourteen years later she was well-known, and there were more women surgeons around; she was no longer the well-informed freak. Still, the events of the afternoon made history painfully fresh. She did not trust herself to confront Giuliano, not with the emotional baggage she carried from the past.

Suddenly the allies Love did have seemed much more attractive. They might have their problems, but at least they were in fundamental agreement about how to practice medicine. When Denny Slamon dropped by Friday's multi conference, Susan greeted him enthusiastically.

"Denny, you came just in time. We've got a Stage 1 woman who's disease-free for ten years, and then comes in with disease everywhere—chest wall, kidney, bones, a nodule in her neck."

"Jeez" was all Slamon could muster.

Love continued, eager to wrap herself up in a nice, complicated patient, one that would distract her from messy politics. The woman's original tumor, diagnosed in 1984, was node negative and under two centimeters. "The only clue to it being aggressive, retrospectively," she said, "is that it's poorly differentiated," which meant that the cells did not resemble normal breast cells.

Barsky showed the new pathology slides—the same breast cancer, throughout the woman's body.

"It makes no sense," said Love. "Why did it take them ten years?" As unpredictable as breast cancer was, early-stage cancer, at least, usually conformed to a handful of general rules.

Slamon and Love were excited by the woman's case. It was the oddball exception that gave them hope. If they could figure out why this patient's cancer lay dormant for so many years, perhaps they could devise an intervention that mimicked her own defenses. Or they could look for whatever triggered the recurrence to see if they could treat it.

"There was some other alteration along the way," said Slamon, "that made the cancer cells aggressive. You see it. You can see patients who, at autopsy, have active breast disease twenty years later, but they died of a heart attack."

"If we could figure out some way to make the cancer cells all quiescent . . ." Love began.

Slamon cut in with an uncharacteristic grin. "We wouldn't need to be here," he said. "That'd be good."

26

NO WAY OUT

GARY WIEMAN WAS FIFTY-THREE YEARS OLD, SIX-FOOT-FOUR AND 270 pounds, most of it in his broad shoulders and heavy chest. His legs were slender, his gait surprisingly light for a big man. Even standing at rest he looked like he was moving forward, his pure-white hair swept back off his brow as though the wind were moving through it. Until this year he had been a supremely happy man. He had no children of his own, and Dee's grown daughter, with whom he did not get along, lived in Seattle. For twenty-one years he had made a comfortable living selling insurance for heavy-duty hauling. He and Dee had a condo that was made for entertaining, with high ceilings and big picture windows that opened onto a little bay. At the center of it all was his wife—the perfect hostess, a fun-loving, sexy woman. She was his vivacious ideal, and he had her all to himself.

On Monday morning, May 23, four days after his wife's lumpectomy, he stood next to her in an examining room at St. John's, waiting for Dr. Giuliano. They did not touch. Dee perched on the end of the examining table, the hospital gown wrapped protectively around her breasts, her hands clasped together.

In the days since the surgery Gary had been acting in an odd manner, at least by Dee's estimation. He had promised to stay home all day the day after the lumpectomy, and yet when she woke at six he was already dressed and ready for the office. All she wanted to do was concentrate on having clean margins, and instead she found herself wondering why Gary was being so strange.

It would all be resolved in a moment, when Dr. Giuliano walked through the door. Dee knew she needed a transplant, but if she got just one bit of good news—if the margins were clean—she would take it as a sign.

She was glad to have a nine thirty appointment. Dee liked to make her appointments early in the day. The notion that someone else had her pathology report—knew her future hours before she did—always bothered her.

Dr. Armando Giuliano was a short, slender man with thinning hair and startling eyes—large, clear, icy jewels that dominated his face. His manner was the diametric opposite of Susan Love's—quiet, formal, controlled. He entered the room and shook hands with Dee and Gary, performed a physical exam, and backed away to a spot near the closed door.

He crossed his arms at his chest and spoke in a low voice.

"I have bad news, Dee. There is tumor everywhere."

Her expression froze, but Giuliano continued. They had taken tissue from across the top of her right breast, to the nipple, and down the middle of her breast to the bottom. There were tumor cells everywhere they looked. He wanted her to understand that this was dangerous business.

Giuliano proposed an agenda: an immediate mastectomy and a transplant, followed by radiation, and finally, reconstructive surgery. If she would agree he would do the surgery tomorrow.

She sidestepped his challenge and asked how large the tumor was.

"Twelve to fifteen centimeters," he replied, larger than even the most pessimistic of estimates she had heard so far.

Gary asked if it was in Dee's chest wall.

"Not yet" was all Giuliano would say.

Gary wondered if Dee would have pain after the mastectomy, and Giuliano looked at him with genuine surprise.

"Physically, no," he answered. "But emotionally, yes. She's going to feel lopsided."

Dee giggled, "I've always been a little lopsided."

But Giuliano refused to yield. Light conversation was the enemy here; it gave Dee a place to hide.

"You're going to feel strange," he said.

"Well," she said, "maybe you could take some out of the other side and I wouldn't feel so lopsided. I don't care."

The surgeon did not respond, so Dee confessed that the doctors at both Hutchinson in Seattle and City of Hope had recommended a bilateral mastectomy.

Unexpectedly, Giuliano replied, "That might not be a bad idea." Until now he had tried only to get her to accept a mastectomy on the right side, where the cancer was more advanced. If she was finally ready to consider more aggressive surgery, he would encourage her to have both breasts removed. But simultaneous reconstruction was not part of the plan. The one thing Dee's various doctors did agree on was that she needed the stem cell transplant to fight systemic disease—and it would not be wise to delay the procedure while she recovered from plastic surgery.

Dee had not expected Giuliano to endorse the suggestion. She began babbling about having scans and blood tests to look for metastatic disease, and he just let her go on until she ran out of steam. He leaned back against the door.

"It's bad news, Dee," he said gently. "I'm not happy I had to deliver it."

She looked at him through watery eyes and managed a wan smile.

"Oh, I'm all right," she said. "I've had a lot of time to think about it. Are you okay?"

"Yes," he said, and left the room.

After four months of evasion and denial, Dee and Gary Wieman were alone in a room with a nightmare. The cancer was everywhere; there was not a moment to lose; prudence demanded postponing the reconstructive surgery; and even Giuliano liked the idea of a double mastectomy.

There was to be no more shopping around. The world had suddenly shrunk down to a narrow hallway with a single door at the far end, no side exits, no windows, a stifling, still vacuum. The only way out was to them an agony, not a solution, and worst of all, they had to hurry to get there.

Neither of them could handle it. As Dee started to get dressed she had an inspiration. If Gary's schedule could accommodate it they could call the plastic surgeon Dee had seen last week, and perhaps go right over to talk to her. She ought to see the pathology report. She might disagree with Dr. Giuliano. Dee could call Dr. Shaw at UCLA, too, and fax over the pathology report. She had not yet seen him, and had no idea if he would even work with a breast surgeon from another hospital, but such practical considerations never entered her mind.

So they went downstairs and called the first plastic surgeon from a pay phone. She was booked all day. Gary pressed Dee to call Shaw instead. He was not impressed with the woman surgeon. She had instructed Dee to have Gary look through some copies of *Playboy* magazine, looking for the kind of breasts he liked, an idea that offended him.

"But these are perfect," he had moaned to his wife. "Can't someone just make a matched set exactly like these?"

Besides, he had to get to a meeting that he had postponed twice. He left his wife at the valet parking desk, waiting for her car. Dee was not ready to go home; the day stretched ahead of her like a desert. She decided instead to drive over to the biomedical library at UCLA, to see if there were any new research articles she ought to read.

Susan Love wrote Dee a short note, wishing her well, but she held out little hope. With twenty-six positive lymph nodes, the likelihood that Dee would develop metastatic disease was very high—and there was no way to tell in advance if the transplant would help. Dee might have done just as well taking that trip to Italy—spending what time she had on a life rather than a plan.

It did not matter that most women never developed breast cancer, or that two-thirds of the ones who did died of something else. A woman with breast cancer knew that she could die of it, and the descent could be sudden, and by surprise. Anyone could end up like Dee. Many of the younger patients developed a glib fatalism. What was going to happen was going to happen.

In May, Shirley Barber finally got bored with biding her time and decided to go back to work. So she signed up for a flight and donned her dress blues, the meticulous upswept hairdo, the impenetrable flight attendant smile.

The only concession she made to the DCIS was to go braless, because any pressure on her breasts increased the pain. She was standing in the aisle watching some guy load his case into the overhead bin when he flung his elbow back, hard, without looking, and jabbed her in the chest.

He apologized profusely. She wondered, through the pain, if her smile looked convincing. She thought to herself, okay. That was as bad as it can get, and it's over. She checked all the overhead bins and strapped on her shoulder harness—right side first, for the first time, to make sure she was comfortable, and then the left.

Shirley had to admit that it was fun to be back in the air. She teased Mitch that he missed her only because she took the family car and left it at the airport. Kim was glad to have the run of the house again. Tracy confessed that he liked the occasional nights alone; it was hard to come home every night to what his wife called the "honey do" list—could he fix this, could he help with dinner, could he put the wet clothes in the dryer.

Still, it had been nice, for the first time in their marriage, to pick up the phone at any time of day and call his wife for a chat. He was sorry to see that end.

The daily press challenged Shirley with two bits of news: *The New York Times* reported that smokers had an increased risk of dying of breast cancer, while the *Los Angeles Times* cited a British study on the relationship between tamoxifen and uterine abnormalities. Shirley ignored them both. She smoked with a plastic filter, less than a pack a day when she was home and even less than that when she was flying the nonsmoking skies. If her family's entreaties had failed to make a dent in her habit, a single newspaper story was hardly going to make a difference. As for tamoxifen, she had made her decision when she signed up for the trial. The news about increased risk of uterine cancer had not budged her, nor had the NSABP scandal. She was not the type to second-guess.

She intended to be fine. That was all there was to it.

There was evidence to support Shirley's position. A study published in the late 1980s had divided breast cancer patients into three categories: the ones who denied they had a problem, like Shirley; the ones who believed they could fight their disease into submission; and those who succumbed to fear and perceived themselves as victims. The researchers found that women who gave up hope fared most poorly. The patients who survived were the fighters—and the ones who refused to accept that there was anything wrong with them in the first place.

Susan Love identified with what she called "the deny-ers," because she shared their approach to life. She proudly told people, "It takes an awful lot to rattle me; I've always been on an even keel," and was pleased to see the same imperturbable air in her daughter, Kate. Life was too short to get upset over little things. Days after her encounter with Dee and Dr. Giuliano, the wound had closed and begun to heal.

The problem with denial, though, was that sometimes its devotees failed to acknowledge real dangers in the road ahead. Shirley smoked as though she had some special immunity. Susan Love assumed that she would prevail over Denny and Zinner's replacement, whoever that turned out to be, because she wanted to, and because she was doing important work. She continued to ignore their complaints about her travel schedule. They wanted good numbers; now, with an estimate for May of 360 patients, a record high, they had good numbers. That ought to buy her some independence.

Laura adjusted to her new set of circumstances with grim determination—six weeks of chemotherapy for the premalignant condition in her uterus and a nine-week delay before she could have her mastectomy and reconstruction. Just as she felt she had got things under control, though, reality shifted again. Her blood levels dropped so dramatically after only one cycle of chemotherapy that her doctor decided the risk of a uterine malignancy had subsided. He canceled the rest of the treatment. Laura was back to square one.

She called the Breast Center and Shaw's office immediately to see if they could move up her July 19 surgery date. This time life worked in her favor. Love and Shaw were both available on June 28, just thirty-five days away, not much of a wait at all given what she had anticipated. She would not have to bother with a prosthesis after all.

Laura knew she ought to be pleased at the news, but instead she felt herself slipping. She was beginning to feel suffocated by cancer. She followed the news about Jacqueline Kennedy Onassis checking into the hospital and assured herself that the former First Lady, who suffered from non-Hodgkin's lymphoma, must be all right. Hadn't she been spotted in Central Park just four days before? When Mrs. Onassis died, on May 19, Laura was devastated, convinced she was part of some terrible, dark trend.

Death lurked everywhere. What she had to do was not become one of its casualties. She had to pick herself up, as she had countless times since her first diagnosis in 1988, and get ready for a happy life.

She began to make a list of things that she could not change and would not allow to upset her anymore. She stopped worrying about being lopsided and ran around in T-shirts without a bra. She blamed the laparascopic procedure for a newly soft stomach, and the chemo and her iron supplements for making her bloated, but she was not going to put so much energy into fighting. None of it mattered. By fall this would all be over.

In the meantime, Laura had a few souvenirs of easier times—a treasured diamond bracelet, a heavy gold necklace—that she could sell if she still had not found a job.

She heard about one opportunity that sounded perfect for her. The president of what she considered a very cool production company was looking for a vice president, and all she had to do was write him a letter explaining why he ought to hire her.

She spent a day staring at her word processor, trying to remember what she liked about herself.

"Come on," she scolded. "Sound like you're a happening broad."

Draft after draft, and nothing that sounded convincing. What if he wanted her to start right away? How was she supposed to make plans when her body kept playing tricks on her?

Finally she got up and went into her bedroom to meditate. When she was finished she marched back to her desk, finished the letter, and called a messenger to take it away. Then she fell to her knees and offered up a little prayer for some good luck.

Ann Donaldson did not have to have her labor induced. She began to have contractions while she was in the middle of her first chemotherapy cycle, and the doctors tried to hold off her labor with drugs until she finished the course. When that failed, they performed a caesarean delivery. On Monday, May 30—nine weeks early—Ann gave birth to a baby girl, seventeen and a half inches long, weighing only four pounds, one ounce. The baby was put on a ventilator for twenty-four hours and then transferred to the UCLA neonatal intensive care unit to be monitored for apnea, a potentially fatal interruption in an infant's breathing pattern.

It was the first of many separations the family could expect to endure. Now that Ann had given birth, it was time to schedule her transplant.

In May, Jerilyn Goodman went to Wisconsin to see some friends and went for a whole day without once thinking about her breast cancer.

She was tired of being a prisoner to it. Over the Memorial Day weekend she and one of the other women from her support group went to Home Depot, a large do-it-yourself home improvement store, to buy a shelf for Jerilyn's increasingly neat kitchen. It was a madhouse, and when they were ready to leave they got stuck in the parking lot. There were people weaving between the cars with their paints and their plywood, a line of cars trying to move out and another trying to get in, and it seemed an eternity before they could escape.

Jerilyn turned to her companion. "You know," she said, "if these are the last two years of our lives, I'm not sure I want to be spending my next-to-the-last Memorial Day Sunday in the parking lot at Home Depot."

Dee and Gary no longer felt they had the luxury of denial, or resistance. Their visit with Dr. Giuliano had robbed them of the hope that informed such feelings. Gary understood for the first time that Dee might become a casualty of breast cancer, despite all her efforts.

He was furious. The day after Memorial Day, his lunch turned into a rage fueled by five glasses of wine and endless cups of coffee. He felt only sympathy for his wife. He no longer saw her as a traitor. Gary had switched allegiance on the morning they got the lumpectomy pathology report from Dr. Giuliano. All the doctors were evil, and he and his wife, their hapless victims.

He found himself doing what his wife had always done, replaying scenes over and over again in a desperate attempt to make sense. All he came up with was greed and self-interest. He believed absolutely that if Love and Giuliano had only talked to each other they could have come up with another treatment regimen, although he had no idea what it might have been. Love had given his wife false hope. Giuliano had walked away from UCLA. It was clear, at least to Gary, that the two of them were enemies—and that their unwillingness to cooperate had cost his wife her future.

He saw ulterior motives everywhere. Gary was convinced that more surgery would not help—all it would do was destroy their happiness and make a handful of doctors a nice fee. Dee still intended to have her transplant at UCLA; it had to be there or City of Hope, and she nursed the faint hope that Dr. Love might drop in to see her if she was at UCLA. But Gary did not think the transplant was going to do his wife any good. He considered it nothing but a profit center, meant to pad the coffers of UCLA's Medical Center and impress gullible patients who actually thought it would make a difference.

He understood his wife's indecision. Dr. Love was right about one thing: the best that medicine had to offer boiled down to slash, burn, and poison. No wonder Dee had balked at having to make a choice.

The university had an advertising agency to promote its cancer services, and that agency had a mandate from Denny Slamon: Sell the Breast Center first. He had a responsibility to all the oncology programs, but circumstance dictated that he make sure the community knew about Susan Love. She was the celebrity, the competition was already advertising, and other UCLA doctors had their eye on Slamon's expensive, high-profile experiment.

It was not an easy commodity to sell. Referring physicians were the traditional target for UCLA's advertising. A woman went to her internist or Ob-Gyn, who referred her to a specialist he had gone to medical school with, one who lived down the street from him, one he had seen in the hallways and at department meetings for years. The patient who ignored the internist's suggestion and went shopping for a specialist on her own was the exception.

Managed care promised to strengthen the connections among doctors even further, since the primary care physician would now take on the role of "gatekeeper," deciding whether additional care was necessary. But Susan Love's practice was based on the exceptions—women who had read her book, seen her on television, or heard about her from a friend. As interested as she might be in the managed care future, at present most of Love's patients came to her because they chose to. Any ad campaign featuring Susan had to speak to the woman, not her doctor.

At the end of May two representatives from the advertising agency and the two UCLA marketing staffers assigned to the project came to the Breast Center to present their first idea, a television commercial designed to appeal to women who liked to make up their own minds about the doctors they saw. There would be a real patient who talked about something she liked to do, like travel, followed by an announcer who talked about all the options available at UCLA.

All the agency needed to get started was a patient, which was where Sherry Goldman, who kept track of all the multi patients, came in. She had a suggestion right away, a woman who had come to UCLA as a high-risk patient and went through the diagnostic program when a mammogram revealed a suspicious mass. She had breast cancer, so she attended the multidisciplinary clinic, had a lumpectomy with a node dissection, chemotherapy, and radiation. She was doing fine.

"How old is she?" asked one of the marketing people.

"Fifty, fifty-five," said Sherry, and then she realized what they were looking for. "Very attractive."

The ad man hesitated. "Sounds like she's still in treatment."

"Just coming out the other end," said Sherry.

"What's the prognosis?"

"Good. Do you want somebody who's all done?"

"Well, let's just say, we're doing commercials and we're talking to this woman, and God forbid she takes a turn for the worse." He did not want to launch a campaign for UCLA's cancer services featuring a patient who was likely to die.

"Okay," said Sherry. "I hear you."

"Does she have hair?" asked one of the women from the marketing department.

"Yeah."

They discussed a few other candidates. One sounded too ill. Another had been through a bone marrow transplant—and the agency people worried that if she appeared in an ad more women might ask for an expensive experimental treatment that their medical insurance did not cover. They kept coming back to the first one Sherry had suggested. Did she look her age?

Sherry smiled. "I don't think *any* woman in L.A. looks her age. She's very outgoing, social, a country club kind of woman, plays golf. . . ."

The ad man brightened. "Perfect," he said. "Just the kind of woman we need. Golf."

"And she still works," said Sherry. "She's very active."

She sounded like the sort of person who could deliver the commercial's message with sincerity.

"The last thing we want to do is put words in their mouth," said the agency executive, "but we do want to guide them toward our message."

"Which is?" asked Sherry.

" 'When I found out I had a lump, I was scared to death. I looked around until I found UCLA. Then I felt I had options.' "

"And we may not want to get too deep into specific treatments, a this-ectomy or a that-ectomy," he concluded. "We want to focus on the less sad side of breast cancer."

Sherry shot him a cool look. "I don't think there is a less sad side to breast cancer," she said evenly, "but if you want women who have come through and look okay, these do."

27

CROSS-TALK

W HEN DAVID MCFADDEN ARRIVED AT UCLA IN AUGUST 1992 TO BE
the chief of general surgery at the Veterans' Administration Hospital, he faced a practical dilemma. UCLA
was world famous for its gastrointestinal surgeons, "senior states-
men," as McFadden called them. He was just starting out, eager to
establish a clinical presence, build up a patient base, and start paying his way. That usually took about two years—but he could
hardly compete with the other, older surgeons in his specialty. So he
took a popular sidestep and did breast surgery while he waited for
his GI practice to grow.

Lots of doctors came to breast surgery that way. It was unde-
manding, unlikely to surprise, and there were rarely the late-night
emergencies associated with invasive procedures. Breast surgery
was a predictable, dependable source of income—general surgeons who were just starting out or about ready to retire often
included it in their repertoire.

Love had just arrived at UCLA that summer, determined to
recruit doctors for the multidisciplinary program who were committed to quality breast cancer treatment. She and McFadden got
along well from the start, despite their dissimilar personalities. He
was a good foil for Love and an asset to the clinic.

Lately, though, he had missed the clinic several times, either because a GI surgery ran long, or because he had an emergency. Once he forgot and scheduled a conflicting meeting. He had been heard to complain about long afternoons that failed to generate any revenues, and Love worried that as his GI practice grew his interest in the multidisciplinary program would wane.

She arranged to meet with McFadden after her surgeries on Monday, June 6, and she arrived in a buoyant mood, expecting merely to remind him of his responsibilities and be on her way. She was not prepared for his response: McFadden had decided that he could no longer participate in the multi because of the financial unpredictability of the arrangement. A solemn man, McFadden believed in the work ethic; effort should yield reward. He had a wife and children to support, and had to devote his energies to making a living. The multi was not a healthy source of revenues.

Love went from McFadden to the conference room for the monthly meeting of the Breast Center Steering Committee. The entire membership rarely attended, given their scheduling conflicts. This time Slamon was out of town and McFadden had an emergency surgery, so only five members showed up—Mary Bading, the Division of General Surgery's administrator; Leslie Laudeman and Tamara Dobson; Dr. Bob Bennion, a surgeon; and Dr. Love. When she walked in, the others were huddled together discussing the latest news: Dr. Zinner's replacement as head of the Department of Surgery was Dr. E. Carmack Holmes, a surprise choice, and to this group, a worrisome one. Holmes was an unknown commodity, a fifty-four-year-old thoracic surgeon who was considered part of the university establishment—not a vocal critic of the Breast Center, but not an avid supporter either.

Holmes might be perfectly satisfied to go back to the old days, when each specialist—the surgeon, the oncologist, the radiation therapist—saw his patients separately. Or he might decide that the Department should play a more active role. If Holmes picked a crony to run the Division of General Surgery, the largest and most lucrative of the nine disciplines that made up the Department, there could be even more resistance to the Breast Center concept. When Zinner held both posts, Love was certain that the

Center was protected—their arguments were always about how best to run the program, not whether it ought to exist. Holmes did not have a vested interest, as Zinner had; there was no guarantee he would cut the Center any slack.

Love tended to see things in extremes—she understood heroes and villains better than she did politicians. All she wanted to know was, "Are they going to leave me alone with my vision, or try to impose theirs?"

It would depend on the numbers, which were the topic of the current meeting. For the 1993–1994 academic fiscal year, to date, the Center was $62,000 below its projected profit figure of $170,504; for the most recent third quarter, $44,000 below projected profits of over $67,000, in part because people were late paying their medical bills.

Mary Bading, a trim, tailored woman with a reserved, almost scholarly air, found reason for optimism regardless. Yes, revenues were down, but so were costs. There was a benefit to seeing fewer patients—the Center had a favorable rental arrangement based on volume, not a flat rate, so lower numbers meant lower rent. As late payments came in, the picture would improve.

Bading was prepared to take good news where she could find it. "We're not doing as bad as we thought," she said happily.

The question was how to make next year's figures look even better. A standard rule in medicine was that a new doctor or a new program would likely take two or three years to show a profit. If a practice was still in the red after that, something was wrong. Managed care made it more difficult for doctors to generate the kind of profits they were used to, though. A multidisciplinary clinic that depended on donated time seemed the generous vestige of an earlier era, when doctors made so much money that they could contribute an afternoon a week without a second thought. Ironically, the multi might have fared better in the old, private practice structure that Mike Zinner had worked so hard to dismantle.

Thanks to Denny Slamon, the Center had one important asset the committee could use to strategic advantage. The Department of Medical Oncology made a $50,000 annual contribution to the Breast Center out of Slamon's departmental discretionary fund.

Slamon had from the start given the steering committee permission to spend the money in whatever way it thought best.

In the first year the Center had asked to delay the payment until the second year, to make the numbers look like progress; less of a loss in the second year than the first. Now Bading suggested holding off again until the new fiscal year, which began July 1. If they dumped the entire $150,000 into the program then, it would look even better.

Revlon was prepared to invest $500,000, separate from the proposed $7.5 million expenditure, as a matching grant with UCLA to facilitate the Breast Center's move down to its own dedicated center in the basement, but as far as Love was concerned that money meant a new set of problems. The fact that she did not like the space was beside the point. The rent downstairs was a stiff $2.80 per square foot, a fixed rate for the space no matter how many patients moved through it. Even consistent performance was going to look bad on paper, which was why she wanted to use Revlon money to defray operating costs. Slamon still refused even to consider the idea. Revlon wanted to spend money on a physical space and research, not on subsidizing what Slamon perceived as the program's weaknesses.

Love did not know what to do. The new arrangement virtually guaranteed worse numbers, and Revlon's involvement would exacerbate what she felt was Slamon's imperious attitude. Ronald Perelman was, after all, Denny's donor. All Susan could do was make suggestions.

But Revlon was a useful buffer between the Center and the university. Everyone on the steering committee agreed that UCLA could decide to shut down one of its own programs. The Revlon/UCLA Women's Health Center would have a more public profile. It would be hard for a university to turn away private funds.

In a way, Love faced the same dilemma Bernie Fisher had faced. He had been expected to function as part of a layered bureaucracy—the NSABP, which answered to the National Cancer Institute, which answered, in turn, to the National Institutes of Health, the Department of Health and Human Services, and Congress. Yet Love was convinced that he never would have accomplished what he had if he had behaved as an obedient bureaucrat.

Bernie Fisher had run the NSABP as though it were his personal fiefdom. That was how he got things done, but it was also what finished off his career. His arrogance had enabled him to do groundbreaking work, just as it kept him from acknowledging his public responsibility.

Not for the first time, she reminded herself that she could always go somewhere else if UCLA did not work out.

There was nothing to do but wait and see. Everything was up in the air—the UCLA hierarchy, the Revlon proposal, even the way the Center did business. Managed care providers had changed forever the definition of reimbursable expenses, and because of that every experience with an HMO patient was an adventure in fee negotiation.

Reimbursements at the Breast Center were, as Love put it, "all over the place." Some managed care groups balked completely if the multi doctors were not part of their network, while others dismantled the $350 to $800 charge and paid for only a single consultation with a specialist. Patients felt they had the right to have their bills adjusted. Laudeman told the steering committee that she was regularly accosted in the hallway by people who considered a fee to be a starting point for debate.

Follow-up care, which traditionally had been a dependable, relatively easy source of income, was also up for grabs, as insurers tried to trim costs. Love wondered if the Center ought to "unload" some of its follow-up patients back to their primary care physicians, but Bennion warned her not to move too quickly. UCLA's managed care staff spoke of the city's wealthy Westside with the reverence an archaeologist might reserve for a priceless relic. There were still plenty of wealthy patients who had third-party indemnity insurance, the kind that reimbursed doctors more liberally. There were rich women who would gladly pay out-of-pocket if they had to, just to have Dr. Love's blessing. There was no reason to send them back to their internists or gynecologists.

* * *

Dottie was one of those women. She swung from one biweekly Wednesday morning appointment to the next like a trapeze artist in the circus—she got her bearings and took off into space, secure in the knowledge that safety waited on the other side.

In between, depression came calling. One Sunday morning she and Joe were in the bedroom when she gave in to a black mood.

"Oh God, I don't care," she said. "Let the cancer grow and let me die in a year or two. I don't want to go through this. I can't take this hassle anymore. It's just too much pressure, too much, too much. Let me die in peace."

He looked at her, terrified.

"I don't want to hear you talk that way," he said, and walked out of the room.

She felt terrible. She and Joe had grown up together; she had seen him become a husband, a father, now a grandfather. She could be down on the floor in her sweat clothes doing her exercises, and when he came into the room he smiled at her as though she were her old self, dressed in some coordinated outfit with her hair done and her makeup on. Joe did whatever Dottie needed—brought her breakfast on the weekends, brought her things when she was too tired to walk—and never complained. But now she needed something different, and she had to figure out how to ask for it.

She wrote him a note: "What I need is someone to put their arms around me and hug me."

The note bewildered him. Joe kissed his wife good morning, and he kissed his wife good night, and he adored her. After all this time, didn't she understand the depth of his devotion?

At the beginning of June she had an idea. Before the fibromyalgia Dottie had been an avid gardener. She might not be able to work in the yard herself, but she could still design a landscape that would give her pleasure.

Roses. She wanted rosebushes to wind around the back of the house behind the master bedroom. She could start her research now and over the summer order the bare-root bushes she wanted, before the varieties she favored were all gone. There would not be many roses the first season, but by the second spring, in 1996, the yard would be in bloom.

A rose garden required two things—planning, and renewed faith. If Dottie undertook the project it meant that she expected to live for at least two more years.

She ordered a catalogue so that she could study all the different varieties that were available on the West Coast. Dottie intended to plant old roses, heirloom varieties from the dignified past. She was not seduced by the new hybrids. She would have a classic garden, of eternal style.

O n Tuesday, June 7, Love delivered her annual lecture to the third-year medical students on the surgical rotation. She relished the opportunity to disabuse them of certain notions, to see their fledging professional egos deflate as they realized that surgery was not the solution, not to this disease.

She rattled off the most popular misconceptions she encountered. Fibrocystic disease was "background noise," not a challenge for an overeager surgeon. Women with lumpy breasts could drink coffee if they wanted to, because the warning against it was based, she said, "on a horrible study done ten years ago."

She smiled when one enthusiastic student suggested a bilateral mastectomy as the answer to DCIS or even the benign condition that sometimes preceded it, atypical ductal hyperplasia. The aggressive surgeon's mentality was alive and well in the next generation.

She appealed to the class. "Does it decrease her risk of breast cancer?"

The student who had suggested it answered first. "Yeah," he said, smugly. "She doesn't have breasts."

"Uh-uh," said Love. She told them about the rat study and watched his face fall. Just to make sure that no one else had any illusions, she repeated a set of statistics that always surprised students. Chemotherapy decreased the mortality rate by about one-third in premenopausal women, and by one-fourth in menopausal patients. Tamoxifen decreased mortality by twelve percent in premenopausal patients and by twenty-nine percent in older women. It still was not clear whether transplants raised the odds of survival; although as many as seventy percent of metastatic patients showed an initial response, median survival was only twenty-three months, which was less than some studies of conventional drug therapies.

This was what she liked to do—not split hairs with Denny Slamon, but incite the next generation of doctors to think about what they were doing.

"In the global scheme of things," she said, "we're not making a major dent. The answer's going to have to come from looking at it in a different way. *That's* the exciting part."

A dozen doctors and researchers attended the first meeting of the Los Angeles Breast Cancer Research Group—the group Love had conceived weeks ago and Connie Long had implemented—on Tuesday, June 7, in a private dining room at a hotel across the street from UCLA's main hospital. Although most of them had worked in Los Angeles for years, they had never met each other, which was precisely the reason for the event. Love hoped that synergy might take medicine farther than individual enterprise could—that the paradigm shift she talked about eluded doctors and scientists not because breast cancer was beyond their comprehension, but because they were cut off from each other.

They were hardly used to collective endeavor. Clinicians were in constant competition to attract new patients and keep the old ones. Researchers were divided by the promise of a new prize: whoever made any kind of inroad in breast cancer care, whether it be in basic science, a better treatment or an effective prevention strategy, was guaranteed adulation and quite probably a great deal of profit. Altruism was a romantic luxury that none of them could quite afford. The same ambition that drove them to fourteen-hour days also guaranteed a proprietary air about the knowledge they accumulated.

They approached any group encounter with a certain wariness. The early talk that evening was intended not to forge alliances but to establish the relative valor of the participants—who was doing the most against breast cancer, and against what odds.

The private doctors envied the academics for the financial and personnel support a university provided. The university doctors in turn taunted the private doctors for charging high fees and offering less comprehensive services. Three doctors from the Breast Center, the large private facility in Van Nuys, countered that they had funded ten years of clinical research out of their own profits—and had recently delivered 150 tissue blocks from women with DCIS to Denny Slamon, so that he could test them for the HER-2/neu oncogene and for P53, a tumor supressor gene that in its mutated form inhibited normal genes and enabled cancer to grow.

Dr. Mel Silverstein, a breast surgeon and cofounder of that center, was a tall, imposing man who prided himself on having devised a private practice version of the multidisciplinary clinic thirteen years before Susan Love blew into town. Women who came to his center could see anyone they needed, from a surgeon to a mammography specialist to a plastic surgeon—and if the doctors did not set aside a specific time to meet as a group to discuss the patient, as UCLA did, if a woman still had to set up a string of individual appointments, at least the doctors were in the same suite of offices. They talked to each other all the time. He believed that the service provided was of equally high quality.

A UCLA geneticist listened to him and asked if the Van Nuys Breast Center counseled family members and worked with high-risk relatives. Silverstein said that the center's psychiatrist had until recently seen every cancer patient, over two thousand of them since the center opened. The problem now was managed care, which often did not reimburse for psychological services.

Love asked Silverstein if he had a statistician, since she was having trouble setting up a computer database, but he mistook the question for a challenge.

"We have a $7 million building to run with no outside help," he said. "If we want a statistician we have to pay for it."

"So do we," said Love.

"You guys get grants."

"Nah," Love shot back, still smarting from her track record with the DOD. "We just write them."

Her willingness to make fun of herself slowly put the others at ease. She told them about the "funny grant" she was working on to counsel women who had BRCA-1, even though there was no gene yet and a test to detect it might take years. She told them how hard it had been to get approval for her ductoscope study—and she willingly confessed her disappointment at being rejected on her biggest DOD grant application, which would have provided information on patients of diverse ethnic and environmental backgrounds.

"I don't know if we would have had enough numbers to generate answers," she said, wistfully, "but perhaps it would generate hypotheses."

Malcolm Pike, a USC epidemiologist who was studying the link between hormone levels and breast cancer risk, tried to reassure her. He had heard on the grapevine that he was getting a grant from the DOD, but he had not yet been formally notified. Perhaps she was still in the running for the big grant and did not know it.

She shrugged. She could always file the grant with the state of California. But Pike was indignant on her behalf. He agreed with Denny Slamon. What was the DOD money, he said, if not "Susan's money"?

Malcolm Pike was even more of a renegade than Susan, a man who reminded his dinner companions that night of his peculiar celebrity among breast cancer researchers—that he was "singularly unable to get an NIH grant," and had yet to receive a scientific merit rating in the top half of eligible grant applicants, on any of his applications. He wore his rejection like a badge, proof that what he was doing was so ahead of its time as to be incomprehensible to the research establishment.

As an epidemiologist, Pike was at the opposite end of the spectrum from Love, focused on large populations rather than individual patients. What interested him was the theory that breast cancer was related to a woman's lifetime estrogen production. Pike and USC oncologist Darcy Spicer believed that early menarche, late childbirth, and fewer children conspired to raise the risk level of American women by increasing the number of times they ovulated. They also thought that progesterone might be dangerous, because most breast cell proliferation occurred at the point in the ovulatory cycle when progesterone was being secreted.

It made historical sense. Women who had an oophorectomy, the surgical removal of their ovaries, had a decreased risk of breast cancer. Pike wanted to mimic that effect without actually removing the ovaries, so that a young woman could decide at a later date to get pregnant.

He and Spicer were studying a drug called a gonadotropin-releasing hormone agonist (GnHRA), which prevented the production of estrogen and progesterone, in the hope that it would reduce the incidence of breast cancer in high-risk women. They were conducting a clinical trial involving fourteen high-risk women, to see what GnHRA would do.

Each woman received a monthly injection of GnHRA—and took a very small daily dose of estrogen and progesterone, what Pike called a "fraction" of the amount in birth control pills, just enough to protect the bones and heart from what was otherwise an induced menopause.

The researchers had already found that they could alter a pre-menopausal woman's mammogram—diminish the breast density and make her film easier to evaluate. Pike believed that the drug dramatically shrank the epithelial tissue lining the breast ducts, making it resemble the tissue of a woman who had had her ovaries removed. If Pike and Spicer could fool a younger woman's body into thinking it had no ovaries—if she produced neither estrogen nor progesterone—perhaps she would not develop breast cancer.

He predicted dramatic results: lifetime risk reduced by thirty-one percent after five years of treatment, forty-seven percent after ten years, and seventy percent at fifteen years.

The only trouble, he admitted glumly, was that "nobody else thinks we know what we're talking about." Pike's scenario had its problems. Depriving a young woman of hormones put her at risk for osteoporosis, which required Pike and Spicer to add testosterone to their chemical mix. No one yet knew what the long-term consequences might be.

Worse, they had been at it for so long that their peers had begun to doubt their credibility. Pike's career was tied up in his hypothesis; if it started to go sour he might not be able to recognize the signs. At the moment he was looking for other researchers willing to repeat his studies—in the hope that they would get the same results and restore faith in his findings. Studies were getting under way at Harvard, Johns Hopkins, and the University of North Carolina, and he hoped for more sites. He desperately wanted to be taken seriously.

"We're regarded as extremely passionate and no longer objective," he said. His eyes twinkled mischievously. "And they're absolutely right."

Of all the people at the table, Pike was Love's spiritual kin—impatient, outspoken, critical of a national research effort that seemed to him to be standing on its head. He was tired of coming up against scientists who were more interested in getting credit than sharing information. Pike was eager to talk about his project to anyone who would listen—and about his primary interest, which was to figure out how and why breast cells divided.

In a way he agreed with NIH director Harold Varmus. Breast cancer research was too often a cart-before-the-horse effort. Varmus sought a basic understanding of the human body; Pike, fundamental knowledge about how the cells in the breast worked. Without it, everything was speculation, millions of dollars spent on second-generation ideas before the proper foundation was laid.

"I desperately want to understand cell division in the breast, but here's the tremendous problem," he told the others as the evening wore on. "How do you figure out what's going on in the breast without cutting it open?"

"There's no intermediate test," Love admitted.

Pike's watery eyes fairly popped with indignation, and he ran his fingers through a wayward head of graying brown hair. "It's like eighteenth- or nineteenth-century medicine," he said, his voice rising uncontrollably. "It's a desperate problem. *Figuring out what goes on in the breast is the most important problem in breast cancer today.*"

"It's the major problem," agreed Love. No one else spoke.

In his isolation, Pike had begun to assume that people who were part of the research establishment had some of the information he wanted—they just would not part with it. He was upset at his inability to get his hands on the NSABP's data on how tamoxifen affected the breast. "I bloody well know Bernie Fisher has it, but he won't give it to me," he complained.

He went on. There were too many randomized trials and they took too long. He was not sure that estrogen receptors mattered, although they were part of the standard evaluation of any new patient. He wanted someone to figure out if simultaneous tumors in both breasts were separate cancers or part of the same tumor. There was so much basic work to be done. And yet that evening's dinner was proof of what scared him most, that breast cancer researchers, even ones who lived and worked in the same city, were not aware of the others' efforts, nor of the gaps in knowledge that had to be addressed.

The most urgent question was the status of the gene hunt. Like Alison Estabrook, the surgeon from New York's Columbia Presbyterian Medical Center who had visited Dr. Love, Malcolm Pike had heard troublesome rumblings about Mary-Claire King's efforts—in his case, from King herself.

"Mary-Claire says they don't know why they haven't found it," he said. "She's said if it were straightforward they would have found it by now. She's worried."

Love allowed that she had heard another rumor—that Mary-Claire was starting to think that the gene pertained only to women with both breast and ovarian cancer, or to a specific age group. What everyone had hoped would be a door flung wide might in fact be just a thin crack of light, a glimpse, but not the complete picture.

Pike leveled his gaze at his silent colleagues. "What the hell? There are nine million people here," he said, referring to the population of southern California. "We're twice the size of Sweden. We should be doing twice the work. But we're not organized."

He wondered how many of them even knew about Dave Heber's interest in nutritional intervention with high-risk women. Heber and Love had decided to apply together for a grant to study the connection between soy, dietary fat, exercise, and estrogen levels, and if they got money they would need patients. Everyone else was surprised, and eager to refer women who qualified.

"It's going to require real community effort and support," said

Pike, visibly pleased by the response. "This is why Chinese and Japanese women have less breast cancer—because in premenopausal years they produce little estrogen." That, he believed, was because they exercised, ate a lot of soy and fish oil, and did not consume the corn and safflower oils found in a Western diet.

One geneticist asked if the only dietary component was low fat.

"And soy protein," said Love. "It's very in right now."

"Actually," said Pike, wincing, "it's all the chewing you have to do."

Silverstein, who considered himself a practical man, doubted that healthy women would bother to stay on such a restrictive diet. He believed they would choose a subcutaneous bilateral mastectomy and a flap reconstruction, a finite agony, over the endless discipline of a tough diet.

"Maybe not," said Love. "Women are used to long, arduous tasks." She liked whenever possible to remind her male colleagues that women were tougher than men. Pregnancy, childbirth, menopause; they could handle the discipline Heber's diet required. Besides, there was no proof that a prophylactic mastectomy worked.

Silverstein said he still would try it. It was beginning to sound to him like this group had given up on the old surgical solutions— and yet he had not heard anything that sounded to him like a reasonable alternative.

Love could not resist the chance to try out her "criminal analogy" on her peers—that perhaps not every breast cancer cell required the death sentence. If scientists could figure out instead how to make a cancer cell dormant, to make it "go to sleep," that might be a better solution than surgery, chemotherapy, and radiation, all of which came with their own host of side effects, none of which worked often enough to suit her.

Susan preferred the idea that they could simply lock up the criminal for life.

"Now, do I know the details of this?" said Love, with a big laugh. "Not a bit. I'm the vision person. 'The Love Paradigm: the rehabilitatable criminal.' "

She dismissed surgery. "It'll hold until our retirement, Mel, but it's not a long-term career."

Silverstein raised an eyebrow and said nothing.

"Oh, yeah," insisted Love. "Ten years."

No conversation was complete without reference to cost. One doctor had heard a rumor about a new cost-benefit study that discussed the possibility of not doing mammograms at all. It might turn out that waiting until a woman had a palpable lump, and giving chemotherapy to all patients, was a cost-effective alternative to mammography.

It was hardly a scenario that would find favor among patients who had to endure the toxic drugs, but that was not the issue. In the long run, it could save money.

The guests at the table found the idea almost too horrific to contemplate. How could anyone consider submitting a woman to chemotherapy if a mammogram might catch a malignancy early enough to avoid toxic drugs? The only sane reaction was laughter.

"Well, wait," said Charles Haskell, the medical oncologist with whom Love had worked on a textbook. "The most cost-effective thing is for the patient to *die*."

"Early," said Love.

"Without treatment," said another doctor.

"Without that bone marrow transplant," said Silverstein.

Pike had one serious comment to make. He reminded the others that mammograms found small lesions in premenopausal women, all right—but finding them did not seem to make a difference in mortality. The bean-counters' suggestion about abandoning mammography sounded awful, until they analyzed what, exactly, they were losing. A woman under fifty gave up a false sense of security, and that was all.

"Then I should go home and just watch TV," said Silverstein. He was offended at the suggestion that what he did made no difference, however many studies there might be to suggest it.

"No," said Love. "Think about prevention."

"No," said Pike, in a loud voice. "We should figure out what's happening."

Silverstein agreed with that. He said that a really good study of women under fifty had not yet been done. Someone needed to follow a large number of those women—say five hundred thousand—and track what happened to them each year. A large, coordinated effort was the only way to get definitive answers.

The evening ended—as did almost any conversation between breast cancer specialists—with shop talk about tricky cases. Every clinician had a story about a patient whose disease did not behave predictably. Change was essential, but in the meantime individuals suffered, and were lost. Their doctors, ever hopeful, talked about their cases on the chance that someone else would see an answer they had missed.

28

RISK/BENEFIT

I T WAS DUSK. THE CREAM-COLORED WALLS ON THE EIGHTH FLOOR OF THE Century City Hospital were shadowed in faded gray and the hallways were empty. Most of the rooms on the surgery floor were vacant, and the nurses' station was quiet. At the end of the hall, with a wasted view, was Dee Wieman's room. She lay in the bed against the inside wall, her face turned away from the waning sunlight. The vestiges of the morning's anesthesia dried her mouth and made her eyes loll. She licked her lips and tried to focus on the empty room.

On the morning of June 9, Dr. Armando Giuliano had performed a bilateral mastectomy on Dee. Having lost Susan Love, fearful of losing her way entirely, Dee had become the most cooperative of patients. If Giuliano thought a bilateral mastectomy was best, that was what she would do; she had dutifully scheduled the surgery soon after her last appointment. If he wanted her to wait until after the transplant for her reconstructive surgery, she would wait.

At the end of the day Dee was alone, prepared for any surprise visitors. Her wig was back in place. On the side chair next to her bed was the box that contained a lacy bra contoured with a temporary prosthesis.

Dee had spent most of the previous afternoon on the 405 freeway, going to and from the office of the woman who was going to make a customized prosthesis to get her through the next six months. In the meantime, she had made a temporary model—not as perfect a fit as the final design, which would be contoured to Dee's healed body, but a necessary interim solution for a woman who refused to get out of bed unless she looked like her old self. Dee had insisted on picking it up. She would not go to the hospital without it.

Gary had driven his wife to the hospital for the double mastectomy and spent that first day and night with her. He wondered how to make sense of what had happened. He had come to think that there were three stages to the process—three phases anyone would have to go through if they faced this kind of surgery, or loved someone who did.

The first reaction was the selfish one; that was how he now categorized his initial response, of not wanting Dee to lose her breasts. The second phase was vanity, when they talked about simultaneous reconstruction and took comfort in the notion that Dee would still look great in clothes. The third stage—a door he had walked through when Giuliano told them how bad the lumpectomy looked—was life. Gary had come to a cold place, where all he wanted was for Dee to survive.

The next morning Love had a farewell meeting with Mike Zinner, who was scheduled to leave on July 1. Zinner tried one last time to get Love to listen to reason. He entreated her to make an effort to fit in. He wanted her to attend the weekly mortality and morbidity conference. Love never visited her office in the main hospital building, and she never attended the M & M's. The other doctors considered her behavior a slight, and Zinner urged her to correct the impression.

She sighed. There was one M & M conference from eight to ten on Saturday mornings, which was one of the few times she got to be with Kate. The other conference was at seven thirty on Wednesday nights, after a day of patients, the multi clinic, the journal club, and dictation.

She agreed to try. In return he offered her a glimmer of hope. One of the candidates for General Surgery division chief under Dr. Holmes was Dave McFadden, who would presumably be a valuable ally.

Denny Slamon seemed to have an uncanny instinct for trouble; he came looking for Susan whenever she was not around. He dropped by the multi that afternoon, just after she had left for Irvine, where she was scheduled to deliver the commencement address at the University of California, Irvine School of Medicine.

Denny took every absence as a personal affront. After the multi conference he escorted Sherry Goldman into the consultation room and closed the door. He wanted to explain to her what was at stake, so that she would appreciate, not resent, his concern. More to the point, he wanted Sherry to keep him apprised of how things were going.

She bluntly refused to be his "go-between," and the following Monday reported to Susan the contents of what Sherry called Slamon's "tirade." Love called Slamon and asked him to keep Sherry out of it.

John Glaspy had been trying for months to add what he called "an attractive product line" to the Breast Center program—general gynecological care, provided by two young internal medicine specialists. Dr. Jodi Friedman and Dr. Mitzi Krockover finally became available for the diagnostic clinic in mid-June, once the overlapping departments involved in their participation cleared up issues of hours and priorities and schedules and salaries. As soon as Krockover showed up, Love dragged her into an examining room and began a crash course in the unexpected.

The Breast Center saw twenty to thirty patients with benign problems for every one who eventually landed in the multidisciplinary clinic, and Love spent much of her time with these women undoing excess. She railed against an overzealous infectious disease specialist who had put a woman on long-term antibiotics for a subareolar abcess, a chronic infection that could be resolved easily with minor surgery. She made sure Krockover understood that the endless tests one woman had undergone were "private practice stuff," her favorite euphemism for a lucrative, padded agenda prescribed when a patient's insurance covered it.

Love told her new recruit that eighty percent of the surgical biopsies for calcifications done in the United States were benign, compared to forty percent of the biopsies done in Europe. It did not mean that there was more cancer in Europe, but that there were fewer biopsies. American doctors did them too often—as a defense against malpractice claims and, Love believed, because they mistakenly equated more with better.

"This is an entrepreneurial system," she told Krockover. "We have lawyers, we do tests, we tell the patient they're fine, they think we're great, and we get paid."

By the end of the afternoon Krockover was reeling. The patients she had seen were the lucky ones, the ones with benign problems. But what an assortment of odd symptoms and elusive complaints— and what confusion, trying to sort them out and provide the patient with a little peace of mind.

"What we need," she said, with surprise in her voice, "is a better diagnostic tool."

"Right," said Love. "The easy way out is to talk about breast self-exam and mammography. It's harder to say that early detection doesn't work."

Coincidence worked strange patterns. Love often observed that a particular multi clinic would have a distinct personality— most of the women were young, or everyone needed a mastectomy, or lots of transplant patients showed up. The teacher in her made her look for similarities, so that the conference became instructive.

Several of the June 15 multi patients had lots of positive nodes, but no evidence of distant metastases. They forced a philosophical question: Once they had finished their treatment, what was the best approach?

Love had a simple answer: Let them live their lives. She was far more concerned with the quality of a woman's life than with tracking the development of a disease she could not arrest once it began to spread. She tried to discourage women from having either of the two blood tests currently in use to determine whether cancer had spread into the bloodstream, the CA-15-3 and the CEA. Other variables, including whether a woman smoked, or was a diabetic, could affect CEA test results, and neither marker was very specific. She weighed the terror of a false positive result against the benefits of a true positive, and saw no reason for doing the test. As for scans, they might reveal metastatic disease before a woman felt symptoms, but still there was nothing a doctor could do to keep the disease from killing her. Why spend extra time knowing you were sick? Love thought it far preferable to spend it feeling well.

Sometimes women refused to listen. Dee had endless tests. Dottie halfheartedly inquired about them from time to time. One of the women at the June 15 multi brought a battery of test results with her—blood tests that contradicted each other, chest X rays that showed spots on her lungs.

Glaspy was curt. The tests were useless—and he fully expected the woman to keep having them.

"You can tell her it doesn't help to diagnose metastatic disease, but it won't matter," he said. "She needs precision and she can't get it. She thinks a degree of certainty accompanies a good test result, and it doesn't."

A recently published study in the *Journal of the American Medical Association* came to the same gloomy conclusion. GIVIO (Interdisciplinary Group for Cancer Care Evaluation), a cooperative group of investigators at twenty-six Italian hospitals, had in 1986 randomly assigned 1,320 patients with Stage 1, Stage 2, or Stage 3 breast cancer to one of two groups. The first group received intensive surveillance of bones, liver, and lungs, as well as laboratory tests to detect metastases. The second group saw their physicians as often as the other women, but were tested only if clinicians determined that there was reason to do so. Both groups received mammograms.

The study was designed to look at overall survival rates and quality of life, which the researchers defined as "overall health and quality-of-life perception, emotional well-being, body image, social functioning, symptoms, and satisfaction with care." The results were the same, except that a patient who chose surveillance outside a clinical trial faced higher medical bills. Twenty percent of the women in the intensive group and eighteen percent of the ones in the control group died while the seven-year study was under way. Quality-of-life measurements were equivalent at six months, one year, two years, and five years.

"Results of this trial," read the *JAMA* article, "support the view that a protocol of frequent laboratory tests and roentgenography after primary treatment for breast cancer does not improve survival or influence health-related quality of life. Routine use of these tests should be discouraged."

On that same Wednesday, June 15, the House Subcommittee on Oversight and Investigations that had first met in April reconvened for its second hearing. The witnesses called to testify included Dr. John Patterson, the international medical director of Zeneca Pharmaceuticals Group, the sole supplier of tamoxifen in the United States, accompanied by two Zeneca executives; J. Dennis O'Connor, the chancellor of the University of Pittsburgh, and Dr. Thomas Detre, the senior vice chancellor for Health Sciences; as well as Dr. Ronald Herberman, the interim chairman of the NSABP; Dr. Bernard Fisher; and NCI director Dr. Samuel Broder.

It was an irresistible political opportunity for Congressman Dingell, who opened the proceedings with a provocative attack on Dr. Fisher and the NCI's Dr. Broder, accusing Fisher, the University of Pittsburgh, the NCI, and the Office of Research Integrity of "multiple and serious failings" in their handling of data in the lumpectomy and tamoxifen trials.

In the two months since the first hearings, the House committee had received letters that Dingell said came from "some of Dr. Fisher's top colleagues at the University of Pittsburgh, under the cloak of anonymity," demanding both an investigation of the NCI's culpability and Fisher's reinstatement. They only served to further polarize the participants. Zeneca Pharmaceuticals was prepared to defend the benefits of tamoxifen, but pointed out that the NCI and the NSABP were responsible for the prevention trial; Zeneca was merely the supplier. The NCI wanted to reassure patients and protect its clinical trials program, and was willing to end its relationship with Fisher if that was what it took. The members of the House subcommittee saw their mandate as the defense of American women against unresponsive scientists. Fisher's camp continued to take the position that the data was sound, that no one at the NCI had seemed particularly upset about it until the newspapers got hold of the story.

In April both Dr. Varmus, director of the NIH, and Dr. Broder had apologized for the NCI's passive acceptance of Fisher's delays in reporting the fraud and reanalyzing the data. In June, as though to compensate for the public embarrassment, the NCI took an aggressive stance, suggesting to the ORI that the University of Pittsburgh look further into Fisher's actions, to see if a formal investigation of scientific misconduct was called for.

Dingell complained about high-handedness in all quarters, the "inappropriate deference to the superstars of science" that Dr. Detre had observed, suspicious financial contributions from Zeneca—with the accompanying implication of compromised ethics—and sloppy reporting by the researchers of deaths from endometrial cancer.

As with the disease itself, nothing was that simple. Dr. Patterson, representing Zeneca, was quick to point out that tamoxifen was "one of the most studied drugs in the world. . . . With over six million patient-years of experience in more than twenty years of clinical use around the world, tamoxifen continues to be a key weapon in the battle against breast cancer." In addition to reducing the risk of recurrence after ten years and the mortality rate for women with early-stage disease, it reduced cancers in the other breast. It seemed to decrease cardiovascular disease and stabilize postmenopausal bone loss—the benefits of estrogen without the increased risk of breast cancer.

It also caused an indisputable increase in the risk of uterine cancer, but Zeneca defended its actions on that front. The company had changed its label four times since 1989 to reflect new risk figures and reported all new data to the FDA. As far as Zeneca was concerned the potential benefits of tamoxifen far outweighed the risk. The NSABP scandal was about bad behavior, not a bad drug.

"We are concerned that public confusion over these issues could lead patients with breast cancer to be afraid of tamoxifen," said

Patterson in his prepared statement, "a medication with the demonstrated ability to delay recurrence of their disease and prolong their lives."

After reviewing the data, Patterson presented his most compelling statistic, that "the increased risk of uterine cancer associated with tamoxifen is approximately twenty times smaller than the more deadly risk that breast cancer will recur or spread if patients do not take tamoxifen."

He insisted that everything else paled in light of that risk-benefit ratio—the fraudulent data, which was not Zeneca's fault; the delays in notifying patients; the funds paid to the University of Pittsburgh and the sponsored entertainments, all of which, Patterson reminded the panel, was "entirely consistent with both the letter and spirit of FDA policy and the codes of conduct adopted by the American Medical Association and the Pharmaceutical Research and Manufacturers Association, not to mention our own stringent internal corporate guidelines. . . ." Zeneca's position was simple: the company had behaved properly, and breast cancer patients needed tamoxifen.

His position on the prevention trial was more cautious. Zeneca had twice been approached about a prevention trial, and the first time, in 1985, had decided against it, despite being "strongly encouraged by a significant number of scientists within the medical community." Five years later the company agreed to cooperate—but Patterson wanted the congressmen to understand that Zeneca was only a guest at the party.

"I want to make it clear," he said, "that Zeneca is not sponsoring or endorsing the tamoxifen breast cancer prevention trial. This trial is sponsored by the National Cancer Institute and is being conducted by the NSABP." Any criticisms ought to be directed at them.

The NCI's Samuel Broder was not the only one who had fallen under Dr. Fisher's potent spell. J. Dennis O'Connor, the chancellor of the University of Pittsburgh, made a conciliatory statement in which he acknowledged that stronger mechanisms were needed "to ensure that even our most experienced, tested, and accomplished faculty are responsive to administrative imperative." He was no longer willing to accept Fisher's diversionary explanation, that the data was valid despite the fraud and subsequent delay.

"Charges of deficient administration," he said, "are not adequately answered by merely asserting that the research findings remain valid."

From now on the University of Pittsburgh would take a more aggressive stance. "All honor that is due Dr. Bernard Fisher and his colleagues for their achievement in pathbreaking breast cancer research is their, not the institution's, honor," O'Connor said. "We fully recognize, however, that the responsibility for competent research administration ultimately rests on the university."

He thanked the committee for working with the university and the NCI to "get the NSABP research back on track," and establish a "healthier partnership between NSABP and NCI than sometimes prevailed before."

Fisher was not prepared to go quietly. If he was going to be a casualty of the falsified data scandal, he intended to take others with him. Bernard Fisher had spent over thirty-five years studying breast cancer, twenty-seven of them as chair of the NSABP. He was not going to let this incident, however unfortunate, eclipse a lifetime of achievement.

The deposed director of the NSABP testified before the House panel for over two hours. He did not dispute the falsification. What he did contest was the chain of events following the discovery of the lumpectomy data discrepancies. Fisher had been notified about the discrepancies in November 1990, but "at that point," he said, "no fraud had been identified." He told the House panel that the NSABP had suspended Dr. Poisson and notified the NCI as soon as its own investigation turned up falsified data, in February 1991.

The intervening months were not a delay, but a necessary safeguard. In his prepared statement Fisher insisted that he had obeyed the rules, not flaunted them: "We believe that the detection and reporting of the St. Luc Hospital fraud was carried out according to the 1988 Clinical Trials Cooperative Group Program Guidelines, which state that, 'In more serious cases, it is the responsibility of each Group to define the gravity and degree of potential problems, and to be consistent and fair in the actions and sanctions it applies when significant problems are uncovered.' The time spent by the NSABP investigation was used to ensure that fair action was taken."

Once the NCI got involved, Fisher said, his group was "embargoed from further discussions of the matter" until it was resolved. After a year of reanalyzing the remaining data the NSABP informed the NCI, NIH, and ORI that the conclusions held. The falsified data represented 0.3 percent of the 33,885 women enrolled in the NSABP studies. From a scientific standpoint, they made no difference.

"Neither we, the NCI, the NIH, nor the ORI perceived that the Poisson falsifications had resulted in a public health problem," said Fisher. "If the NCI had considered this to be the case, they could have issued a 'clinical alert.' " They had not. Women did not learn of the problem until the *Chicago Tribune* unearthed the results of the federal investigation.

Fisher apologized for the inadvertent consequence of the delay in releasing the lumpectomy data, "the unjustified concern that women with breast cancer were receiving inappropriate therapy." He would not budge from his position on tamoxifen, regardless of the public anxiety over reports of increased uterine cancer risk: the benefits of tamoxifen for women with breast cancer far outweighed the risks. Fisher maintained his position that some of the patients in the tamoxifen trial may have died with endometrial cancer rather than from it. He had not withheld information about possible treatment-related deaths because he remained unconvinced that endometrial cancer had killed them.

"When a death occurs in a woman who had both breast cancer and endometrial cancer," said Fisher, "it is extremely difficult to be sure which cancer caused the death. It cannot be assumed that the death occurred as a result of the endometrial cancer. She may have died of breast cancer." When Fisher did learn of deaths from endometrial cancer among tamoxifen patients in the fall of 1993, the NSABP, the NCI, and Zeneca were notified.

"In retrospect," said Fisher, "it might have been possible to collect and report information about these deaths sooner, but there was never any intent to withhold information."

He blamed overwork for any delay in reporting and auditing.

The prevention trial for high-risk women, which had begun in 1992, caused a jump from twenty-five thousand patients in NSABP studies to forty-one thousand in 1993. The NSABP simply could not keep pace.

That was an administrative error. The current solution—the suspension of the trials by the NCI—was a grievous overreaction.

"Clinical trials must be restored at once," said Fisher. "If clinical trials are eliminated, we have no good alternatives. We cannot return to the system where treatment is based on physicians' intuition."

Dr. Broder agreed with Fisher that the trials needed to continue—but like Chancellor O'Connor, he envisioned a future in which Fisher did not play a role. He spoke of "new scientific leadership." He announced that the NCI's advisory boards and the Oncologic Drugs Advisory Committee of the FDA had recommended renewed accrual for the prevention trial, which had so far signed up only eleven thousand of its sixteen thousand target population.

He was ready to start again without Fisher, with the continued help of the oversight committee and a new administrative plan. The government was prepared to turn its back on Dr. Bernard Fisher, but not on his work.

29

SEEKING REFUGE

D R. DAVID HEBER REFERRED TO HIMSELF AS "THE PROVERBIAL TREE in the forest that falls and nobody hears," a man who for twenty-five years had toiled in happy isolation. He knew that most scientists considered nutritional research a frivolous endeavor, one step removed from the advice doled out in the aisles of health-food stores. He agreed about the quality of much of the research, which was poorly conceived and inconclusive, but not about the subject itself. Heber believed the axiom *You are what you eat,* and had devoted his professional life to finding out what you might become, in terms of disease risk, if you ate something else.

He could often be seen striding down the halls of the medical center, deep in thought, oblivious to anyone walking by. When he did talk, it was difficult to get him to stop. Heber had already defied his own destiny, as the son of two obese parents, on a diet rich in pasta and garden-grown vegetables. He was eager to wean others from their traditional high-fat, high-cholesterol American diet—and used lower disease statistics from other countries as his ammunition. He was a principal investigator on the government's Women's Intervention Nutrition Study (WINS), which looked at fat levels in women's diets, and a member of the committee that had analyzed the design of the Women's Health Initiative.

On the afternoon of Monday, June 20, he met with Susan Love

and nutritionist Dr. Karen Duvall to figure out how to translate his ideas about lowered estrogen levels into a grant proposal for a clinical trial.

Despite the difference in their personalities, Heber and Love shared one common trait, a tendency to fall in love with an idea and then stumble over the details involved in pursuing it. He was adept at grantsmanship and had trouble translating his scheme into clinical reality, while Love was great at working with patients and weak on the details of funding. All Heber wanted to do was pour Ralston-Purina's soy protein fruit drink mix down the throats of high-risk women, to see if his high-soy, low-fat diet and lots of exercise decreased their estrogen levels, and so their breast cancer risk. But he was having trouble designing the pilot study to determine whether women could comply with the difficult regimen. He was there to ask Love and Duvall to review the three essential aspects of the study—how to set it up, how to evaluate the results, and how to make sure women obeyed the admittedly difficult dietary rules.

Heber wanted to watch the subjects in his pilot study for three months to see if the diet caused their estrogen levels to drop, but Love insisted that he needed at least six months to get a sufficient response. Heber was trying to be practical, since grants came with time constraints, but Love insisted that three months was a pointless exercise.

"Okay," he said, "we'll do six months, good work, and forget about our deadlines."

At the end of that time he wanted to do a mammogram, a fine-needle aspiration of any suspicious lumps, take a sampling of duct fluid, and if Susan's ductoscope had by then been approved for more general use, sample cells from the lining of the duct as well. The women in the study were supposed to be on an exercise regimen as well, so that Heber could check their cardiac strength, but the biggest question to Love and Duvall was how to get them to stick with the diet, since the slightest deviation would skew the results.

The diet was such a radical departure that Heber intended to supply prepared meals to the participants. Absolute compliance meant no between-meal snacks, no taste of someone else's real food at a restaurant, not even a sip of a friend's cappuccino. Susan wondered how Heber was going to make sure that a patient had not sneaked a single piece of popcorn at the movies.

"You mean, do they throw the prepared food in the sewer?" he replied.

"Gorge at McDonald's on the way home," suggested Love.

"That's my concern," said Duvall, who often counseled women in the Center's high-risk program on how to maintain a low-fat diet. "Eating between meals."

"I don't know," said Heber, shaking his head in sudden despair. "I just don't know."

"On these first ones," said Love, "we've just got to let them know how important it is." She regarded her colleague, who was fumbling with his reading glasses and seemed quite distressed.

"Here's a question," she said, with a teasing note in her voice. Heber looked up. "What if you used liposuction to get rid of fat?"

Karen Duvall broke in with a laugh. "You'd get more candidates."

Heber still looked like he had been run over, so Love told him about the Love Paradigm—the rehabilitatable criminal, the breast cancer cells made dormant by changing the environment. Heber paid attention in spite of his frustration. This was what Love did best—goaded her patients and colleagues by reminding them that answers had to exist somewhere. Heber's research was just the kind of imaginative work that might lead to a prevention strategy. It was important that he not be defeated by logistics.

Dee Wieman was scheduled for an EKG in mid-June, about a week after her bilateral surgery, and by all rights she should have been pleased that the technician was someone she knew. He previously had done one of her bone scans, and he was a perfectly pleasant young man. But as he walked over to place the EKG leads on her chest she began to cry. She could not let him see the incisions. He had to find a woman to run the test instead.

A week later, on June 23, she had an appointment at Belle-Amie, Inc., a discreet suite of offices on the first floor of a two-story business park adjacent to the John Wayne Airport. The waiting room betrayed the owner's dual history as a breast cancer patient and a creator of special effects for Hollywood. There were turbans for women who had lost their hair to chemotherapy, a display of Joe Blasco theatrical makeup, and a comforting array of coffee and cold drinks—as well as movie posters and, atop a pillar, a huge statue of Mickey Mouse.

When Dee arrived the owner, Jan Thielbar, was waiting for her. This was Dee's third appointment. She had come here twice before her mastectomy to have plaster impressions taken—one, a cast of her torso when she was wearing a bra, and one, a cast of her naked breasts. Those were the models Thielbar would use to shape Dee's two prostheses. This appointment was for a third impression of Dee's chest, now that the surgery was over. If Dee had to wait six months for reconstruction, she wanted Thielbar's custom prostheses, which fit against the contours of an individual's body.

Dee stepped just inside the doorway and crossed her arms protectively over her chest.

"I don't fit so well today," she said, referring to the temporary prostheses Thielbar had provided. "I feel like I've got oranges sticking out in front of me."

Jan Thielbar smiled and held out a welcoming hand. She was a small, vivacious woman with a soft honey-blond pageboy and a sweet, slightly weary expression on her face. Jan had made her first custom prosthesis cast for herself—and though she ended up having only a lumpectomy, she could not forget the anguish she had felt at the prospect of losing a breast. She was all too familiar with how Dee felt.

"You've had something there all your life," said Thielbar quietly, "and then there's a void."

Dee quickly changed the subject. "You got a haircut, didn't you?" She pulled up the top of her wig to show the one-inch stubble that covered her head. It was black stippled with gray, and she was not at all sure she was happy to see it.

"I know it means that other things are growing," she said. "I ask, 'Don't I need some drugs?' but they say I'll get such a blast with the transplant that it'll kill everything."

Thielbar ushered Dee into a softly lit dressing room, complete with a mirrored vanity table, to show her some of her wares—two prostheses, one large, dark-skinned breast and a tiny pale one. She applied glue to the smaller prosthesis, affixed it to the skin on the back of her hand to show Dee how snugly it fit, and explained that many women liked to use the adhesive so that they could comfortably go swimming. Dee wondered aloud if she might just glue the breasts in place every day, but Thielbar dissuaded her. These prostheses fit so well that she would not need adhesive.

"So then I'll just wear any old stuff—bras—at night," said Dee. She had already decided to wear the prostheses twenty-four hours a day.

The technician, Candace, was waiting for Dee in the laboratory down the hall, ready with a goopy batch of plaster she had just mixed. It was time for Dee to get undressed, to surrender even the large elastic bandage she had refused to remove since the surgery. She slid out of her linen sheath, an ivory camisole and a fuschia brassiere, down to the wrap that covered her from her armpits to her waist, talking nonstop as Thielbar carefully hung her clothes on a hanger.

"I apologize for babbling," said Dee. "I know I'm doing it, and I can't stop it, but I do apologize."

"You babble away," said Jan.

Finally she was ready—a turquoise plastic apron to protect her half-slip, plastic covers for her shoes, a white towel draped over her naked shoulders. Dee held her head up and at an angle, as though she were trying to avoid looking at the two incisions that ran across her flat chest. Two weeks after her surgery there was still a row of Steri-Strips running across both incisions, though some of the thin bandages had begun to come loose. Dr. Giuliano had told her she could take them off by now, but she could not bring herself to do so. Jan removed the loose ones and trimmed the others, before Dee could resist.

It took about fifteen minutes to cover Dee's torso with a layer of thick liquid that hardened into a backing for the impression. The technician slathered it on with a spatula, from shoulders to waist, and then Dee stood motionless for five minutes while it dried. Jan took a marker and wrote Dee's name and the date on the cast, and drew a little heart.

Dee talked throughout the process. The next day she was going to UCLA for surgery to install a portable catheter in her chest, for the stem cell transplant, and Gary was being his usual skeptical self. He wanted Dee to call Dr. Glaspy and ask what her chances of recurrence were now that she had had the double mastectomy. At diagnosis she had a seventy percent chance of recurrence. Wouldn't removing her breasts reduce the risk to zero? He preferred not to think about systemic disease. Gary refused to regard micrometastases as a real threat—and he chose not to recall that even such extensive surgery left some breast cells behind.

"He's saying, 'In two months you'll be just like you were,'" said Dee with a rueful grin. "I'll never be like I was."

When Jan and the technician began to pry the drying cast off of Dee, her voice got shaky with fear. What if the pressure caused her wounds to open, and she began to bleed? "I'm sure nothing's open," she said, sounding unconvinced.

"Oh, Dee, nothing's open," said Jan.

She quickly cleaned the extra bits of plaster off of Dee's skin. Once she was clean, Jan pulled back a sheet on the lab table to reveal three very fancy, lacy bras, two mauve and one ivory, a 44 DDD—Dee's usual size was a 44 FF—and two 44 DD's, which Jan thought might make for a better look, since Dee had lost about thirty pounds to stress and chemotherapy.

Jan picked up the ivory bra and put it on Dee, empty. Dee stared heavenward. "This is weird. So weird. What a strange sensation this is."

"How's it feel?" asked Jan.

"OK. Do I really want to look?" She walked over to the mirror and twirled, just a little bit.

"It's a very pretty bra," said Candace.

Dee managed a wistful smile. "It is, isn't it?"

There were four half-round molds on the table, two exactly the shape Dee was before her surgery, and two a bit smaller, with the sides trimmed in.

"The projection is the same," explained Jan, "but you don't need that fatty tissue on the side."

These were measuring forms. As Jan fit two of them inside a bra she warned Dee that they were heavier than the final product, which had an air pocket in the center to lighten it.

"Oooh," said Dee, when the bra was fastened, "I've got bowling balls against my chest."

She stood in front of the mirror and studied every view: front, side, front again, the other side. Jan draped a T-shirt over Dee so that she could see how she would look with clothes on. She looked smaller than she used to—but this was fine for now, until she could have her plastic surgery.

Next, Jan produced a plastic bag that contained a little vial of liquid.

"We have your *nipple* color," she announced.

Dee slumped on a stool. "I don't even remember . . ."

"That we did it?"

"No. What they looked like."

Thielbar ignored the comment. "And we measured your areola."

"I know. I just haven't thought about all this for two weeks," said Dee. "About what's gone."

The answer came in a firm tone. "But we're moving on, Dee. Moving forward."

"Right."

"You'll wear these beautiful bras, Dee. I'm excited for you."

The technician mixed another color sample, this time to match the skin on Dee's chest, and then it was all over, time to get dressed. The prostheses would be ready in a couple of weeks.

"Well, you can leave," said Jan brightly. "We're done."

"I hate to leave," said Dee. "I feel so safe here."

It was the intimacy of shared experience, the comfort of being with people who understood. A woman like Shirley Barber was lucky; she was surrounded by family, by a husband and children who if anything seemed to pull more closely together when one of them was in trouble. Dottie had her family and friends. Barbara Rubin had made up a new family for herself, of friends and various therapists, when her past caved in to divorce and geographical distance.

But Dee had trouble confiding in Gary, and Jerilyn and Laura were cut off by their own sense that they were different. Jerilyn had begun to make friends at her support group, where they joked derisively about normal people, the ones who had no appreciation of what they had gone through, or of how precious a single carefree day could be. A lower life-form.

Laura yearned for that clubbiness and had not yet found it. In the days before her June 28 surgery she did not feel safe at all. She had not won the job she had wanted, which made it difficult to feel that she had a career at all. It had gone to a younger woman.

Laura's preoperative appointment with Dr. Shaw was early in the morning on Thursday, June 23, and what should have been a brief meeting became instead a marathon review of the advantages and disadvantages of each potential flap site. Laura still wanted him to promise that he would remove the left implant and lift that breast at the same time, although he reminded her again that he could not make that decision until he saw how long the reconstruction took. She complained about the iron pills she took to keep her blood healthy enough to donate, in case she needed a transfusion. She worried that her left breast would turn out to have cancer. She fretted over being crooked.

After Laura went through her litany of questions, she got to her real terror. She had endured several surgeries, but she did not tolerate anesthesia well, and she had never been out for an entire day.

"You ever had a patient die on you?" she asked.

"No," said Dr. Shaw. A nurse came in to escort Laura across the hall, where a photographer took a series of photographs of her naked—"Arms up," "Face the back wall," "Just part your hair and put it in front," "Turn to the forty-five-degree mark, now turn to the ninety."

Her next stop was the flap ward in the main hospital. Laura worried about the environment. Her home was testament to her belief in the impact of inanimate objects. If she had to spend five days in a drab hospital room, in one of those limp hospital gowns, she knew she was going to feel worse.

The surgery facilitator was an attractive, stylish woman who reassured Laura immediately. Yes, she could see a room. No, she could not redecorate it—but truly, it would not matter. She was going to doze her way through the first few days. The most important part of the decor would be the automatic dispenser that sent a premeasured amount of pain medication into Laura's veins when she pushed a button.

The facilitator took Laura over to one of the rooms, where three patients rested in the soft, curtained light of afternoon. She pointed out a woman who had had a bilateral simultaneous reconstruction only the day before, and when the patient saw them in the doorway she raised herself up slightly and beckoned to Laura. Hesitantly she walked over to the woman's bedside. They spoke in low voices for several minutes, and when Laura came back out into the hallway there were tears running down her cheeks.

She finally had found someone who knew from experience what she was about to go through. Susan Love could joke that Laura was going to feel like she had been run over by a truck. This woman had felt it. Laura was visibly relieved, and grateful. She had made the connection she had been looking for since the day Carol Fred told her not to come to the support group meeting. One emphatically busy weekend, full of appointments and dinner parties to keep her mind off the surgery, and she would be on her way.

For her part, Shirley Barber preferred to keep her relationship to breast cancer purely professional: she took her pills, kept her appointments, resented the calcifications, and tried to live a normal life despite them. It was summer, the season when the Barber family indulged its wanderlust. The day after school let out they packed up their recreational vehicle for an annual week-long camping trip north to Yosemite.

It was Shirley's favorite outing. They started with a leisurely drive—the standing joke was that the length of the trip depended entirely on how many mom-and-pop fruit stands Shirley wanted to visit. Once they got to the campground, the kids and their friends set up tents wherever they wanted, while Shirley and Tracy slept in the camper.

The good mood lasted even after they had returned home.

Somehow in the summer there was always time to goof off, even with Shirley flying again and Tracy running his own business. They went out to dinner; they went to the movies and ate junk food. One night Tracy wolfed down a hot dog so fast that he started to choke, and he had to leave the theater in search of a water fountain.

After a minute Shirley got up to look for him, but it was a ten-screen multiplex, and by the time she found him he was fine. She, however, was not. For a sudden instant she could not see out of one eye—briefly, but long enough to scare them both. She glared at her husband.

"If you try to choke yourself to death and make me have a stroke and go blind," she said, "I'll kill you."

By the time they got back into their seats they had missed a good chunk of the story. Shirley teased Tracy about that crucial scene whenever she got the chance. What a relief, for once, to have him interrupt the rhythm of their life instead of her.

The office Dr. John Glaspy came to at five thirty every morning was, like Glaspy himself, weighted down with information. There were books and magazines everywhere, not just on the shelves, but on his desk and on the floor. It was almost impossible to see the desktop, for all the phone slips, handwritten notes, copies of journal articles, and patient files. The office was tucked into the far corner of the Bowyer Oncology Center, as though cancer, over the years, had backed Glaspy against the wall.

After all the false starts, Dee Wieman had finally come in to start the transplant procedure. A surgeon implanted a portable catheter in her chest. She had her bone marrow harvest, an hour-long surgical procedure to collect marrow from her pelvic bones. The next step was the growth factor injections to stimulate the stem cells, followed by pheresis, to collect those cells from her bloodstream. Once her defenses were safely stored away, it was time for the high-dose chemotherapy.

Glaspy took little pleasure in the victory. All this bought Dee was possibility, nothing more.

Faith in transplants for patients like her, women with positive nodes but no demonstrable metastatic disease, rested on a shaky tripod: the theory that the earlier a woman received treatment, the better her chances; data from metastatic patients that showed improved survival in the first years following the procedure but said nothing about long-term results; and emotion, the willful desire to do something big, rather than sit around and wait.

Proponents of the transplant pointed to Duke University's compelling statistic for this new group of patients—a seventy percent disease-free survival rate after three years. Skeptics were quick to point out that Duke carefully screened its transplant candidates, but did not compare them to a control group. It could be that these women were healthier than the general population of breast cancer patients, and so likelier to survive no matter what treatment they had.

Glaspy felt he had a moral responsibility "to debunk this whole business, debunk it right away," whenever a patient came to him for treatment. He had told Dee about the limitations of transplants, although he was not sure she had heard him. Glaspy had one transplant patient who was still alive eight years out. He also had a patient who was diagnosed with metastatic disease in her liver in 1982, did not have a transplant, and was still alive twelve years later. And there was the transplant patient UCLA had lost just three months after the procedure. He could hardly give Dee a guarantee.

The one thing Glaspy did know was that a transplant did not cure women with demonstrable metastatic disease. It might shrink the tumor and buy them some time, but the cancer always came back. There was no way to tell how Dee would turn out. Patients with more than ten positive nodes but no distant metastases were relative newcomers to the procedure. It would be years before anyone knew if transplants improved their survival rate.

He was frankly not interested in buying time; there were plenty of drugs that might purchase months, or even a couple of years, but the stated goal with transplants was to eradicate disease, not stun it temporarily. With that as the criterion, the procedure had failed.

"The goal of this treatment is to have more cures," Glaspy said, "and if it does not cure more people it's a failure, in my opinion. There are people who would say, 'No, if it prolongs life it's a success,' but I think the goal we had going in was to cure people. You can't change your goal and then declare a success.

"It's more often a repudiation of standard therapy than it is an affirmation of this wonderful new therapy." Transplants only proved that some patients failed to respond to chemotherapy no matter how high the dose.

Three weeks after her daughter was born, Ann Donaldson picked up the front section of the *Los Angeles Times* and saw a headline that left her paralyzed with fear: PREGNANCY AND BREAST CANCER POSE LETHAL RISK: A NEW STUDY SAYS EXPECTANT WOMEN WHO HAVE THE DISEASE ARE THREE TIMES AS LIKELY TO DIE.

Epidemiologists from Houston's M.D. Anderson Cancer Center had studied 407 breast cancer patients who were treated between 1978 and 1988, all of them in their twenties, some of them pregnant, and found that expectant mothers were likelier to die of the disease than other women. There was no explanation—perhaps hormonal changes did spur on an existing malignancy, perhaps a weakened immune system made it harder for a pregnant woman to fight the disease—but the findings seemed to have nothing to do with the accepted notion that pregnant women fared poorly because their cancers were detected late. This study showed that a pregnant woman in her twenties who developed breast cancer was likelier to die of it regardless of how advanced her disease was.

Worse, doctors assumed that the heightened mortality risk applied to all pregnant women, regardless of age. The newspaper reported that both Dr. Vincent Guinee, one of the authors of the study, and Dr. Eugenia Calle, of the American Cancer Society, agreed, "the results with the young women should hold for pregnant women of all ages."

What Dr. Love had told Ann was partly right: no one understood exactly how pregnancy affected breast cancer. But whatever the connection was, it could kill her.

30

THE OPERATING ROOM

LAURA'S SISTER AND HER TWO BEST FRIENDS HAD BECOME HER SURGERY support team since her 1988 diagnosis. They were working women whose schedules were not flexible enough to accommodate Laura's doctors' appointments, but they always banded together for her surgeries—the implants, the first surgical biopsy and lumpectomy, the recent biopsy and re-excision, the abortion, and now the mastectomy and reconstruction. On Monday, June 27, the night before the operation, they slept at Laura's house to keep her from being nervous—and did so well that all four of them slept peacefully through the four thirty alarm. Luckily, another friend called at four forty-five to make sure they were ready to leave at five.

They were resourceful beauties who were used to looking their best on schedule. Somehow they managed to get in and out of the bathroom in record time, find a predawn cappuccino on their way to UCLA, and land in room 213 of the university's main hospital by six, looking as composed as if they had spent a languid morning anticipating a stylish lunch. They were insistently lovely—perfectly groomed, well-dressed, nails polished, hair burnished to a healthy sheen. They clustered around Laura's bed as though they could, by their very presence, will her to return to them, and to her old, fashionable ways.

Dr. Love appeared just before seven to accompany Laura's wheeled bed to the elevator that would take her to the basement, where the inpatient operating rooms were located. She rarely came over to the main hospital these days. All the surgical biopsies and lumpectomies were done on an outpatient basis in the Medical Center building where the Breast Center was located, and she intended soon to start doing simple mastectomies there as well. She expected eventually to come across the street only for surgeries like Laura's, or for women with other health problems who needed more extensive care. The twenty-three-hour stay—less than a day, easily covered even by managed care—was going to be a staple of the medical future.

She stood in clumsy counterpoint to the other women, shuffling along in her hospital scrubs and shapeless cover gown, a dowdy disposable hairnet on her head. As they and the orderly made their way to the elevator behind Laura's bed the three women ganged up on Dr. Love, entreating her to take the very best care of their friend. "Are you sure she'll get her Zofran?" asked one, referring to an expensive antinausea medicine that had kept Laura from getting sick after her most recent surgery. "She gets sick from anesthesia. She'll throw up for thirty-six hours. I mean, one time the anesthesiologist had to come to her house."

Love looked confused. "Why wouldn't she get it?"

Laura's friend said that the anesthesiologist had told Laura it was too expensive—that other, cheaper drugs would be good enough. Love scoffed at the idea, and promised to make sure Laura got the drug.

When the elevator opened, the orderly rolled the bed in, and Laura's friends quickly crowded around her. There was no room left for Dr. Love, who shrugged and headed for the stairs.

At seven fifteen in the morning the pre-op holding room looked like some demented airport lounge. Knots of people studied a television monitor that listed the day's procedures, crowded around their departing loved one, held babies up to be kissed good-bye, and offered good-luck wishes in a half dozen dialects. At the appointed moment orderlies appeared to whisk each traveler away—for he or she was at that point halfway to happy oblivion, premedicated, chemically calm. It was the relatives and friends who felt the frenetic anxiety of the place, and anticipated a long, blank morning awaiting word. One little boy distracted himself with a video game; his father comforted his crying baby sister.

Nurses and doctors bustled about, dispatching patients to one of twenty-one operating rooms, maneuvering beds out of their berths and rolling them down the hall. One tall, slender doctor with a melancholy air approached the man with the crying baby and gently took her from her father's arms. He shuffled down the hall, his footsteps muted by the cotton surgical slippers that covered his athletic shoes, and as he escorted his tiny charge to the room where doctors would open her body, he cooed to her. He held her against his shoulder, her tiny, sleepy face nestled against his neck, and bounced her ever so gently, up and down.

Love shuddered as they passed. "I hate pediatric surgery," she said, to no one in particular. "The good news is that they get well really fast, but . . ." She had never gotten over her initial resistance to pediatrics. It was hard enough to inflict pain on adults who could understand why they had to have a shot or a surgical drain, let alone on some little kid who had no idea why the doctor was being so mean.

Laura did not have to wait in the holding room. Simultaneous reconstructions took as long as eight hours, so they were always scheduled for the first slot of the morning. By the time Love got downstairs Laura's bed was parked in the cold, bright hallway outside of Operating Room 9. Her friends could not accompany her that far, and left alone, in the uncompromising light, Laura quickly lost her confidence. Her lower lip began to quiver. Her eyes darted around, as though she were looking for an exit. Love laid a hand on her shoulder to steady her, and Laura confessed that her last visit to Shaw had made her very nervous. She did not see how he could possibly make her a new breast to match what the other one would look like once the implant was gone.

The anesthesiologist, a cheerful, fresh-faced woman, came up behind Laura's bed and overheard her anxious patter. As she pushed Laura into the OR she leaned over and whispered, "Okay. Now we're going to give you some good stuff."

* * *

A few moments later Dr. Shaw arrived, and he and Love huddled in a corner to review Laura's case, out of her earshot. But as soon as she noticed him she raised her head and called out. One last time, she implored him to remove the implant in the healthy breast and perform a lift, to make her two breasts match.

"The lift?" He was so focused on the reconstruction that he had forgotten about the other procedure.

"I'm trying to get a handle on what my psyche will be when I wake up," said Laura, in her most efficient voice. "Will I be small on the right side and big on the left, lopsided like I've been for four months, or what? Do you have time to take out the implant and do the lift?"

Love came over to help. She knew it was unlikely that Shaw would do anything beyond the delicate reconstruction. "Depending on the tailwind," she joked, trying to break the tension. "On how long we sit on the tarmac. It's too soon to tell."

Shaw sat on a stool alongside Laura, and she sat up and dropped her gown to her waist. He picked up his pen and began to draw on her breast, to show Love what he needed her to do before he began the reconstruction. Love watched in awe.

"This is the most important part," she said. "The surgery's easy."

More and more people drifted into the OR, and Laura made a vain attempt to keep a running tally of who worked with Susan and who belonged to plastics. By seven fifty she was on her left side and Shaw was drawing the incision lines on her buttocks. The premedication continued to drip.

"Laura, are you feeling relaxed?" the anesthesiologist asked.

"A little relaxed. Not completely relaxed."

"You could still use a little something?"

"Yeah," said Laura. "To help me acquiesce."

Love flipped through Laura's chart with mounting impatience, looking for a number she could not find. She knew that her facilitators and Shaw's office must have allowed at least three weeks between Laura's last chemotherapy and this surgery, but she could not find proof of it in Laura's records. She was not going to embark on a day-long procedure without hard proof that Laura's system was strong enough to handle it.

"When did you have your last chemotherapy?" she demanded of Laura. "Do you know your numbers?"

Laura could not recall her white blood count, and she had great difficulty figuring out how many weeks it had been since her last chemotherapy treatment. She was starting to get foggy.

"I'm not worried," said Love, "but if your white blood count was low you'd be in increased danger of infection."

Laura dreamily suggested that Love call her oncologist, but the surgeon doubted that anyone would be at work this early. She dispatched a nurse to fax up to her office for the results.

There were now ten people milling about the room, and Laura's body was shrouded in white. The anesthesiologist raised Laura's head slightly to tell her that she had given Laura more drugs twice, both times she had asked—and in a little while, if Laura felt the need, she could have some more. In the meantime, Shaw took photographs with a big Nikon for his before-and-after study, and Love waited for the white blood count numbers. By the time she got them from the Breast Center and reported the news to her patient, Laura was too relaxed to care.

Just after eight o'clock, with nineteen people in the OR, Love stepped over to Laura's side and took her hand. Most surgeons would be scrubbing at this point. But Love insisted on being with a patient at what she called the moment of greatest fear, just before the anesthesia was administered. A woman was most vulnerable then, and did not need to be abandoned to strangers. It was an unusual practice. The surgeon usually arrived after a patient was asleep, and Love frequently had to remind the anesthesiologists not to get started without her. Now she rubbed the back of Laura's hand with her thumb, and gazed into her patient's slightly glazed eyes.

"I think there's hope for you," was the last thing Laura heard her say.

From behind Laura's head came the anesthesiologist's soothing voice: "You know, Laura, we're going to give you some oxygen, and then some medicine, and you're going to go to sleep. We're going to take really good care of you, so take a few deep breaths."

Love held Laura's hand and watched the anesthesiologist as she placed a mask over Laura's face. Moments later, Laura's hand went limp, but Love continued to massage it gently. It took two people to pry open Laura's mouth and insert a breathing tube down her throat; only when they were finished did Love relinquish that hand.

The anesthesiologist looked up and asked, "How'd she find it the second time?"

"Mammography," said Susan.

The anesthesiologist shook her head pityingly. "And she's a nice lady, isn't she?"

"A nice lady," said Susan. "Not a very good luck lady."

Once Laura was unconscious she began to disappear. The nurses worked quickly to prepare her naked body for surgery. They pulled socks up to her knees and put boots on over them to massage her calves and prevent phlebitis. They pressed EKG leads onto her chest to monitor her heartbeat, and inserted a Foley catheter into her bladder to enable her to urinate. Her left arm was stretched out on a padded board with a blood pressure monitor attached to a fingertip.

There was tape over Laura's eyes to hold them closed, and around the tube that went into her mouth. At eight twenty the anesthesiologist carefully tucked the patient's mass of thick black hair into a pale blue cap. All the while Laura's mouth was frozen open, as though she were appalled, even in her chemical sleep, by these physical humiliations.

The nurses struggled to arrange her limbs in the proper position for the surgeries. They heaved her onto her left side and strapped her legs into place, her right leg slightly in front of the other, as though she were taking a walk. A white blanket covered her up to her thighs, but her buttocks, hip, and pelvis remained uncovered.

The nurses pushed her torso down flat and pulled her right arm up and out of the way, wrapped first in an ivory sock and then a taped fabric cover, positioned on a metal frame over her head. Much of her pain that evening would be from muscle cramps, from lying so long in a torqued position, but there was no choice. The plastic surgery team had to get at her right hip while Dr. Love and her resident worked on her chest.

By eight thirty it was time to begin cleansing Laura's body. Plastics started at the bottom, the breast team at the top, and in a few minutes her entire torso was wet with Betadine, a coppery red disinfectant. From her upper thigh to her neck, front and back, up her right arm, her skin no longer seemed like skin, but rather like some fragment of an ancient bronze sculpture.

Only then did Love leave the room to scrub.

She had once observed a breast surgeon in Sapporo, Japan, and had been delighted to find that the surgical ritual was the same there as it was in the United States. All this draping and cleansing was a comforting tradition, for it enabled the surgeon to put some distance between herself and the woman she had been talking to only minutes before. By the time the nurses and residents were finished with Laura Wilcox, she would be invisible—a technical exercise, not a person. Love defined surgery for her residents as a terribly intimate act between strangers. Ritual took the raw edge off the intrusion.

When Love came back into the OR she held out her arms so the nurses could help her into her operating gown and gloves. One of them spun her around to tie the strings of the gown around her waist. Having stepped on her eyeglasses the day before, Love donned large plastic goggles over her contact lenses, to protect her eyes from any spurting blood.

While she was scrubbing, Bill Shaw came back into the room to survey the body. Silently he placed a blue fabric drape over Laura's face and attached it to her neck with a staple gun. He placed a second drape under her left breast and brought it up along her torso, over her crotch, to a line just below the drawing of her hip incision. For a long moment the only sounds in the room were the bleep of the heart monitor and the *ke-thick, ke-thick* of the staple gun. Shaw stapled a third blue drape over Laura's outstretched right arm just as Love came back into the room.

She looked around. "The operation is so anticlimactic after all this," she said.

"Yes," said Shaw. "After all the planning and discussion."

He moved the last drape into place—a large piece hung verti-cally in front of Laura's face, to separate the anesthesiologist's domain from the surgeons'. Laura was completely gone, and they could begin.

Love quickly stepped into place behind the operating table. "I need a knife," she said. "A knife. Skin hooks. Let's get going."

Next to her the plastics resident who would begin to prepare the flap site rested his hand for a silent moment on Laura's right hip—as though in prayer, as though trying to make peace with a woman he had never met.

Ever the teacher, Love glanced over and murmured to her resident, "Never touch the body until you check with the anesthesiologist."

A moment later the acrid smell of burning skin filled the air, as Love made her first skin incision with a knife and then used an electrocautery, a delicate, penlike instrument, to simultaneously cut the tissue and cauterize the wound. Smoke rose from the cut. Simon & Garfunkel floated into the room, courtesy of the hospital sound system, singing their 1970 song "Keep the Customer Satisfied": "And I'm one step ahead of the shoeshine / Two steps away from the county line / Just trying to keep my customers satisfied / Satisfied."

A mastectomy was simple enough surgery, a matter of cutting the breast tissue away from the skin and then peeling it off the underlying muscle. Love's resident, Mike Walker, worked alongside her, and she kept up a running commentary on what she was doing. They worked up to the collarbone, down toward the bottom ribs, in to the breastbone and out to the latissimus muscle. Breast tissue extended far in each direction, and while Love knew she could not get it all—it looked just like other tissue—she wanted to get as much as possible.

There was plenty of time to kibbitz with the plastics team, and she tried to keep them entertained. They were going to be there most of the day; she wanted them to be in a good mood. So she taunted them about doing free flaps—"I didn't think you guys in plastics did anything for free"—and inquired frequently about their progress.

One of the surgeons complained that Laura was too fit. They needed fat, not lean muscle, to make this work.

"Buns of steel," he muttered.

"That's it," said Love, referring to a popular exercise videotape. "She's been doing *Buns of Steel*. Only in southern California would you find buns of steel."

"Right," said Dr. Christina Ahn, a colleague of Dr. Shaw's who oversaw the preliminary work. "In most places—"

Her male colleague interrupted, "It would be buns of Jell-O."

An hour and twenty minutes after she began, Susan Love handed the results of her effort to Mike Walker, who placed it on a blue cloth held out by a surgical nurse: Laura Wilcox's right breast, removed from her body in a single piece, the nipple and the scar from her 1988 surgery still attached. All that remained—and the most difficult part of the procedure—was to locate the vein and artery that had kept this tissue alive, and would now supply blood to Laura's reconstructed breast.

Love could not find them. Laura's body was tilted just enough to make the blood vessels hard to find under any circumstances, and the scar tissue from her 1988 surgery made it even harder.

"It's socked in," she complained to Dr. Ahn. "I haven't seen it. I started to poke, but it could be a little deeper."

Ahn took Mike Walker's place and peered at the open wound. Shaw stepped up and Love moved out of the way. Moments later, Ahn announced that she had found the blood vessels, and Love was visibly relieved.

"Now I feel better," she said. "Christina's made me happy." She and Walker could head over to Operating Room 18 to see if their next patient was ready. She had done everything she could for Laura.

Love was an hour late starting her second mastectomy of the day, but before she began her next operation she dashed upstairs to the lobby, where nervous friends and relatives waited for news. Laura's friends were not there. The volunteer at the visitors' desk called out, "Wilcox. Wilcox," in the hope that they might magically materialize. The others in the waiting room looked around too, knowing that Wilcox's friends, wherever they were, would be upset to have missed the surgeon's report. Love waited a minute and then ran back downstairs to the pathology lab to see if they had yet received a breast tissue sample to look at, on her way to hold the next patient's hand.

An acrid smell filled the operating room again, as smoke rose from Laura Wilcox's hip. The plastics team had freed the wedge of tissue that Shaw would reattach and fashion into a breast.

At eleven two orderlies wheeled a Zeiss Universal S3 Super-Lux 40 microscope into the operating room—a hulking seven-foot-tall T-shaped piece of equipment with eyepieces that hung down from each side of the T—and centered it over Laura's chest. Dr. Ahn took a seat behind Laura. Dr. Shaw sat down facing Laura. The Zeiss allowed them to see the tiny blood vessels, one set from her armpit, one set from the flap, that had to be joined for the tissue to survive. What they saw also appeared on a large color monitor in the rear corner of the room, and as they got ready to work three middle-aged doctors suddenly appeared and crowded in behind the staff working at the operating table. The man whom Susan Love referred to as "the king of flaps" was about to go to work; anyone who thought about performing the operation wanted to observe.

Shaw surveyed the others' handiwork. Love had made a dauntingly deep excavation in Laura's chest. The ends of Laura's ribs showed under the skin, just at the edge of the hole.

"All right," he announced. "Let's do this now."

The plastics team severed the flap's blood supply and lifted it out of Laura's body. It lay on a sterile blue cloth on a small steel table, next to where the breast specimen still lay.

"Could I have a picture with my camera?" asked Shaw.

One of the visiting doctors accommodatingly picked up the camera and photographed the empty flap site, as well as the flap tissue.

It was time to close the hip, reconnect the flap, and shape it into a breast, stitching the flap skin to the loose skin that had covered Laura's breast. Shaw worked on the hip for half an hour before turning it over to another of the surgeons to complete the stitching. At noon he stretched and secured Laura's right arm, to open the armpit area even more and make sure there was no movement. The monitor showed a mass of dark tissue with a small, pulsing area near the center—one of the blood vessels that Shaw had to connect to the flap.

One of the plastic surgery nurses hoisted the flap and handed it over to him, and he placed it on the empty space where Laura's breast had been. He took his seat at the Zeiss and began to look for the single vein and artery he had to free from the flap tissue. It was an odd, disjointed exercise. Shaw sat rigidly upright, staring into the eyepiece, while his hands did his bidding. He never looked down at Laura—only at the magnified image that guided his hands.

The procedure went on for over five hours, slightly longer than they had expected, because the scar tissue from Laura's node dissection made it hard to connect the blood vessels. When it was done Shaw stitched the skin that had covered Laura's breast to the skin on the flap tissue. Finally, in the late afternoon, it was over. They turned Laura onto her back and placed her on an air mattress, put surgical dressings on her hip and thin rows of Steri-Strips across her new breast. A temperature probe was attached to the reconstructed breast to make sure the temperature did not dip below 32 degrees Celsius, a signal that there was something wrong with the blood supply, and Laura was taken up to the flap unit that she had visited the week before, the specially staffed unit for patients who had reconstructive surgery using their own tissue.

By six in the evening Laura began to regain consciousness. As she stirred, her friends and her sister reappeared at her bedside, finished with work for the day, fully intending to stay with her through the night to make sure she was all right. For all her determination, Laura feared and hated surgery, and her system was easily thrown out of whack—as though all her carefully managed anxiety welled up and demanded physical release. They were not going to let her go through the first night alone.

At 6:15 P.M. Mike Walker, the surgery resident, came in to see Laura. Her face was puffy from all the tape, her eyes shut, her features vague from the pain medication. But she managed one question.

"Did they do everything on the left?" she asked. She still hoped that Shaw had removed her other implant, and in the process discovered that that breast was free of cancer.

"Everything?"

"They get all the cancer?"

"As far as we know."

"And did they do the . . ." She stopped herself. He wouldn't know about the implant. "I guess I'll ask plastics."

"Can I take a look?" asked Walker. He peered at her right breast, a swollen, reddened mound with stitches marching across it. "Looks great."

A moment later Love walked in. The surgical process never failed to amaze her: an anesthesiologist put the patient into a comatose state, paralyzed him, and then doctors did outrageous things to his body—held a heart in their hands, transplanted a liver, moved tissue and made it live again. That same night the patient was up and talking. No matter how many surgeries Love performed, the process still seemed magical.

Laura was not in any state to appreciate the transition.

"So," said Love, "you feel like a truck ran over you?"

"Yeah."

"Okay. It did. Ran right over you. But it's done. Now you just have to get your nipple." Love peeked at the new breast. "It looks great."

"Oooh, I did get hit," mumbled Laura, from the far side of her medication. "Gonna throw up."

Love grabbed a pink tray and handed it to Laura. "Okay. Turn your head."

Laura slumped back onto the pillow. "Maybe not. Oooh."

"Okay, where's your bell?" Love rang for a nurse. "See you tomorrow." She was out the door. Laura was still too woozy to appreciate her doctor's patented optimism, but there was another patient in the next room who was already two days out and eager to talk.

At two in the morning Mike Walker walked down the deserted hallway, hoping for a catnap, when Laura Wilcox's three friends rushed out of the flap unit and grabbed him. Something was wrong, beyond Laura's usual postoperative distress.

"We've been through nine surgeries with her," one of them said, "and she never looked like this."

When Walker got to her bed Laura was thrashing around, her legs twitching, not quite in seizure but shaking, and very agitated. Someone had paged Dr. Shaw at home, who insisted on trying to speak to Laura to calm her down, but all she could do was scream into the receiver that she wanted a gun to end her misery. She was tugging at the socks on her legs, trying to pull them off, and Walker noticed that her hands were beginning to curl inward, almost like claws. That was a classic sign of calcium deficiency—and when he tested her blood her other salts were low too. He turned her over to check the incision on her buttock, and that looked fine.

It must be a calcium deficiency—perhaps all the intravenous fluids had flushed her out too well, washed the calcium she needed out of her system. Laura was sobbing about the pain in her legs, and her terror only increased when she saw Walker preparing an injection. It was more than she could stand.

First he gave her a shot of Valium in her thigh, to calm her down, and then set up an intravenous drip of two grams of calcium gluconate along with other salts. The shot and the fluids took effect quickly, and enabled her to sleep through the rest of the night. When Love stopped by early the next morning to see her patient, unaware of the night's drama, she found Laura sitting up in bed and eager to talk. The magic Love depended on had worked, with a slight late-night assist from Mike Walker. Her patient had returned to the living.

Love and Mike Walker were both a bit punchy all day, the aftereffect of Laura's surgery and her scary first night post-op. The free flap was proof that doctors could manipulate nature; the surprise calcium deficiency, a sharp reminder not to get too cocky. Still, Laura had got through it all right. It was hard not to be just a little impressed with modern medicine.

When Love walked into the facilitators' office that afternoon she asked Shannon who the first diagnostic patient was.

"Young woman with a grape-size firm lump," came the reply.

Love snorted derisively. "Fibroadenoma," she said, referring to the kind of benign tumor usually found in young women. "Soon I'm going to get to the point where I can stay home and do this by phone."

31

STALLED PROGRESS

THE LARGESSE OF THE EARLY 1990s WAS START-UP MONEY, REALLY. The Women's Health Initiative was the first attempt to elevate the level of research on women's health issues, with long-range trials, and the Defense Department program was the government's first concerted effort against breast cancer. The National Action Plan on Breast Cancer that Clinton had announced in October 1993 was meant to create an ongoing strategy that exceeded the scope of either of those programs.

The focus of breast cancer research had shifted, thanks to an infusion of money and the NSABP scandal. What had been an elite enterprise had become a populist concern, driven by activist demand as well as scientific inspiration. The problem, now, was to make the new model work.

The two cochairs of the National Action Plan, Fran Visco and Dr. Susan Blumenthal, faced a daunting task, given the institutionalized disregard that had preceded their efforts. They supervised a six-month effort to catalog existing and proposed government programs and identify gaps that needed filling, and by June had a list of six "priority action areas" and nineteen "short-term priority action areas" that required immediate attention.

Blumenthal—the NIH alumna, the congressman's wife—was the consummate insider. Visco was edgier, more impatient, quicker to take things personally. She understood that the stately pace was appropriate to the task of defining a national agenda, but the longer the process wore on the more frustrated she became. She had learned Donna Shalala's lesson well: In politics there was no such thing as a heartfelt ally; only expedient rapport. She was doing her best to get along, but Visco did not need a list of action items to tell her that not enough women had good access to breast care, no one knew what clinical trials were available to them, and the available methods of early detection were seriously flawed.

Like Love, Visco was looking for a new paradigm. If this was what it meant to be a Washington insider—overseeing a plodding bureaucracy that took an inordinate amount of time to state the obvious—then she was happier on the outside. Making trouble was far easier than making policy.

On July 8, 1994, Dr. Bernard Fisher filed a federal lawsuit against the University of Pittsburgh, seeking reinstatement as chairman of the NSABP. He charged that the university and the NCI had acted illegally when they demanded that he resign—and he continued to insist, as he had at the June 15 congressional hearing, that NSABP staff members had informed the NCI of the falsified lumpectomy data as soon as it was discovered. He claimed he was not responsible for the ensuing delays. If NCI director Dr. Samuel Broder had truly considered the matter an emergency, Fisher asserted, there were steps he could have taken.

A week later Susan Love got another phone call from Dr. Ronald Herberman, the interim director of the NSABP who had invited her to join the oversight committee. This time he wanted to know if she was interested in heading up the NSABP. It was certainly a flattering inquiry, but she turned him down. The last thing she needed was more administrative responsibility.

Depending on how bad a day they were having, doctors and researchers guessed that it would be another five, or ten, or fifteen years before there was a breakthrough in terms of breast cancer prevention or cure. Visco and Love had to strengthen the

NBCC for the long haul. The Coalition's short-term strength was its handful of leaders. If the group was going to prevail over time, there had to be a national network of trained activists. The NBCC had to live up to its reputation as a grassroots organization—but at the moment it was a loose-knit group, buoyed over the last year by petition-drive volunteers who needed to know what to do next.

Growth took money. The Coalition had been working for months to ensure a second two-year appropriation from the Defense Department, pushing this time for a $150 million appropriation. That effort took travel, and time in Washington, and orchestrated pressure from women around the country. Revlon raised more money than any of the Coalition's other corporate donors because it underwrote the group's annual fund-raising dinner in New York, but the NBCC had a healthy list of other donors, including Wellcome Oncology, Bristol-Myers Squibb, Co., and several financial institutions and philanthropic organizations. There were angels within the NBCC ranks as well, wealthy patients who expressed their gratitude by paying for Visco's travel expenses or underwriting part of her salary.

It was never enough to subsidize Visco's ambition. On Saturday, July 9, she and Love attended a fund-raiser for the NBCC at the Coral Casino, a private beach club in Montecito, California, an exclusive enclave just south of Santa Barbara.

At sunset, a handsome woman in a tasteful silk dress stood next to the buffet table, chatting with a friend.

"No one in *my* family has it," she said, loud enough for those nearby to understand that she was there purely out of charity. "But I guess this has to start somewhere."

Her friend answered in a low voice.

"*You* had it?" said the first woman in a startled tone. "I didn't know."

While the guests circled the food, Love and Visco huddled on the small stage platform to work on Love's speech. Visco, who had already prepared her remarks, knew what points she wanted Love to address, and as she rattled them off Love frantically scribbled notes on a small pad.

Visco wanted Love to mention statistics, and they both agreed that she had to refer to breast cancer as an epidemic.

"And I'm going to talk about activism," said Love.

"No," cautioned Visco, looking around the room. There were over one hundred guests, clearly a wealthy crowd, and probably a fairly conservative one. They would be likelier to write a check than to pester a congressman or collect petition signatures. "I don't think this is a crowd that wants to hear that."

"They *do*," replied Love. "They're coming up to me and talking about being obnoxious. They do."

"Okay," said Fran, unconvinced. "You say that, and then introduce me."

"Right," said Love. "I'll say, 'And here's the most obnoxious person I know.'"

Love gave her usual rousing speech, and Visco followed with an inspirational history of the NBCC. Then she paused for a moment. How many times had she stood in front of a roomful of strangers and exhorted them to get involved? How many weekends away from her husband and son? She was on sabbatical from her law firm that year, and even so, she never seemed to have a moment for herself. Breast cancer had not killed her, but it had claimed her life.

When she spoke again her voice had a sorrowful edge.

"If I had been given a choice I wouldn't be here. I'd be a lawyer in Philadelphia with my husband and son," she said. The casual chatter in the crowd stopped abruptly. This was Susan Love's career, but it was Fran Visco's fate. She was there because of a blip on a mammogram, and every other woman in the room could be one exam away from the same surprise. For all the statistics, the governmental neglect, it was the plight of the woman behind the podium that seemed to evoke the strongest response.

"But I wasn't given a choice," she went on. "I was given an opportunity, and I seized it, to use my energy and resources to solve this problem."

She made a pitch for funds, but she did not need to work very hard. There were new sounds in the room—handbags being opened, checkbooks being pulled out of suit jacket pockets, pages riffling, pens clicking open.

* * *

Medicine marked time in decades. To the patients, eternity could be ten minutes long. Monday, July 11, was Dee Wieman's BCNU day, and it made the three days of high-dose chemotherapy that preceded it seem like a holiday. All morning Dee's father and stepmother waited in chairs set out between the elevator banks. Gary ferried between them and Dee's room, where he could sit for only five or ten minutes before he had to come out to the makeshift waiting area to collect himself.

They had been warned. Linda Norton had told Dee and her family that BCNU elicited dramatic reactions. Nothing could have prepared Gary for what his wife was doing.

She was like a wild woman—agitated, restless, whiny and angry by turns, nauseated, and then, a split second later, seized by racking diarrhea. The medicine that was supposed to turn her back into his charming wife had for the moment transformed her into a bald, sweaty, bilious monster. Gary tried to stay in the room with Dee. He sat in the chair at the foot of her curtained bed and studied his jingling car keys and his kneecaps, but he was able to look up at her only briefly. After a few minutes he got to his feet, slowly, heavily, and lumbered out into the hallway. He looked confused, as though his eyes could not adjust to the light, and when he emerged his father-in-law called to him, softly, to guide him over to a chair.

"It's going okay," Gary said. There were tears in his eyes. He sat down, he stood up, he looked down the long hallway for no reason at all, and then he went back into his wife's room.

Dee's stepmother reached over to hold her husband's hand. Maynard Smith and his wife, Rita, had driven in from the desert to be at his daughter's side. He intended to stay in town until she was through the worst of this—but he could not bear to go into his daughter's room, not today.

When she regained her sanity—and it would be two weeks of fevers and pain and paranoia before she did—Dee swore to anyone who would listen that the transplant experience was a thousand times worse than she had expected. She had forgotten most of the details, a common side effect of the combination of drugs, disease complications, and isolation, but in a way that was the hardest thing. Everyone else knew what had happened. Her husband had been there when the nurses had to change her soiled bedclothes; he had seen her without her wig. She had lost control of what was left of her body, and instead of looking forward toward health she kept glancing back over her shoulder in embarrassment.

In the last days of the transplant she had started making early morning phone calls to her friend Suzy, begging her to come help Dee pack up and go home, entreating her to sleep over in the hospital room to see how awful it was. She told Suzy everything: how hard it was to swallow, how much her chest hurt, how she hated the smell of food and the tray it came on and the perfume she was sure the inconsiderate nurse was wearing. Her stomach hurt. The only one who understood what she was going through was Dr. Boasberg, who a couple of times had come to visit her early in the morning, around six thirty, before he went to his own office at St. John's. The UCLA doctors were not listening to her—or rather, they were not responding in the way she wanted them to.

She told them she was going to die if she had to stay in that hospital room a day longer. The only way she would survive was to get back home. Instead, they suggested medication to calm her down and warned of the increased risk of infection outside the hospital halls. She thought she would lose what was left of her mind.

There were the women who suffered, and then there were the ones who wondered: Am I next? Dee Wieman had a sister and a grown daughter. Laura had two sisters, Jerilyn and Ann, one each. Dottie had a daughter and a granddaughter. Shirley and Barbara, both of them adopted, had no idea how many siblings they might have, but each one had a daughter.

Mary-Claire King had been trying since 1976 to give the relatives of breast cancer patients a better sense of their own risk, but the spring and early summer yielded only disappointment. Her team found differences between the DNA of healthy people and those with hereditary breast cancer in sixteen different genes, but each time they discovered exceptions that forced them to rule out a given candidate. A flaw showed up in a healthy subject, or failed to in a breast cancer patient: the families King was studying simply refused to give up the location of the gene that was making so many of them sick.

Other researchers, including Francis Collins of the National Center for Human Genome Research, faced the same seeming dead end. They were right where the answer was supposed to be, and could not find it.

At the same time, Mark Skolnick's team pushed ever closer to what he was sure was the answer. The first hint of victory for his group came in July, from the offices of the government-funded National Institute of Environmental Health Sciences in Chapel Hill, North Carolina, where two of Skolnick's collaborators were working. The young scientists, Roger Wiseman and Andy Futreal, had narrowed down the list of possible candidates from dozens of genes on the seventeenth chromosome to one particularly promising gene.

Researchers at Myriad simultaneously conducted their own tests, and when they screened the Chapel Hill gene with DNA from the families they were studying, they found the link between disease and an altered gene that had for almost four years eluded researchers around the world: family members with breast cancer had a mutated form of the gene, while their healthy relatives had normal copies.

One of Skolnick's Utah colleagues immediately started looking for the mutations in a larger sampling of breast cancer families— and everyone on Skolnick's team kept their mouths shut. Until they were absolutely certain, any leaked information only gave the competing teams a chance to make the discovery first.

On July 12, *The New York Times* ran a story by the paper's Pulitzer prize–winning science reporter, Natalie Angier, headlined, VEXING PURSUIT OF BREAST CANCER GENE, which noted that scientists had been promising victory "any day, any week, any month now. They have been saying that for the past two years." Mary-Claire King professed her optimism, and divulged that her lab was looking carefully at a candidate gene nicknamed Odo, after one of the characters in the television series *Star Trek: Deep Space Nine*. Francis Collins said he hoped for an answer in the next few months, "but it wouldn't be wise to say that with great assurance, given the fact that I said that a few months ago." Mark Skolnick was not quoted on how much longer the search would take.

As the summer dragged on, NIH director Harold Varmus suggested devoting $1 million of the NIH's discretionary fund to the effort to locate BRCA-1. He planned to decide in September which of the research teams would get the special grant.

Shirley Barber refused to come in for a mammogram unless Dr. Love was available to read the film right away, so she ignored the NSABP's end-of-June mammogram deadline for participants in the tamoxifen study. She finally showed up on July 19, the first day that her and Susan's schedules intersected.

One of the research nurses on the NSABP trial was waiting for Shirley when she got up to the Breast Center from the mammography suite. The NCI had instructed the University of Pittsburgh to have all the 270 participating facilities collect revised consent forms from women in the tamoxifen trials, because of the new risk data on uterine cancer. Shirley had been sent the new form, which the nurse wanted to discuss.

Shirley handed it over already signed; she was not interested in hearing the litany of statistics. Tamoxifen did not scare Shirley half as much as breast cancer did. She proudly listed her symptoms, just serious enough to convince her that she was getting the drug and not the placebo: more hot flashes; what she was sure were circulation problems; and a couple of times, blurred vision. She swore that none of it was chronic, which might make the researchers take her off the trial.

Love found calcifications again, but she insisted that they were the same large ones she had noticed on the last mammogram, in April. They were not suspicious. Shirley could live to be an old lady with these.

Shirley was still disappointed—and unconvinced. She squinted up her eyes and peered at the two spots on the film.

"Aren't these in a different area than the other two?"

"Maybe, maybe not," said Love. "Remember, I've rearranged

things a little. They're probably the same. Don't those two look the same as the other two?"

Shirley wasn't buying. "I'm concerned," she said.

"You're concerned because you're worried that they might be precancer. . . ."

"Um-hm." The first set Love had found had turned out to be evidence of DCIS. Shirley did not want to find another batch like that.

Love sighed. "Right," she said. "Now, can I give you a hundred percent guarantee that these aren't cancer? Of course not. Do I think they're enough to go after surgically? No. They're unchanged. If suddenly there was a cluster around that area, we could go after them. But I wouldn't at this point."

"Okay."

Love regarded her patient suspiciously. "So how are you?" asked Love.

The answer was the same as always: Tired.

"I just want to go to sleep and wake up," said Shirley.

Love smiled at her. "You're pretty demanding. I can put you to sleep where you *won't* wake up."

Shirley laughed in spite of herself. "No, I don't want the Kevorkian sleeping pills, thank you."

"They're cheaper."

"And you don't need a refill." Shirley glared at her surgeon. "You're sick."

"That's why we like each other," replied Love.

Dr. David McFadden was named chief of the Division of General Surgery at the end of July, an announcement Susan Love greeted with great enthusiasm. This would be as good as having Zinner in place, maybe even better. Zinner always acted like her boss. McFadden was her contemporary, her friend, and a friend of the Breast Center, the perfect emissary to his boss, Department Chairman Dr. E. Carmack Holmes.

Her response made him uncomfortable, and he resolved to talk to her about it as soon as he had time. Being friends was not enough, not in the current economic climate. As division chief, Mc-

Fadden was in charge of what he called "an eight-million-dollar corporation." He intended to warn Susan: If she did not have all her ducks in a row, someone else was going to step in and line them up for her. Those were the words he would use. "Susan," he was going to say, "you have to get your ducks in a row."

McFadden's familiarity with the Center's operation worked both ways—he was sympathetic to the concept, but more aware than an outsider of just what was wrong with it. As far as he was concerned it all boiled down to Love's headstrong personality. She continued to behave as though she operated in a splendid vacuum, insulated from the mundane concerns of doctors who were merely involved in maintaining a practice, not a crusade. Despite a genuine admiration for Susan's energy and skill, McFadden subscribed to many traditional assumptions about how a surgeon ought to behave, and she did not meet the requirements.

McFadden was used to spending three and a half days a week in the OR, and he thought that Susan ought to be operating more. What kept her from doing so—her political work—was of great concern to McFadden, not just because it made scheduling difficult, but because it was not a dignified activity for an academic surgeon. He shared his colleagues' disdain for doctors who too often showed up on television or in newspapers and magazines. If they were so smart about what they did, they ought to be doing it instead of talking about it.

Like Slamon, he worried that the very activism that enhanced Love's reputation among patients diminished her standing in the professional community and distracted her from the Center's problems. He had to take that into consideration. If he was going to defend a staff-heavy, money-losing operation to the university, it had to work better. McFadden felt that Love's outside political work had to come later, with specific constraints. "Not on company money," he said, "and not on company time."

It was for her own good. In January 1995, the Department of Surgery intended to change the way it paid its doctors, including Love, along lines that Mike Zinner had suggested before his departure. Not a flat salary, but a partial incentive plan tied to an individual's clinical revenues. McFadden had seen it happen before; it could mean as much as a $100,000 cut in pay for a surgeon who didn't operate often enough.

Slamon, who had been trying for almost two years to rein Susan in, was happy to have a new ally, but at the same time he was determined to maintain his own emotional equity in the Center's operation. Together he and McFadden laid out an orchestrated presentation—what McFadden called a "planned onslaught"—designed to force Love to accept certain administrative changes. It was not intended as a punishment. Both McFadden and Slamon, like Zinner, believed that everything they suggested was for Love's own good, part of her continuing education as a university physician.

Love brought a proposed organizational chart for the Center to the July 27 Steering Committee meeting, at Slamon's and McFadden's request. It reflected her assumed alliance with McFadden, since it showed Love, as director of the Breast Center, reporting directly to him and bypassing the Steering Committee. Slamon objected immediately. He insisted that she continue to report to the entire committee, which included all her financial benefactors—his own department, as well as surgery, radiation oncology, and radiology.

"All of the groups in the steering committee have a financial interest," he said, because of the time they volunteered at the multi. "That's the only arrangement I'm comfortable with."

Love was caught off guard by Slamon's tone, which was harsher than usual. Before she could reply he questioned her diagram of how the Center itself should function—the facilitators, volunteers, and Connie Long reporting to Leslie Laudeman and everyone involved in the clinical programs, research, and education reporting to Love. Slamon would not stand for it—Susan lacked the time and temperament to run the whole show—and since he had organized his allies beforehand he could afford to be blunt.

"I thought Leslie was going to be the administrator of the whole Center," he said, "for anything that was paid for by the company ticket." He wanted Leslie directly under Susan on the chart, so that even Sherry Goldman would report to Laudeman.

Love studied the paper in front of her for a long moment before she replied. Surely the medical students should report to her, and she ought to be the one to evaluate Sherry's clinical performance.

"That should be true," said Slamon, "and you evaluate the facilitators' performance too. But I've got to tell you, when I voted to get a full-time administrator, it was with the idea that she would run the whole shooting match."

Love was not adept at handling this kind of confrontation, and it was clear from the silence in the room that no one was going to take her side. She was the outcast again, although not by choice this time, and for a moment her usual bluster betrayed her.

"Okay," she said, her eyes downcast, her voice tight. "I'm just new to this. I'm just feeling my way through."

At that, McFadden spoke up. However sympathetic he was to Slamon's views, McFadden did not want Love to come out of the meeting feeling that she had been ambushed.

"Look, the more people you can trust, the better off you are," he said gently. He gestured toward Laudeman and Mary Bading, the Division of General Surgery administrator. "You have two very trustworthy filters here."

Slamon wanted Love to see that he was in fact doing her a favor. "Trust me, Susan," he said. "You don't want to deal with this stuff."

"Okay, okay," she said, sounding unconvinced. "I trust you."

Slamon had one more thing to say. With Mike Zinner gone, Denny Slamon perceived himself as the Breast Center's primary guardian. The new Department of Surgery chairman might prove sympathetic, and McFadden's heart was in the right place, but Slamon had been in this from the start. He wanted to put McFadden and McFadden's new boss on notice: if their enthusiasm ever began to lag, Slamon was prepared to step in and take over.

"There has been a feeling," he said, "that the Department of Medicine wants to take over the Breast Center, and I'm here to say in front of this forum that that is not true. We don't want to do that—but if you guys don't want it, we'll take it over. It's hard to start up, it's going to need more infusions, it's going to take a while.

"We're not interested in taking it away from Surgery—but what I won't let happen is let it go under the waves because nobody's looking after it. So if you guys don't want it, we'll be happy to take it over. I think it's a good thing."

McFadden smiled. "That's an interesting diversion," he said.

While they talked Love scribbled the words *Is this it?* at the top of a clean sheet of paper. Underneath she sketched a revised organization chart, based on what Slamon and McFadden had said. She would report to the Steering Committee, which would report to McFadden, who kept Mac Holmes apprised. Leslie would report to Mary Bading, who would also have McFadden's ear—a concession to Slamon, who clearly wanted Laudeman to have more authority. Love would control the physician staff, including the students, while Laudeman was in charge of the facilitators. She could not quite figure out what to do with Sherry Goldman. Love was not going to cut her line to a woman who was a staunch ally, and a link to the high-risk and follow-up programs.

It looked unnervingly like a traditional program, administered by a woman who had been handpicked by Slamon. If this was it—if this was the structure Slamon and McFadden wanted—Love was not at all sure how she felt.

Having sat through a discussion of what she was doing wrong, Love wanted to address the ways in which the university had disappointed her. She complained about the interminable delays in promoting the Center. She and her staff had sat through endless meetings on how to sell services to a managed care provider, and had cooperated with the advertising agency that was trying to devise a campaign. They had worked up a script for the first television commercial, but it had yet to be produced. In the meantime patients were choosing other breast programs.

"This is as far as we can get on my book," she said. "We need to take the next step and do some marketing. I've heard that the word on the street from our competition is, 'Don't even bother, they're too busy there, you'll never get an appointment.' "

She walked right into a trap. This time McFadden took the offensive, with the same argument Slamon had so often made before. They could not market the Breast Center until it was in better shape. He asked her to lay out her weekly schedule, and when she did so Slamon took it apart. She was not performing enough surgeries. She ought to be at both multi clinics, Wednesday and Friday. He wanted to remind her that members of his department took four weeks of vacation; he had never been able to stomach the fact that she took six.

Love claimed that Zinner had promised her six when they were negotiating.

Mary Bading spoke up. The extra ten days were supposed to be the national holidays that everyone took off, not added time.

Susan zigzagged. What about the medical fellow she had been promised? No one had written the ad to recruit one, and now it was too late in the academic season.

McFadden told her she could not hope to get a medical fellow on her staff until she established a curriculum. "You can't just have someone hanging around the multi," he said.

Weakly, Love changed the subject and started to describe her first attempt to insert the ductoscope through a patient's nipple without damaging surrounding tissue, an effort that had gone better than she had expected. There certainly was no point in debating the substantive issues that had been raised that afternoon. The new order was quite clear: a cautious endorsement from the Division of Surgery, on condition that the Breast Center implement the changes that Denny Slamon had always wanted to make.

HOPE

32

BIG BUSINESS

E VERYONE WAS WATCHING MARY-CLAIRE KING, WONDERING WHEN SHE
would discover BRCA-1, a gene so closely identified with her
that she joked in a proprietary manner about its initials,
which she said stood not for breast cancer, but for Berkeley, California, the location of her research laboratory. Mary-Claire had
come to embody the search, and the people who wanted her to win
equated her progress with the progress of the overall effort.

They forgot the one central lesson breast cancer had taught
them, which was never to expect justice.

By the end of August, Mark Skolnick's team of researchers in
Salt Lake City and Chapel Hill were convinced they had found
BRCA-1—a single defective gene that showed up in five of the large
families they studied. Donna Shattuck-Eidens, one of Skolnick's
Utah colleagues, had orchestrated a screening effort that yielded
results: the Utah group had discovered what Shattuck-Eidens called
a "frameshift mutation" that disrupted the gene's normal DNA
sequence and prevented the formation of a complete protein. This
time the gene behaved as so many others had not, obediently showing up in altered form in family members with breast cancer, and in
its normal state in healthy relatives. Myriad Genetics and its young
government collaborators had won.

The team planned to submit two articles to *Science* magazine—

one a description of BRCA-1 itself, and one about its possible significance in sporadic breast cancer. In keeping with a research tradition that required new information to be dispensed first by a reputable journal, Skolnick decided to maintain the group's silence about the discovery until *Science* published the work.

He did not reckon with the tremendous hunger for information about the gene. The two papers arrived at the magazine's offices on September 2, and eleven days later Skolnick received a phone call from NBC News science reporter Robert Bazell, who had heard about the discovery. Skolnick refused to comment, as did Francis Collins, who had yet to see the data. Bazell had heard the news from enough sources to proceed, though, and on Wednesday, September 14, NBC News ran a story crediting Myriad Genetics and Mark Skolnick with the discovery. Skolnick's Chapel Hill collaborator Roger Wiseman, who had only just received comments on his paper from *Science* editors, spent that night making revisions. The formal publication date, which was weeks away, had become a joke. With the NBC report, *Science* would have to release the material early.

The next day the magazine formally accepted the two papers and gave them to members of the press. The scientific community scrambled to get organized. Dr. Harold Varmus called members of Skolnick's team to Washington, D.C., for a hastily arranged press conference that afternoon. The National Institutes of Health had funded some of Skolnick's Utah research, and the Chapel Hill laboratory where Wiseman and Futreal had found the likely suspect was funded by the government. As director of the nation's medical research center, it fell to Varmus to introduce the public to the groundbreaking discovery. The Chapel Hill researchers and some of their colleagues flew to Washington for the formal announcement, but Skolnick, two time zones away, had to settle for watching the proceedings on television.

No matter. He owned the future. Skolnick's Myriad Genetics, Inc., had already filed two patent applications, a "composition of matter" patent on the gene and a "method of use" patent for its use in diagnosis and therapy. In the interest of protecting his property, Skolnick had declined to release the actual gene sequence until *Science* published the two papers at the end of September. In the meantime he offered his competitors the chance to become his collaborators. If they gave him their supplies of DNA he would tell them right away what the gene looked like—and Myriad would screen the samples for free as soon as the company developed a comprehensive test. That was the trade-off: inventory for knowledge.

BRCA-1 was an imposing gene, ten times larger than an average gene, long enough to house many different DNA mutations. Skolnick's team had found eight, but everyone expected there would be more. Testing would be a complicated matter, since it involved figuring out the precise mutation that plagued a specific family, and comparing the DNA of healthy relatives to that of family members with breast cancer. The larger Skolnick's supply of DNA, the more mutations he would have access to.

His detractors cried monopoly, and warned that if Skolnick cornered the market he would be able to charge premium rates for a gene screening test, like any exclusive supplier of a product. Access to the latest medical advance would be defined by economics, not need. Skolnick replied that he was acting in a responsible manner: he had a small public company that depended on investors to grow, and the only way to attract those investors was to deliver a return on their money. He pointed out that he did not intend to charge for the test when used in a research setting; he expected profit only from those who made a profit.

A patent was the best kind of protection, in a field increasingly driven by entrepreneurial effort. It promised seventeen years of unassailable profit from all BRCA-1 diagnostic tests and associated treatments, an irresistible clear shot for investors. Skolnick argued that investment money would, in turn, enable Myriad to develop a reasonably priced screening test. If the women of America were truly interested in getting a test for BRCA-1 as soon as possible, then good business—not scientific altruism, which made a lot of friends but ate away at profit—was the way to proceed.

Mark Skolnick's credentials as a geneticist stretched back as far as Mary-Claire King's did. The difference was that King was dedicated to finding the gene for heritable breast cancer, however long it took, while Skolnick had a more pragmatic commitment to results.

After an early failed collaboration with King, Skolnick had gone on to work on simpler hereditary diseases, as well as on other cancers that seemed likelier to yield answers. He and his colleagues published papers in 1985 and 1988 on genetic predisposition to colon cancer, and in 1987 he was involved in the discovery of a gene for neurofibromatosis, a skin cancer. It was only when King announced the narrowing of the search for BRCA-1 to the seventeenth chromosome, in 1990, that Skolnick was encouraged to rejoin the effort. He continued with his other work as well, discovering a gene for familial melanoma in the fall of 1992.

The only question was, how to pay for the pursuit of BRCA-1. Since 1984 Skolnick had been looking for funding in the business community. By the late 1980s he had come to believe that there was no room for him in the upper echelons of government-funded research. He had already been beaten out on the discovery of one disease gene by two colleagues who were now competitors in the BRCA-1 race, and he felt that the grant money he had received since 1980, over $12 million from the NCI, about $5 million specifically for breast cancer research, was not enough to subsidize a more aggressive pursuit of BRCA-1. The only way for him to compete was to find private or corporate funding.

After two failed attempts to start up a biotechnology company, he formed Myriad Genetics, Inc., in May 1991. Two years later a public offering raised $10 million to continue his work.

The funds enabled Skolnick to chase the gene the way he thought best, with enough money to support researchers at his Salt Lake City headquarters and collaborators at Chapel Hill and the University of Utah, as well as in London and Montreal. By the summer of 1993 Skolnick had over twenty people working in Salt Lake City alone.

The losers in the race expressed admiration for Skolnick's prescient decision to open shop in the midst of a genealogical gold mine, and respectful envy at the size of his purse. The only problem was that he had beat out King. Francis Collins set aside his own disappointment to tell *The New York Times* that he was sorry King had not prevailed: "It was her reason for getting up in the morning," he said.

King insisted in a *Science* magazine article that she was fine. All she cared about was that someone had finally found BRCA-1.

Mark Skolnick was too tired, from the last months of the search and from a lingering case of bronchitis, to even think about celebrating. People kept calling to congratulate him and ask if he had broken out the champagne, but he felt none of the elation they assumed he was feeling. Relief was the overwhelming emotion—that, and a rueful appreciation of his role in the drama.

Skolnick felt he was being depicted as the "evil villain," his reward for besting King, who was portrayed as "the most wonderful individual in the world." Winning had made him instant enemies—and the fact that he had turned his back on academia after two decades, in favor of a faster track and private funding, which probably accounted for some of the venom. A lapsed academic who had chosen instead to build a business, Skolnick imagined that some of his ex-colleagues considered him "doubly evil: I was King's scientific enemy, and then I went and used the biotechnology industry."

As far as Skolnick was concerned, all this talk about purity was just hypocrisy. " 'We work for the purity of the world,' and then out there, there are the exploiters, who come in the form of commercial people," was the way he characterized his detractors' position. "But academics, and people who buy into this idea, forget that we're using telephones. That's a commercial invention. Almost all progress in computers in the last twenty years has occurred in the commercial area. They ride in cars and work in buildings that have fax machines, that use the Internet. Commercialism is part of our life."

He resented being portrayed as a spoiler. He suggested instead that he ought to be spoken of as a hero, "galloping up on a white horse with a white hat." But he did not engage in public debate. To Skolnick, the question of how he had found the gene was a digression. The crucial news was that his group had found it. He saw himself as a political activist, not unlike King, except that his cause was to overthrow the tyranny of disease. With the discovery of BRCA-1, the revolution could begin in earnest.

*   *   *

The advocates, who until now had held the franchise on change, were not feeling generous. To Visco and Love it was as though a big bully had roared into town and swiped something that rightfully belonged to their friend, Mary-Claire King. King's allegiance was clear; she wanted to improve the wretched state of breast cancer detection and treatment. Skolnick was a less dependable ally—and if his current behavior was any indication, he felt no responsibility to the advocates at all.

Visco was furious that Skolnick refused to publish the gene sequence immediately, and she called him twice over the next week to try to convince him to change his mind. He had received some NIH money, even though the bulk of his funding was private; as far as Visco was concerned that made the government part-owner of the gene sequence. It was public information, and Skolnick had no right to behave as though it belonged to him. What about the women who literally gave their blood for his research? Visco figured the gene sequence belonged to them too.

She did not like the fact that Skolnick was trying to tie up DNA supplies, which only confirmed her suspicion about his profit motive. She thought it was greedy, and worse, she thought it set a bad precedent. A few weeks might not make a substantial difference, not after a twenty-year search, but the time frame was not the issue. Secrecy was.

What if the next researcher who came along decided to hang on to his information for a whole year, until he could develop a genetic test? An unlikely scenario, in an age of e-mail and the Internet, but Skolnick's refusal to cooperate inflamed Visco's imagination.

For the first time since she got involved in breast cancer research, her will made no difference. Visco arrived in Los Angeles for a September 21 meeting of a local group called Women in Business, looking distracted and irritable. She and Love were the evening's featured speakers, but as the guests filed into the banquet room the two women held back, just for a moment, to compose themselves.

It was almost a year since they had stood at President Clinton's side as he announced a new assault on breast cancer. Now, unexpectedly, they were on the sidelines, while a man they considered an interloper took credit for a bright future. They were temporarily at sea, reduced to swapping rumors and complaints.

Love's one-time Boston colleague, Dr. I. Craig Henderson, had scheduled a breast cancer symposium for September 24–26, sponsored by the University of California, San Francisco, where he now taught. All that anyone wanted to talk about was the gene. Love's third partner at Dana Farber, radiologist Jay Harris, debated the issue with Helene Smith, the chair of the DOD Integration Panel, a career breast cancer researcher and a recent patient herself.

Harris said that he found Skolnick's behavior "appalling," but Smith, a small, self-effacing woman with a gentle manner, tried to calm him down. What Skolnick was doing, after all, was no different than what a drug company did when it developed a new drug and then sold it.

Harris remained unconvinced. The idea of making licensing agreements with other researchers was, to him, "so offensive."

Harold Varmus greeted the news that BRCA-1 had been found with a certain academic reserve. He found it mildly amusing that everyone was running around talking about the first breast cancer gene, when he could rattle off a list of ten other genes involved in that and other cancers. This was proof, to him, of the gap between scientists and the public. Varmus wanted knowledge; advocates wanted results. What they refused to accept was that science was not a set of linear problems. BRCA-1 was not the key to all breast cancer. It was a marvelous piece of information in a puzzle that had yet to be solved, part of the multistep process that turned normal cells into malignant ones.

On one point he and Visco were in agreement, although they came to it from opposite sides: it was hardly time to pack up and go home.

Varmus regarded with weary frustration Skolnick's refusal to release the gene sequence immediately. Waiting until *Science* released its October 7 issue at the end of September was not going to matter in terms of public health, but it was bad politics to keep the sequence a secret. As long as the discovery had been announced, however prematurely, Skolnick ought to file his patent claim quickly and release the information.

Instead, Skolnick waited. The director of the NIH watched from the sidelines as many researchers "got in bed" with Skolnick, as he put it, and agreed to provide the Utah researcher with their DNA samples in exchange for the sequence and free testing. "My objection," Varmus said, "is that I think he is using the leverage of having gotten the information out, and not feeling required to release the sequence, to develop a lot of collaborations which otherwise would have been competitions."

Varmus knew the rationale: collaboration would enable the scientists to develop a test more quickly than if they worked independently. An interesting position for a man like Skolnick, who had spent the last three years in secretive isolation.

The government encouraged scientists to patent their discoveries; the reward for successful effort was ownership. The sequence for BRCA-1 was no different than the formula for Coca-Cola, kept secret for 108 years because there was no way to patent a recipe. A gene for heritable breast cancer and the ingredients in soda pop—both were valuable commodities, endless sources of revenue. A patent was the only way Skolnick could protect himself. Varmus was not about to argue a researcher's right to safeguard his discovery, and thought Visco naive to suggest that Skolnick hand out the gene sequence before his patent claim was in place.

"We're in the real world here, boys and girls," he said. "This is a country that honors the profit motive."

What Varmus did dispute was Skolnick's contention that Myriad should own the patent exclusively. Skolnick had received NCI grants, two University of Utah researchers who worked with him had received between $1 million and $2 million from the NIH, and Futreal and Wiseman at the NIEHS were paid by the government. Varmus felt strongly that the NIEHS researchers ought to share the patent as coinventors.

But Myriad Genetics insisted that its Utah lab, not the North Carolina team, was responsible for satisfying the two basic requirements for a gene patent: identifying the gene's structure and explaining its function in the body. A top Myriad researcher dismissed the two NIEHS scientists' identification of what proved to be BRCA-1, telling *The Wall Street Journal,* "We would have found the gene exactly when we did without their help."

Varmus was not convinced. On October 6, 1994, the day before the two articles on BRCA-1 finally appeared in *Science* magazine, the government decided to file a competing patent claim that included Wiseman, Futreal, and seven Utah scientists.

While the others argued politics and profit, the gene hunters got ready to go back to work. Embedded deep within the excitement was a sorry little truth: identifying a gene for heritable breast cancer was not the end of a quest, but the beginning. There would be more waiting—for screening tests and for a clinical response.

BRCA-1 was a puzzle inside a revelation. Francis Collins told a reporter for *U.S. News & World Report,* "You can think of the gene as a whole chapter in a book, and a single misspelling can cause disease. If you want to find a misspelling, you have to read the entire chapter."

Mary-Claire King was more succinct. "Of all the sorts of genes BRCA-1 might have been," she told the magazine, "this one is as difficult to work with as we could imagine."

Denny Slamon was determined to alter Susan Love's behavior. What he did not realize, as she began her third year at UCLA, was how profoundly he, too, had changed. In the 1980s Slamon had operated on his own, hamstrung by how little money the federal government had to spend and how hard it was to acquire. Since 1990 he had been protected to a great extent by his patron at Revlon, Ronald Perelman, whose contributions enabled Slamon to complete the preliminary research he needed to compete for government grants.

Love introduced him to a larger universe: young researchers who could not get started, established researchers who could not find the money for ambitious projects, government studies that were canceled because it was too expensive to do them right. She complained about the old boys' network at the NIH. Slamon came to understand that his predicament was part of a larger problem.

Then he hit the jackpot, and reaped the very real benefits of Love's and Fran Visco's activism: Slamon received two major DOD grants, an $800,000 grant to continue his HER-2/neu research and a four-year, $899,000 grant to establish a state-wide tissue bank with Dr. Michael Press of the University of Southern California. It was a dream come true for Slamon, the end of an era when researchers had to go begging in the pathology lab for tissue specimens that otherwise would be discarded. Slamon and Press planned to collect three kinds of breast tissue samples—malignant tissue from cancer patients, biopsy tissue from high-risk women, and tissue from healthy women with normal risk levels who elected to have breast reduction surgery. They would take fat tissue and bone marrow tissue samples from all three groups as well, to study environmental factors.

It was the sort of fundamental project that should have existed long ago—what the DOD referred to as an "infrastructure" grant, designed to help build a proper foundation for future research. Slamon loved the idea. Years from now he could find out the fate of the women whose samples he had collected, and perhaps learn something new about the disease. He might see a trend based on a variable no one had yet thought to consider.

The army had bought him an expansive future. Slamon found himself spouting just the sort of rhetoric Fran Visco used, about what a difference the price of a single B-1 bomber would make if applied to the war on breast cancer. It cost $1 billion to build and deploy a B-1 bomber, he told his colleagues. Imagine what that money would do spent on the national medical defense.

He had become politicized in spite of himself.

His benefactor, Col. Irene Rich, released the first official grant award list for the Defense Department's breast cancer research program on Friday, September 30, 1994—444 grants that covered everything from vaccines to digital mammography. There were training programs for the next generation of researchers, and continuing aid like the HER-2/neu grant for established researchers like Slamon. Rich riffled through the pages of the list with barely restrained glee. This was the future, and she had been instrumental in making it happen.

She was as certain as a newcomer could be that this group of grants was going to make a difference. There were sixty-seven grants in genetics alone, sixty-seven researchers about to be set loose to change the direction of breast cancer research. It was impossible to be restrained on a day like this. It was her dream to conquer breast cancer—and like any good soldier, she had absolute faith in the army's ability to prevail. She was already hard at work on a computerized questionnaire for the researchers who had received the 1993–1994 grants, so that she could get a sense of where the gaps were in the overall research program. For Visco and the politicians who had engineered that first $210 million appropriation had managed what the army had always insisted was impossible—they had convinced Congress to continue the program with a $150 million appropriation for fiscal 1995. On September 29, House Resolution 4604 had passed in the House of Representatives by a vote of 327 to 86, and in the Senate by a voice vote. President Clinton signed the bill on the same day that Colonel Rich released her list.

Ed Long was too tired to celebrate. The legislative aide to Senator Tom Harkin had just survived a second round of appropriations hearings on the DOD program, and he knew too well just how fragile the victory was. Too many of the "yes" votes were idiosyncratic, based on emotion or personal experience—the senator who supported the appropriation because his wife and sister had breast cancer, the one who voted for it in horrified reaction to the research cuts the NIH faced. The "no" votes were more predictable. There was still a lot of principled resistance to using defense funds for a domestic program.

It was hardly a ringing endorsement. As Long saw it, "There is a mutual collection of self-interests that make things happen." The November 1994 election, barely a month away, could shift that collection of interests. The army could again delay releasing the funds to Colonel Rich's medical command.

The activists had the vote. That was not the same as having the money; not yet. Long might even argue that they were chasing the wrong prize in the first place. Without meaning to, the activists had played into the hands of Republican budget-cutters. The DOD was a delightful diversion, an embarrassment of riches, while in the background the real mayhem, the attack on next year's NIH budget, continued unchecked.

On Sunday, October 9, *The New York Times*'s "On the Street" photo feature showcased fashion designer Ralph Lauren's FASHION TARGETS BREAST CANCER T-shirt, which his employees had worn the Saturday before to usher in Breast Cancer Awareness month. In the largest photograph two young employees posed wearing their shirts, carrying bottles of water and brandishing cigarettes. Lung cancer killed more women than breast cancer did; awareness, it seemed, was an incremental process.

October was an endless parade of designers using clothes to raise awareness and money. Various well-known models wore Lauren's shirt in a national magazine advertising campaign; shoe manufacturers staged a tent sale in Manhattan's Central Park, offering chic footwear at discount prices; and the First Lady invited Lauren, Donna Karan, and a handful of prominent designers and fashion editors to the White House.

If Breast Cancer Awareness Month in 1993 had been about political activism and changing the system, in 1994 it was a tribute to private money—a vibrant, stylish distraction from apprehensions about what a Republican victory in the congressional elections might do to the future of government support.

The October 19 announcement of new national guidelines for mammography went almost unnoticed, but it was a solemn reminder of how much work was yet to be done. Among Donna Shalala's goals were improved quality and a strategy to make sure women actually got their results. That was how basic the plan was: too many women still needed access to mammography centers that took decent images and notified women of the results within ten days.

Susan Love made her usual hectic round of appearances—and was diagnosed that month with an ulcer.

On October 13, Fran Visco attended the final meeting of the army research program's Integration Panel to review what the group had accomplished with the first batch of grants, and to plan for the next round of applications. It was a bittersweet afternoon. The scientists and doctors who at first had kept their distance had become precious allies.

Along the way several of them had approached Visco to let her know how much they valued her contribution, but two members of the panel had said nothing until this day. At the end of the meeting they both came over and embraced her. All three of them began to cry.

"Now I understand how you feel," said one of the doctors. Visco had the same heady feeling she had had in the East Room of the White House almost a year before. No, they did not have the answers, but they had intent and momentum, and she believed they would prevail.

By the first week in November, Lilly Tartikoff was working out the final details of the fifth annual Revlon Fire & Ice Ball, a $1,000-a-plate benefit for the Revlon/UCLA Women's Cancer Research Program, scheduled for Wednesday, December 7. The 1993 ball had brought in over one million dollars from ticket sales and donations, a figure Ronald Perelman had matched. The 1994 event promised to be even more of an extravaganza. Instead of the standard formula—lots of celebrities and a lovely evening—Tartikoff had joined forces with the designer Giorgio Armani, who had agreed to come to Los Angeles for the first time in six years. Construction workers were already busily transforming a soundstage at Twentieth Century Fox Film Corp. into a replica of Armani's Milan runway showroom, down to the upholstery on the chairs. Armani was going to stage a fashion show of three hundred pieces from his upcoming spring 1995 collection, followed by a dinner on a second soundstage dressed to look like an Italian garden.

The press coverage would dwarf anything that had come before. It would be the perfect moment to announce that Perelman was going to fund a new center—except that Revlon had yet to respond to UCLA's $7.5 million proposal. Tartikoff had waited as patiently as an impatient woman could, through an entire silent summer. It was time to ask Perelman for an answer, in the hope that they could tie the news to the Fire & Ice Ball.

She went to New York for the November 7 National Breast Cancer Coalition dinner honoring Hillary Rodham Clinton and Donna Shalala, and the next day had an appointment with Perelman and his chief counsel, Jim Conroy.

Tartikoff had become used to Perelman's style. Much as she wanted an answer, they never talked about business first. They chatted—and when there was a lull she tried to steer the conversation to the UCLA proposal.

"Well," she said, "I'd like to maybe talk about the Center now."

"Yes," said Perelman.

For an instant Tartikoff wondered if he was saying yes to the topic or yes to the Center.

"Do you want to do it now?" she asked.

"Yes," Perelman replied.

Tartikoff could not believe that it was going to be this easy. She turned to Conroy.

"Is he saying 'yes' to the seven and a half million dollar center?"

"Ask him," said Conroy.

Tartikoff turned back to Perelman. "Ronald, is this the seven and a half million dollar center?"

"Yes," said Perelman.

Then Lilly Tartikoff did what she always did when it was no longer necessary to be controlled and disciplined. She burst into tears.

She could hardly wait to tell Slamon the news. Over the years she had called him every couple of weeks to ask, "Do you have my cure yet? When are you going to have my cure?"

Now Ronald Perelman had made a public commitment to Denny Slamon, Susan Love, and the rest of the people involved in breast cancer research and treatment at UCLA. Tartikoff intended to take the ribbing up a notch and tell Slamon he had to come up with a cure. It would be so embarrassing if he did not.

* * *

That same day voters elected a Republican Congress, which fairly ensured a fight over the budget. Everyone who depended on the government for sustenance—the Defense Department breast cancer research program, the National Institutes of Health, the National Cancer Institute, the Department of Health and Human Services—prepared for trouble. Their intramural disagreements were insignificant. If they did not get the money they needed, philosophy would be beside the point.

33

THE WILL TO SURVIVE

SOMEDAY THE WOMEN WHO CAME TO SEE DR. LOVE IN 1994 WOULD BE ancient history, relics from an era long since past, carrying odd souvenirs of how things used to be—surgery scars, a lingering cough from radiation to the chest, hair inexplicably curly after the chemotherapy. Their daughters and granddaughters? With luck they would not have to settle for such an undependable arsenal.

At the dawn of a new era, anything seemed possible. At the end of an old one, it was hard to see anything but limitations. Love's patients were time's hostages. They could only learn to live with what they had—or in spite of it.

Dottie figured she had room for twenty-one rosebushes. Susan Love had decided to wean Dottie slowly from her biweekly schedule to a monthly appointment, and the move had had the intended effect: Dottie began to rely on herself again. She debated hybrids versus old roses with anyone who would listen; she wondered whether she had room for climbers and bushes, or whether she had to stick to lower shrubs. She gave great thought to color; she could not tolerate true orange.

The planting would take place in December.

Often she thought to herself, "Oh, God, will I be alive to see them when they're full grown?"

In the meantime, she pushed herself, as she always had. She decided it was time to abandon the clumsy cotton batting she had been stuffing in her bra, and bought a silicone prosthesis in a lingerie shop in Beverly Hills run by a breast cancer survivor. She started going out to lunch again at the Beverly Hills Tennis Club, and looked forward, maybe in the spring, to doing a little shopping. She and Joe went out for an early dinner every Saturday night, and to a movie matinee every Sunday afternoon. Next fall it would be time for her grandson to spend a year with them.

As far as she was concerned, Susan Love was right. There was no point in wondering when she was going to wake up with a symptom of metastatic disease. Maybe this time she would get lucky, and be one of those women with positive nodes who sailed on for years and years. Worrying was not going to change the outcome, nor was depression.

Better to plant roses. At the last moment, with an optimist's abandon, Dottie increased her order from twenty-one to thirty rosebushes, and added a half dozen other varieties of flowers. Let the gardener take out more of the lawn to accommodate the extra plants. Dottie could not pass them up.

She debated whether to tell people, "I have breast cancer," or "I had breast cancer," and decided to use the past tense.

Laura was experiencing a euphoria specific to Hollywood deal makers, whose future could turn on a lunchtime conversation or a serendipitous phone call. Autumn was a giddy hash of networking and unlikely good fortune. She met a novelist who was just finishing a promising property and got him to let her option it, as she described it, "for a tiny fee." Her producing partner, an older woman much wealthier than she, offered Laura the use of her house in Sun Valley, Idaho, known as a favorite getaway spot for many movie industry executives and stars. Laura packed, happily imagining herself walking down the main street and bumping into deals.

She was wearing a regular bra and her old clothes, and was eager to show her new breast to anyone who expressed the slightest curiosity. She watched people carefully to gauge their reactions. If they were horrified by the way she looked, then it was no better than a prosthesis—and for all her insistent good cheer, she was frightened that she might in fact look strange. She joked too loudly about the faint hairs she saw on the flap skin ("My breast has *butt* hairs on it!") and waited to see if anyone winced. Behind the jokes she wondered if she ought to wax the skin, to remove those almost invisible hairs.

Dr. Shaw performed a second procedure on most of his reconstruction patients, once the swelling went down and he could compare his work to a woman's other breast. In Laura's case, that effort came with a laundry list of other considerations. The left implant had to come out, the left nipple had to come up, and she insisted on liposuction to reduce her left buttock until it matched the right.

Shaw also had to create a nipple on the right breast, by pulling up a small section of skin and shaping it to look like her other nipple. Once Laura was healed a nurse would tattoo the nipple and areola in the proper shade. That would be the end of it.

Until then, Laura concentrated on putting her business life in order—but Hollywood obstinately refused to obey. Laura's novelist defected and sold his book outright to someone else for a million dollars. She was devastated. She had had a studio and a big-name director interested in that project, and it had been all too easy to imagine a solid future built on nothing more than expressions of interest. Instead, she was back to nothing and her severance pay had run out. Laura had a dozen other projects in development, so she quickly started making appointments to pitch them, only to experience a week of Hollywood hell: five pitch meetings five days in a row, and a rejection each time out.

It was hard to keep a bright face. One morning she decided to take a stroll down Rodeo Drive. When she got to the Giorgio Armani boutique she could not help but stop. She stood frozen in front of the window, staring longingly at a deep brown tweed suit, imagining how wonderful she might look in it, her broad shoulders in that double-breasted jacket, her long legs swathed in effortless wool.

For the first time in a year Laura Wilcox felt like doing a little shopping—which is to say, she was prepared to get undressed under the watchful eye of a salesperson. Being naked in front of Dr. Shaw was easy. Being naked in front of someone else was still far harder than she liked to admit.

In fact, she had not yet been naked with anyone, for all her willingness to show off Shaw's handiwork. That was bravado. Intimacy was more difficult. Some days she could not even be naked alone; she got out of the shower in the morning and began to weep. It was a great relief to stand in front of a store window like a regular person, thinking about how great she would look in that suit, for once not thinking about the details of how she had got there.

Barbara Rubin often reminded herself of what her boyfriend had said to her way back in the beginning, when she had to have a biopsy—about how it was only her body, a container for the more important stuff.

The more time passed, the more the breast cancer seemed an aberration to her. She was certain she had done the right thing by refusing to let Love perform a lymph node dissection or put her through radiation therapy. At the end of August she traveled to Oregon for a spiritual retreat taught by Ram Dass, born Richard Alpert, the Harvard University psychologist who had conducted psychedelic drug experiments alongside Timothy Leary. The eight-day program required three days of silence, an unnerving prospect for some of the participants. Barbara reveled in it.

She had come to believe absolutely in the connection between the mind and the body—in her ability to heal herself—and if someone like Susan Love required more data, well, that was what being a Western doctor was all about. Barbara did not require any more proof.

*   *   *

Dee had given up on everyone—the doctors who had supervised the transplant, her family. No one could give her any respite. The symptoms that had plagued her in the weeks following the transplant had subsided, so she could taste her food and get through a day without collapsing in an exhausted heap. But her body's silence was just as frightening. What was going on? Susan Love would have said not to go looking for trouble, but Dee no longer had access to Susan. And in her own way, Dee liked data as much as her one-time surgeon did. She wanted information. She told her doctors that she ought to have blood tests and scans to make sure the high-dose chemotherapy had done its job, and spent the fall of 1994 commuting between doctors' offices looking for answers. She had scheduled her reconstructive surgery for January 10, 1995. She wanted some proof before then.

She got contradictions instead. One scan showed an infiltrating mass in her right lung, but her blood marker levels were down, suggesting that the cancer had not spread. A CAT scan showed metastases on her spine, but a magnetic resonance imaging of the same area came back negative. The back pain she was starting to have might be the breast cancer; then again, it might not.

Dr. Boasberg suggested that she wait three months and have the tests again at the end of December, so she canceled her plastic surgery appointment for January and began compulsively cleaning out the garage. One afternoon she came back indoors to find that her cat, who was diabetic, had missed the litter box and defecated in the bathroom. When Gary heard about the incident his response was blunt.

"That's it," he said. "This cat has got to go."

Dee turned on him. "Well, gee," she said. "I'm glad to see that your response when someone gets very sick is 'That's it, she's got to go.' "

Gary said nothing. The cat stayed.

Jerilyn's summer and fall were full of uncontrollable emotion. The slightest thing upset her—the sight of a neighbor with a heart condition smoking a cigarette, a dream about her ex-lover. She lurched from one freelance assignment to another and chastised herself for not finding a job. She kept reliving the moment she had awakened in the surgery recovery room, which for her was the worst part of the process. One morning she woke up and decided she must be suffering from post-traumatic stress syndrome.

Her escape came not from all the responsible things she was doing to heal herself, but from a perfectly placed golf ball. Friends of Jerilyn's invited her to play hooky one day and join them for eighteen holes, and at first she thought, How can I go? I'm not even playing hooky from a job, I'm playing hooky from looking for a job.

It was the height of irresponsibility. She said yes.

On the thirteenth hole she shot a hole in one. She took it as a sign that she ought to be living her life instead of worrying about how long it would be. Perhaps all her box building—the perfect diet, the exercise regimen, the disciplined life—was a mistake. It certainly was not fun. She wondered for the first time if a bit more spontaneity might be good for her, and decided to modify her diet. She did not really believe that the occasional teaspoon of olive oil was going to kill her, and it surely made eating less of a chore.

November 18, 1994, was the one-year anniversary of her surgery. She decided to go out of town for the weekend.

The day before she left, Jerilyn woke early in the morning and picked up the friend who had accompanied her to get her biopsy results. She carried with her two pages of quotes from the *Jewish Encyclopedia* for a mikvah ceremony, a Jewish ritual bath. She had made an appointment at the University of Judaism, and asked a woman rabbi she knew to meet her there. It was time to move on.

She had to be perfectly clean before she even got into the chest-deep tub, so she took a bath at home, and showered and used a mouthwash right before the ceremony. As she walked toward the tub she handed her friend what she had written.

" 'Tumah is the result of our confrontation with the fact of our own mortality,' " her friend began. " 'It is the going down into darkness. Taharah is the result of our reaffirmation of our own mortality. It is the reentry into light. Tumah is evil or frightening only when there is no further life. Otherwise, Tumah is simply part of the human cycle.' "

She read from Joshua: " 'Be strong and of good courage. Fear not nor be afraid. For the Lord, thy God, will not fail thee nor forsake thee.' "

And from Genesis: " 'For I am on the road on which the Lord has guided me. . . . I have seen a divine being face-to-face, yet my life has been preserved.' "

They spoke together, along with the sixty-year-old woman who conducted the mikvas. " 'Shema Yisrael, Adonai Eloheynu, Adonai Echad. Hear, O Israel, the Lord our God, the Lord is One.' "

It was time for Jerilyn to immerse herself. The idea was to let the water touch every part of her—and for her to float free, curled up in a ball. She did it three times, and then the rabbi uttered the final blessing, first in Hebrew, then in English.

" 'May God bless you and protect you. May the light of God shine upon you and God's grace be with you. May God be always with you and bring you peace. Amen.' "

It was over. She had marked a year of mourning. She was prepared to celebrate her life ahead.

Ann Donaldson had never stayed overnight in a hospital before she checked in for her transplant on August 25, but she was oddly calm about it. Ann had always divided life into two categories, things she absolutely had to do and things she had a choice about. The transplant fell into the first, so there was no point in making a fuss. She preferred to put her energy into getting through it, rather than waste her strength on distress. When she was finished she could debate the relative merits of a mastectomy or a lumpectomy. At the moment she had no time for the luxury of indecision.

She and Rick had a friend who offered to stay with the baby, so that Rick could spend as much time as possible with his wife. They arranged to have a rollaway bed put in her room, and he methodically sorted through their photographs, looking for favorites to pin on the walls—their wedding photo, pictures on the beach, with the new baby, with the dog.

Five weeks later she sat quietly in a chair in her hospital room while her husband perched on the rollaway bed he had slept on every night since she checked in. Between the sedatives and the disorientation of being in one room for all that time, Ann's short-term memory had deserted her; she recalled mercifully little of what had happened to her. Rick answered her questions truthfully, but always with a reassuring edge.

There had been one twelve-hour stretch when he and the nurses changed her bedding and gown eighteen times, between the vomiting and the diarrhea. In his retelling it was a Keystone Kops anecdote about how Ann gave a three-second warning when it always took him and the nurse five seconds to get the bedpan in place. She beat them every time.

He liked to remind her, "As bad as it was, you didn't get any roaring infections, no complications, nothing that was unmanageable from a therapeutic standpoint. We were fortunate that way. Just took a little longer." Ann had hoped to go home in three weeks, not five.

There was the inexplicable fever that spiked at 102 degrees every night and delayed her departure. An equally mysterious rash left her face and arms reddened and coarse. Along the way she had lost the rest of her hair.

She seemed not to care about any of it. Once the worst was over, Ann spent her days in a comfortable bathrobe with a perky little white knit beret on her head, waiting to go home. All she cared about was being with her baby. She asked every woman she knew who had a child if they thought her daughter would remember her after so long. Ann could survive BCNU day because she had to. If her own child did not respond to her touch, her heart would break in two.

When she came back to see Dr. Love in November, what she bragged about most was her little girl's voracious appetite. At five months Lisa was up to fifteen pounds, and she never refused food. Ann and Rick had just started to feed her cereal, and it was as though every eager swallow was a symbol of good health. The baby was flourishing, and Ann basked in her robust reflection.

It had not been easy at first. Ann sported a scar along her right eyebrow from a middle-of-the-night collision with the bathtub that meant a trip to the emergency room and ten stitches; Ann had got up to go to the bathroom and stumbled over the cord from the intravenous stand that constantly dripped a nutritional supplement into her vein. The antinausea drugs had given her tremors, as though she suffered from Parkinson's disease, and the medication she took to eliminate the tremors made her confused. She went back into the hospital, briefly, on the night when Rick found her having an animated telephone conversation with no one on the line.

But it passed. The doctors changed her medication and Ann slowly came back to life. Things still did not taste quite right, and she worried about the hearing loss she experienced—damage to the auditory nerve from one of the chemotherapy drugs, which afflicted about five percent of the women who had a transplant. Rick was always quick to remind her that her hearing was already better than it had been right after she came home. There was no reason to think the damage would be permanent.

Besides, Dr. Love had what qualified as good news. When she completed her physical examination she said that she could no longer feel the lump she had felt at Ann's first appointment. They might consider a "ghostectomy" now rather than the mastectomy they had discussed at first, to see if the high-dose chemotherapy had managed to eradicate all the cancer that had lurked at the margins of the pathology sample. If so, Ann would have radiation, like any lumpectomy patient. If not, they could do the mastectomy.

It would save her another stay in the hospital, since a ghostectomy was a quick, inpatient procedure. And it would buy her time to contemplate reconstructive surgery. As much as Love preferred that women have simultaneous reconstruction, she thought that was asking too much of Ann.

"I'm reluctant to push that on you," she said, "since you've already done your time. My inclination, if we were going to do the mastectomy, would be to say just do the mastectomy. Do the radiation, and then, a couple of years from now, when you're a bit less allergic to the hospital, come and do the reconstruction. Because I think it's a lot. It's a big go, and you've had a lot of big goes. And from talking to you today it doesn't sound like you're eager for any more."

"I could do what I had to do," insisted Ann. "I know I can. The question is, if the reconstruction is elective, do I want it?" She thought not. She wanted not to be around doctors for a while, and more important, she wanted to be with the baby. Reconstruction was not as important as being able to hold her child.

Love encouraged her instead to have a mammogram, and if it looked clean, the ghostectomy. The priority, for this particular patient, was giving her some time to enjoy her life.

For once, there was a medical rationale for Love's emotional preference. Nothing she saw today made her think a mastectomy was necessary.

"Maybe your luck has turned," said Love.

"I need it," said Ann. "I need it, some good news."

"I think that maybe your luck has turned," Love repeated. "I think this is maybe the easy piece."

"Are we doing wishful thinking here, or . . . ?"

Love chose her words carefully. She could promise Ann anything right now and make her happy, and it was such a seductive opportunity. Hard to resist—but Love could not let herself give in. It wouldn't be fair to lie.

"I have had cases," she said, "a substantial number of cases, where it is gone. We've done a ghostectomy and there hasn't been anything." There. She had not promised Ann an escape, but she had offered her a little hope. Nothing wrong with that. It was, after all, the foundation of breast cancer treatment: no promises, but a little hope. The unpredictability of the disease could work both ways— someone who was supposed to falter might in fact get through it fine.

Ann had her surgery a few weeks later, and the pathology report came back negative. There was no cancer in the tissue specimen. Suddenly the horizon was clear. No mastectomy, no debate over reconstructive surgery, no more medical procedures to distract her from her new life as Lisa's mom. She would have six weeks of radiation, and that was it.

When Shirley showed up for her December 1994 mammogram she happened to draw a young resident whose bumbling manner made her hackles go up. She was not in the mood today to obey Susan's edict and help teach the doctors of tomorrow. She wanted a nice, experienced radiologist who could look at her film immediately and say that all the calcifications had magically disappeared.

The young man disappeared to wait for the film to be developed. When he returned he escorted Shirley into a small room, shut the door, and with a vague smile announced, "Well, it's benign."

She shot daggers. "*What's* benign?"

He tried to explain that the calcifications he saw looked harmless to him. But he did not know Shirley's history, and he could not find her July magnification views to compare the spots. From what he could see, these looked like new spots. At that she fairly grabbed the films out of his hands and marched up to the fifth floor, Tracy and the kids trailing behind. Let these youngsters work out their act on somebody else. She would not be able to breathe again until Susan reassured her.

Love slapped the films up on the light board, saw that the two calcifications were the same ones they had been tracking for over a year, and apologized to Shirley for the young resident's confusion. This was one of the reasons she had her follow-up patients come up for their appointments on the same day they had their mammograms, instead of waiting until the radiologist had been able to file his report. In theory, Love wanted Larry Bassett's staff to talk to patients. In practice, she often needed to provide instant backup.

So she reassured Shirley. These were the kind of calcifications she could have until she died of that stroke at ninety.

"Good," said Shirley, with uncharacteristic brusqueness, "because I cannot handle this today."

She had her cigarette in her hand before she left the building, and as soon as she stepped out the front door she lit up. Tracy and the kids let her smoke. The radiologist had meant to reassure her, not scare her, but Shirley had run out of patience for even a harmless surprise.

It turned out that Shirley Barber's life was a rehearsal, not for her future, but for her husband's. The choking incident in the movie theater, and a few similar episodes since, were early signs of hidden disaster. In November 1994, Tracy Barber was diagnosed with Stage 3 cancer of the esophagus, with lymph node involvement and a tumor that stretched like a malicious finger from the base of his esophagus into his stomach. Esophagheal cancer did not flirt and deceive like breast cancer; it ruled. The prognosis was just the kind of flat, unyielding prediction that kept Shirley and other breast cancer patients in anxious thrall, an unspoken terror come to pass. Even with chemotherapy, there was only a five percent survival rate. The specialist Tracy went to see told him that he probably had about fifteen months to live.

Suddenly Shirley's precancer seemed frivolous; her worries about calcifications, peripheral. Fifty-one-year-old Tracy Barber was very likely going to die—before he and his wife got old, before his son graduated from college, before he could walk his daughter down the aisle. He had next to no hope of meeting his grandchildren. Shirley quietly stepped aside and let her husband take center stage. She defied her body to give her any trouble.

A surgeon installed a portable catheter in Tracy's chest, an oncologist hooked him up to a twenty-four-hour-a-day chemotherapy drip, and he went on with his life with a plastic packet of drugs tucked into his pants pocket. It was there the day Shirley encountered the clumsy radiologist. It was there the day Mitch—a wiry, short young man who was too small for football but determined to play regardless—won the David Leidal sportsmanship trophy, his high school's highest honor. His parents sat in the audience and wept, in delight at what their son had accomplished and sorrow over all the things he had yet to do that his young father might miss.

The packet was there for a friend's annual holiday party too. Once the chemotherapy shrank the tumor, Tracy would have surgery to remove his esophagus and replace it with a length of healthy intestine. It was a brutal procedure, but Shirley was adamant. Somebody had to make up the five percent who survived. It might as well be her husband.

34

MONEY

WHAT FRAN VISCO AND SUSAN LOVE NEEDED ON THE EVENING OF December 7, standing in the middle of the cocktail crowd at the 1994 Fire & Ice Ball, was a crib sheet. They were in over their heads. Two days later the *Los Angeles Times* provided a short list of select celebrity guests—models Cindy Crawford, Claudia Schiffer, Veronica Webb, and Linda Evangelista; actors Michelle Pfeiffer, Antonio Banderas, and Laura Dern. The paparazzi stood three-deep along the carpeted walkway outside, shouting out one name, then another. A spotter at the far end of the walkway eyeballed everyone who came by, consulted a clipboard, and then relayed names and descriptions to a greeter at the door, lest anyone with a public reputation be allowed to enter unnoticed.

But Visco, who rarely went to the movies, despaired of figuring out who anyone was, short of Clint Eastwood; and Love, who had a literalist's disdain for fiction in any medium, simply did not care. They were there as honored, if anonymous, guests. Someone might mention their names from the podium, but most of the people who were milling about, bestowing air kisses, did not know that the eager little woman in the black dress was a leading breast cancer activist, or that her companion, whose only sartorial concession to the formal event was the beading on the lapels of her dark jacket, was the legendary Susan Love.

This was one aspect of breast cancer research where they performed only a peripheral role. Private money was idiosyncratic, given out of friendship, sympathy, a desire to do good or be noticed, or some combination of motives. There were no rules about who got it or what for; if Brandon Tartikoff had not come to Denny Slamon for treatment, the fifth annual Fire & Ice Ball might never have happened.

Love admired Denny's work and believed he deserved the money. That was not the issue. What bothered Love was Slamon's seemingly total control over how that money was to be spent. She quietly told Visco about the new Revlon deal. As Love understood it, Denny got money for his research and there would be additional funds for women's health research, as well as new clinical programs. All Love got was $75,000 per year toward operations. No matter how many times Denny explained the arrangement, she felt short-changed.

Visco did not want to hear it. She shoved Love firmly toward the VIP lounge, a small area behind a curtain. Susan had to be gracious no matter how she was feeling. Perelman had taken her under his wing, as he had the NBCC. He had held a press conference the day before the ball to announce the Revlon Foundation's $7.5 million gift to establish the new center and underwrite the program for seven years. In the current political climate, and given the opposition Love faced within UCLA, that protection was worth more than any specific dollar figure.

Lilly Tartikoff, resplendent in a black Armani gown with a black-and-white beaded top, floated regally through the crowd, her alabaster skin and elegant posture a reminder of her dancing past. Her party promised to be quite a coup; even the most jaded members of the Hollywood social circuit had turned out for Giorgio Armani. The maniacal preparations of the past weeks were but a vague memory, hovering at the edge of her consciousness. Tartikoff had met her match in Armani—deferentially referred to even by her as Mr. Armani—a man whose perfectionism rivaled hers. Tartikoff wanted a gala evening to raise money for breast cancer research, and now, happily, to celebrate the birth of the Revlon/UCLA Women's Health Center. Armani wanted what he called an

"Armani event," a glorious evening of fashion and beauty that happened to have a charitable purpose as well. By the night of the ball they were both exhausted.

At eight o'clock the guests were ushered into the first hall, where the replica of Armani's Milan runway had been built, surrounded by twelve hundred copies of the three hundred slipcovered chairs in his Milan studio. Tartikoff sat in the first row with her husband, Brandon, and Ronald Perelman, her face aglow in the soft light of the runway. Denny Slamon and John Glaspy were there with their wives, looking slightly ill at ease. Love and Visco were lost somewhere in the crowd.

The fashion show began. Giorgio Armani, the master of tasteful subtlety, had chosen this season to glorify the bosom. His spring line included a surprising array of jackets worn open with nothing underneath, filmy dresses shown braless, bustiers worn over clothing instead of under it, and a signature smooth silk bra that showed up under otherwise tailored business suits. There were darts pointing at nipples, puckered fabric under the breast, and heavy ribbed bandeau bras. For Armani, the beautiful breast was an essential part of the new season's look.

During dinner, actress Isabella Rossellini spoke publicly for the first time about her mother, actress Ingrid Bergman, who had died of breast cancer in 1982. Hollywood harbored enduringly harsh prejudices about cancer. Ingrid Bergman had lied about her health, to herself and to others, because she was afraid no one would hire her if she were ill.

There had been in recent years a defiant change in attitude, starting with Gilda Radner's failed battle against ovarian cancer and television actress Ann Jillian's 1985 disclosure that she had had a bilateral mastectomy. It was possible to be young and vital—and to fall ill, and to continue to work. Well-known actresses and industry executives stepped forward to say that they had breast cancer, as though daring their industry to reject them: singer Olivia Newton-John, broadcaster Linda Ellerbee, actress Jill Eikenberry.

But the memory of secrecy was so close. It was what kept Bergman and her daughter, Rossellini, silent for so many years—and what kept women like Laura Wilcox, whose ambition outpaced their reputation, from telling the truth.

Two weeks later, on December 21, 1994, Dr. Samuel Broder announced his resignation as the director of the National Cancer Institute. When he left the NCI in April 1995, he would become the chief scientific officer at the Florida-based IVAX Corporation, a seven-year-old pharmaceutical company owned by a friend.

Broder had faced a number of high-profile problems over the last year, including the debate over mammography for women under fifty and the NSABP data scandal. But he and some of his colleagues suggested another reason for his departure—new political constraints that made it impossible for him to do his job. In his six years as NCI director he had seen federal money tighten up, and had weathered the increasingly vocal demands of various activist groups. It was time to defect to the private sector, where he would have fewer masters.

IVAX revenues for the preceding year were almost $1 billion, about half the NCI's budget. Broder could count on money to spend on drug research and a hefty increase over his $120,000 government salary. The only thing he would not have to do was spend vast amounts of time and effort trying to get things done.

"This company can make decisions in five minutes that would take the government probably three to four years to make," Broder told *The Washington Post*.

How to pay for knowledge? The simple, rather exclusive relationship between government and science had turned into a boisterous town hall meeting, with advocates, wealthy philanthropists, angry consumers, lawyers, and insurance companies getting into the act. In July 1994 a jury had awarded $312,000 in damages to a woman who sued Blue Shield of California for refusing to cover a transplant procedure she had in 1992. Several of the jurors said that they were disappointed when the judge would not allow them to award punitive damages, which would have required proof that the insurance company had acted maliciously in withholding approval of the procedure. They wanted Blue Shield to pay even more.

Five months later the insurance company announced a change in its policy. Blue Shield agreed to pay for transplants conducted as part of a clinical research trial.

In a strange way managed care did the breast cancer patient a cold favor. It forced everyone, the clinicians and the women who came to them, to confront the limitations of existing therapies. Finding and successfully treating breast cancer was still a combination of best guess and good fortune, and the days of dressing it up as anything else were over.

Love continued to work on a consistent set of practice guidelines based on data, propelled neither by the greed she saw among private practice physicians nor the penny-pinching mentality of the bottom-line brigade. But other early reformers were as strict about fiscal responsibility as their predecessors had been indulgent. If a treatment cost too much per year of health purchased, it was suspect.

To them, much of what was considered established medical practice did not work often enough to make economic sense. On January 11, 1995, the *Journal of the American Medical Association* published a report from the Rand Corporation, the think tank based in Santa Monica, California, entitled, "Benefits and Costs of Screening and Treatment for Early Breast Cancer: Development of a Basic Benefit Package." Three of the authors were affiliated with UCLA, and one of those, with SalickNet Inc., a managed care group that specialized in cancer treatments; the fourth was affiliated with the Laboratory of Clinical Epidemiology at the Instituto di Ricerche Farmacologiche "Mario Negri," in Milan, Italy.

The authors had reviewed the literature on screening mammography, surgery, adjuvant therapy, and follow-up care from 1980 to 1993, culled survival statistics from the government's Surveillance, Epidemiology, and End Results Program (SEER), and borrowed southern California Medicare fees as representative costs. Their goal was to evaluate the efficacy of each method in terms of "overall survival, disease-free survival, and health-related quality of life."

Their first finding was that screening mammography made cost/

benefit sense only for women between the ages of fifty and sixty-nine. It saved some lives of women younger or older than that, but not enough to justify the cost of screening those populations. Screening the target group every two years cost $11.9 million over a six-year period and saved seventy-three lives, ten years out; screening younger women might not save anyone, or at most, eight lives over a period of seven years—and screening that group cost $11.7 million. Women between the ages of seventy and seventy-four would see no improvement in ten-year survival rates.

The analyzed data showed equivalent survival rates for lumpectomy with radiation and for mastectomy—but mastectomy was cheaper, assuming "that reconstruction therapy is not part of the basic benefit plan." The added cost for lumpectomy came from radiation therapy, which ran $6,752 per person. Without radiation, lumpectomy was a financially competitive option—but early studies had shown an increase in local recurrences with surgery alone, and the issue of whether those recurrences were life-threatening, or simply an indicator that the original cancer had been an aggressive one, had yet to be resolved. The authors warned, "The health care organization could not consider withholding radiation therapy until studies have been performed on the effect of the increased local recurrence on health-related quality of life."

There was no room to negotiate on chemotherapy, because the results were quite clear. "Adjuvant therapy benefits everyone who receives it," insisted the authors, despite evidence that most early-stage patients did not need it, and some would not respond to it. They did explore the range of possibilities, though, from $2 million to treat all patients with aggressive therapy to $200,000 to treat only node-positive patients with a less aggressive regimen.

They dismissed the kind of follow-up testing that Dee Wieman so depended on: "Routine follow-up testing incurs significant excess costs for the health care plan over clinical follow-up ($961,000 vs $343,000 over 5 years) and provides no benefit in survival or health-related quality of life."

Their "hypothetical health care organization" had choices to make, based on a dwindling supply of dollars, and the report served as a hard-line analysis of how the future might look. As indemnity insurance became a thing of the past, women with limited means would find that they had limited options. Statistically it might not make much difference, but that was hard to explain to someone who felt she was being denied comprehensive care.

Health and Human Services Secretary Donna Shalala had insisted all along that breast cancer was a bipartisan issue, that the DOD program would continue because the disease struck Republican families as well as Democrats. Her optimism did not survive the November election. The new Republican 104th Congress was determined to cut expenditures, particularly certain appropriations that the previous Congress had approved. Republicans in the House of Representatives quickly announced their intention to rescind nondefense programs in the military budget—and referred specifically to the DOD's breast cancer research program as a primary target.

Ed Long's more cynical view of politics had been correct. The DOD was in precarious shape, not because the Republicans lacked sympathy for the cause, but because they were offended by an inappropriate expenditure. This Congress did not regard the war on breast cancer as a defense issue, despite the activists' brusque contention that anything that claimed forty-six thousand lives every year qualified as combat.

Fran Visco saw all her hard work going up in smoke. In January 1995 she urged NBCC members to send a message to the appropriations subcommittees as well as to their members of Congress. She composed a sample:

> This year we won another $150 million in the Department of Defense budget for continuation of the Department of the Army peer reviewed breast cancer research program. Whatever the recent election was about, it was definitely not about rescinding that money. Do not take away the DOD breast cancer research money. Women's lives depend on it and we are watching!!!!

On Friday, February 10, the Pentagon's chief budget planner, John Hamre, told the Senate Budget Committee that the Pentagon did not support the fiscal 1995 appropriation of $150 million for breast cancer research. The Pentagon was considering not releasing the funds.

As soon as Visco heard about Hamre's statement she called Hillary Clinton's office to register a complaint. She sent a fax to President Clinton, in the hope that he would act to protect a program that sixteen months earlier he had promoted as one of his Administration's priorities. Donna Shalala was out of town at a meeting, but when she heard of the threat to the DOD she called Leon Panetta, Clinton's chief of staff. The new Congress was not to be allowed to rewrite history.

That afternoon the White House instructed the Pentagon to release both breast cancer and AIDS research funds, a total of $180 million. Leon Panetta released a letter that he had sent to Defense Secretary William J. Perry, reiterating the President's sentiments.

"The President believes that research to combat these deadly diseases is vitally important to all Americans, and it is of special significance to him," said the letter. "The President believes that we cannot afford to allow these tragic losses to continue. And that is why breast cancer and AIDS research is a high priority for this Administration."

The money was safe. Visco immediately started thinking about the upcoming fight for next year's carryover appropriation. Fiscal 1996 was an off-year like 1994, but the NBCC still had to lobby for money to tide the program over, perhaps $75 million this time around.

With a Republican Congress and a presidential election looming, there was another issue to confront. Visco wanted language that formalized the government's ongoing commitment to the DOD program. She knew that the words were only as strong as congressional support in any given year, but it would be harder to dismiss the program if there was precedent for continuing it.

That same week Visco was riding down a Washington street on her way to a meeting, when a car broadsided her cab and sent her to the emergency room with bruised ribs and a gash on her forehead. Breathing was painful, and walking suddenly required conscious effort, but she hauled herself out of bed days before the doctors wanted her to, to attend a February 22 luncheon sponsored by Representative Barbara Vucanovich, a Nevada Republican and herself a breast cancer survivor. This was the first in a Congressional Forum Series the Coalition had devised, and Fran refused to miss the meeting.

The session was about the Department of Defense program, and the invited speakers included Col. Irene Rich and Denny Slamon, out on the stump for his newfound benefactor. Rich had suffered in isolation for weeks as Congress tried to shut down the program, worried about the fate of her marvelous creation and unable to speak publicly on its behalf. She had told herself time and again, "If this falls apart I will wrestle my demons to the ground and go on."

She entered the room like a lonely kid who suddenly found herself the guest of honor at a birthday party, smiling, eager, so pleased to talk to a sympathetic crowd about what she was doing. For her, the lunch was a celebration of possibility, and her enthusiasm was infectious.

Lawyers for the NIH and Myriad Genetics, Inc., determined exactly who would reap what benefits from the discovery of BRCA-1. In mid-February officials at the NIH and at Mark Skolnick's Utah-based company announced an agreement intended to resolve their conflicting patent applications. The NIH would share in licensing fees, and two NIEHS researchers, Robert Wiseman and Andy Futreal, would receive up to $100,000 for their role as coinventors. In return, the NIH abandoned its patent application, and Myriad filed an amended application that acknowledged the government's role.

Money was always news: the skirmish over the DOD, an obvious target for a reform-minded Congress, and the BRCA-1 patent conflict, a fight for dominance between the government and private business. The issue of who controlled breast cancer research was suddenly a provocative one, as activity in the field increased.

But the furor overshadowed a more fundamental problem. Congress was after a balanced budget, and was prepared to hack away at the NIH appropriation to get one. The 1994 cuts that Harold Varmus's predecessor, ex-NIH director Bernadine Healy, had decried as "disastrous" were only the beginning.

Harold Varmus seemed oddly energized by the budget crisis at the NIH, as though the need to prove to Congress the importance of medical research refreshed his own commitment to the cause. On Thursday, March 30, a brisk, sunny morning, he attended a House appropriations subcommittee's hearing on the National Cancer Institute budget. Varmus was not scheduled to speak, but he was there to support Dr. Ed Sondik, who was speaking on behalf of the NCI, substituting for his lame-duck boss, Dr. Broder. Sondik, the deputy director of the Division of Cancer Prevention and Control, was in charge while Varmus and Health and Human Services Secretary Donna Shalala considered candidates to permanently replace Broder. Finding a new director was a delicate mix of diplomacy, politics, and science. Shalala had named Fran Visco to the selection committee, who had already let it be known that the advocates considered Mary-Claire King to be the best person for the job, as though the decision were a test of Varmus's and Shalala's commitment to the cause. In the meantime, Sondik had to fight for funding.

Varmus had already made his position clear to anyone who would listen. President Clinton had proposed a 4.1 percent increase in NIH funding for fiscal 1996 over the 1993 budget of $11.3 billion, basically an inflationary budget and no more. The Republicans had recently suggested a five percent decrease instead, as part of a plan to cut $100 million to pay for a tax cut—and the difference between that and Clinton's "steady state" increase, according to Varmus, was a billion dollars. If Congress maintained the lower funding level, the NIH would lose about ten billion dollars by the year 2000.

The consequences, according to Varmus, would be brutal: "That basically kills medical research," was the way he put it.

For the numbers were deceptive—even Clinton's 4.1 percent increase was really a cut in the basic research budget, thanks to what Varmus called "initiatives," research priorities already identified by the President and the NIH. There was a stated agenda, and only an inflationary increase to pay for it. What would suffer was innovation and inspiration, which had no history and were not part of the funded establishment.

The Republicans proposed cut guaranteed even more radical consequences. In 1995, with a budget of $11.3 billion, the NIH had funded about twenty-four percent of qualified grant proposals. If the Republicans prevailed, only fifteen percent of the qualified grants would get money. Since the NIH was committed to spending seventy-five percent of its budget on existing multiyear projects, the casualty would be the discretionary fund for new basic research.

"If you suddenly yank down our budget line," said Varmus, "we stop awarding grants in a very serious way."

He derisively referred to the Republican proposal as a "flatline" budget, using the term for the straight line on an EKG monitor once a patient's heart had stopped beating.

It made no sense to him. He lived in a country where people prized good health, at a time of tremendous promise for biological research—and yet all anyone wanted to talk about was saving money.

It was the one point on which doctors of divergent philosophies angrily agreed: researchers were being asked to finance a new era in biomedical research on what was not even a maintenance budget. Their bright future was about to be destroyed by misguided politicians who thought that a balanced budget, not medical knowledge, was a proper endpoint for their efforts; by congressmen who dismissed the researchers' call for more money as self-interest.

Sloan-Kettering's Dr. Larry Norton was terrified at what he saw coming. The fact that he had received a $848,925 grant from the DOD to continue his work on tumor growth rates and chemotherapy was beside the point. What mattered was that medicine had an unparalleled opportunity to make great progress—and the government seemed determined to squander it.

"There should be a renaissance," he said. He wanted enough money to pay for basic research, "for the pure joy of understanding," which might not help a patient today but could protect her daughter's generation. He wanted the freedom to explore, for, like Glaspy, he believed in the importance of the grand failure. "If you look at great scientists through history," he said, "they made incredible blunders, along with their great discoveries." Instead, medicine faced an economic depression whose effects would be felt for decades.

"We work in generations of people," he said. "Creative people come in generations. It isn't like you can cut down funding for research now, and in five years say, 'Okay, we got more money, let's step up the research.' Those five years of graduates, from graduate schools and from medical schools and training programs— once you start the ball rolling you not only have cut out the people who are doing the work, but the teacher generations as well. You don't have teachers and you don't have role models. There's enormous danger here.

"It's the worst possible time to be doing this," he said of the proposed budget cuts. "I think the whole thing is tragic."

Norton's colleague, Dr. Jeanne Petrek, got a $157,631 DOD grant to study long-term survivors with lymphedema, an uncomfortable but not life-threatening side effect of a lymph node dissection, in which the arm and hand became swollen. She never filed the application for the large study she wanted to do about the relationship between pregnancy after diagnosis and recurrence rates, because she could not think of any funding body that would consider it. The NIH wanted five-year studies and the DOD had asked for four-year projects, but Petrek remained convinced that she needed ten years to assess whether pregnancy in fact increased a woman's chance of recurrence. Although she could collect data from her own practice, it was not a large enough sample to retire the question once and for all.

Mary-Claire King thought it was wretched, this penurious behavior on the part of the government, and she was not afraid to say so. She was convinced that the systematic drain on NIH resources was going to put science out of business. For the first fifteen years of her work King had depended on the NIH for survival. At that point the NIH was able to fund thirty percent of qualified grant proposals, including speculative work like hers. Now there was less money to spend—just as science entered what she called the "Midas era," in which researchers seemed to find gold in whatever they touched.

"No one can count on being funded, not even me," she said. "It's a crapshoot now. It's not that we're funding excellent work and poor proposals are not getting money. We're funding excellent work—but other excellent work is not getting funded. Another three to five years will destroy us, and we won't be able to rebuild."

Like Norton, she had a story to tell. King liked to remind people about Trofim Denisovich Lysenko, a Russian geneticist who in the 1940s and 1950s managed to paralyze scientific progress in that country with a theory that heredity was not based on genes and chromosomes. Russian biological science lags far behind that of other countries to this day. King shared Larry Norton's fear: if the momentum slowed for a single generation, there would be repercussions for years to come. Bright students would go into private industry or another field altogether. The progress that seemed so possible would stop. King grimly imagined a future society with ever more lawyers and engineers and nowhere near enough researchers.

The price tag for salvation? She estimated that the NIH could happily absorb an additional $5 billion.

Anything less, to King's eye, was tantamount to murder. People would die of diseases that could have been cured or prevented.

"Newt Gingrich is the economic Lysenko of modern biology," she said. "It's genocide."

While she was proud of the DOD program, for which she had served on the Institute of Medicine advisory panel, she did not for a moment think it was enough.

"All we're doing is hanging on by our fingernails with the DOD," she said. "It's absurd. We're not really doing anything toward curing breast cancer."

Donna Shalala had no trouble sleeping through the night. She faced such horrible financial decisions every day that she was numb to the sort of anguish that might have kept her awake. She felt like King Solomon, threatening to cut a baby in half to satisfy two warring parents. Should Health and Human Services spend money on children or women, on Project Head Start or on breast cancer research? What were kids in school going to get for lunch? There were "budgeteers" on the appropriations committees, but advocates continued to make their impassioned arguments to her. Something had to give.

"There's a disaster ahead of us," she said. "And it doesn't have to do with the advocates. It doesn't have anything to do with breast cancer. They just can't protect breast cancer if we balance the budget in seven years. Nobody can. Everything takes a hit."

Breast cancer research was trapped by irony: when there was money back in the 1980s there were other medical priorities. Now that the advocates had made breast cancer an issue—and the scientists saw signs of promise—the funds were drying up.

Just before the National Cancer Institute appropriations hearings began, Fran Visco dreamed that someone was yelling at her because the Defense Department had had to give up a B-1 bomber to pay for the breast cancer research program. She was singlehandedly responsible for the downfall of the United States. Her obsession with breast cancer had made the entire country vulnerable to attack.

The first thing she thought when she woke up was, God, we should only get that much money.

Her second thought was, It is very sad that my life has come to dreaming about this stuff.

But her long-term therapy was to be a moving target, as though cancer could not come back to grab her as long as she was fast on her feet. She fought despair from a speeding train between Philadelphia and Washington, or a cab hastily hailed outside the capital's Union Station; she defied it to find her in the labyrinthine halls of Congress.

Her year's sabbatical was about to end, so she informed the partners at Cohen, Shapiro, Polisher, Sheikman and Cohen that she had decided to resign. She had to devote herself to activism full-time, since she thought about it no matter what else she was doing, even when she was asleep.

After a full day of meetings at the NCI, she had just enough time to grab a quick coffee and snack in the deserted bar of her favorite Washington hotel. She thought about what she had accomplished since that glorious fall day in 1993, when President Clinton had pledged a new commitment to breast cancer research, and she thought about everything that was left to be done. Her eyes filled with exhausted tears.

She thought, I haven't done anything yet.

For all her weariness, Fran had a cause, which was what kept her going. Love, for the first time in her life, had something that more resembled a franchise, and a growing list of people who had a vested interest in her performance: Slamon, Glaspy, McFadden and his new boss, Dr. Holmes; Ronald Perelman and Lilly Tartikoff; the administrative personnel who had been given greater power; and the UCLA main hospital, which was going to bear part of the cost of the new breast center, downstairs in the radiology suite.

What she did not have was her idea of a center—the sunlit suite of rooms up on the sixth floor. The basement might provide private elevators from the Iris Cantor Imaging Center to the Breast Center, so a woman could progress from her mammogram to her doctor's examination without having to get dressed and undressed again, but it did not offer a patient much in the way of hopeful surroundings.

When Love came to UCLA, one of her stated goals was to distance herself from the advocacy movement, which rightfully belonged to the patient activists, not the doctors. She felt she had succeeded too well, despite Slamon's and Zinner's chronic complaints, and in the process had lost a measure of her independence, as well as the pleasure she derived from political work. She had been a pioneer, alongside Fran. The interviews and public appearances she continued to do, the ones that so irritated the people she worked with, were the only vestige of that part of her life.

As a clinician her opportunities were more limited. She could treat patients, and she could strive to do that in what she considered to be a more empathic, enlightened fashion, but she was constantly reminded that her ideal model for care did not make economic sense. She began to feel trapped, like Bernie Fisher, in a world where rules were more important than progress.

It was as though he were a ghost hovering behind her, reminding her again and again of how difficult it was to strike a balance between ambition and responsibility. Fisher got things done because he ran the show. If that was true, what was she doing at UCLA?

Running the Breast Center too often felt like scrubbing the grout in the convent bathroom with a toothbrush—a routinized chore, hardly satisfying, and quite possibly a waste of a formidable energy.

She was enlisted in Denny's passion, not her own. It was the clinician's lot to administer existing treatments while others struck out for the new territories. Love had to figure out whether she could do that at UCLA and still feel that she was leading the relevant life she always talked about. She could not allow herself to become a custodian of the past.

35

A LIFE, LOST

OCTOBER 1995

THE CARS BEGAN TO PULL UP IN THE LATE AFTERNOON. THE BAYSHORE Community Church was a little hard to find, nestled in a residential neighborhood hidden between two main streets. It was not the family's church; they had no church. The minister listened to the little group of strangers reminisce about their loved one so that he could fashion a brief service out of their memories. Some of them wanted to speak, and he had encouraged them to bring along a tape of the deceased's favorite song.

Dena Yvette Smith Wieman died of metastatic breast cancer at Long Beach Memorial Hospital on Saturday, October 21, 1995. It was easy to pick out her daughter and sister as they stood on the front steps of the church—they had the same pale eyes, apple cheeks, pug nose, and dainty chin. Dee's illness had erased whatever resentments had piled up over the past decade. In the days preceding her death they had come to Huntington Beach to sit with her, make her a cup of tea, hold her hand, and wonder why there was no way to save her.

Dee's best friend, Suzy, rushed up, breathless, just as the service was about to start. She slid into a pew next to her husband, her thin hands trembling, her shoulders threatening to give way, and surveyed the seven bouquets of flowers that adorned the small stage. She nudged her husband and pointed to the one she had chosen, a basket of pink and white lilies with pink and white helium balloons tied to it. Just right.

"That's Dee, those balloons," she whispered, and behind her big sunglasses she began to cry.

The service was brief. Gary Wieman sat in the front row next to his mother and father, his face flushed, his arms crossed helplessly in front of him. Next to them were Dee's father, Maynard, and her stepmother, Rita. Dee's sister and niece sat in the row behind the rest of the family. Only Dee's daughter sat apart from the rest, a few rows back, with her father, Dee's first husband.

When the minister began to speak of Dee's sense of humor and generosity, Maynard Smith's reserve crumbled. Rita wrapped her hand around his shoulder, and his surviving daughter moved up to sit next to him, only to drop her head against his chest and begin to sob. Her daughter, Dee's niece, came to sit next to her.

Two banners, one at either side of the church, instructed them all:

REMEMBER

REJOICE

Gary stood outside the church afterward in a daze. How odd: Dee's death was the one definitive event in a year marked by contradiction and confusion. All during the spring of 1995 the tests came back like screaming night terrors, taunting them with worse and worse results. This was a bully cancer, one that sneered at high-dose chemotherapy and continued to romp through Dee's body. She developed demonstrable metastatic disease: the cancer spread to her lungs and her spine, and after a while a glass of red wine no longer made her back pain disappear. A lung specialist at UCLA who tracked the transplant patients said that Dee's lungs had been damaged by the BCNU, and put her on steroids.

By April she was desperate—so she contacted her original doctor in Long Beach, the one who had got hold of her on her car phone an eternity ago, and he put her in touch with a doctor at USC who was involved in a clinical trial. Gary and Dee were so frantic by that point that they never really grasped the goal of the USC study. All they knew was that there was a marker that might identify cancer cells, and Dee's demonstrable disease made her eligible. Action meant possibility: For three months she and Gary lived in what he called "a little thrill box" of hope. But in July the USC doctors found more cancer in Dee's bones. She dropped out of the study, and went through a "demonic dive," so the Wiemans gave up on traditional medicine. So far, it only seemed to have made her worse.

They decided to go to a cancer clinic in Tijuana, where the doctors opened Dee's sternum and took a sample from her bone—diseased cells, they said, that they would use as a vaccine. At their fifth visit Gary was instructed to start giving Dee injections of the drug methotrexate, a standard chemotherapeutic drug, and then the vaccine.

Dee came home each time so exhausted that she often declined to come to the phone to talk to friends—radical behavior for a woman who lived for companionship. Still, Gary allowed himself to be hopeful. He told their friends that the Mexican vaccine was working. Dee was off all the heavy drugs and she felt pretty good.

Gary had changed since the transplant. He had seen Dee suffer so; he could no longer deny the lethal threat she faced. He became her unconditional, if sometimes clumsy, ally, cheerleading, coaxing her to try one more treatment, enticing her to eat. He knew, at last, that he might really lose her, and he behaved as though he wanted to make up for lost time.

He tried to tantalize her with his vision of the future. If she would just keep trying she could recover, and then she could dedicate her life to breast cancer activism, to make the road easier for the women who followed her. She confessed privately to Suzy Drawbaugh that she wished Gary wouldn't say such things. She was having enough trouble getting from one day to the next.

In early October Suzy got a call from Dee, who wanted to know if Suzy could drive her to St. John's to see her oncologist, Dr. Boasberg. It was an unusual request. In the two years since Dee's diagnosis she had never once asked Suzy to do the driving, feeling it was too much of an imposition.

Suzy watched her friend hobble over to the car and thought that if she had not known it was Dee she might have walked right by her. She had changed so. Her hair had grown back in wavy tendrils that she wore short, framing her face. She had lost about fifty pounds, so that her once imposing frame was wearily plump, almost cuddly. She got in and out of the car like an elderly woman, wincing at her back pain, unsteady on her rickety legs.

Boasberg was as close as Dee had come to the shepherd she had so wanted to find, so she asked him the one question she had been unable to ask anyone until now.

"How much time do I have?" she whispered.

He took a long time to answer. Peter Boasberg agonized over what to say when patients asked him a blunt question like that, and yet he felt obligated to give an honest answer. Dee had a right to know. It would be insulting to keep the truth from her.

"A couple of weeks," he said, and regretted the words as soon as they were out of his mouth.

"Well," she said, reflexively. "Then what's next?"

Boasberg began to talk to Dee about pain management, but she could not sit still for that. She thanked him, stumbled out of his office, and maintained her self-control until she and Suzy got to the bank of elevators. Then she slumped against the wall as though someone had punched her.

"I never should have asked him," she said. "Why did I ask him?"

"Oh, Dee" was all Suzy could muster.

Dee was silent until they got downstairs to the main entrance. Then she turned to her friend.

"I thought he was going to say five years," Dee said. She could tolerate the pain as long as she thought she had enough time for someone to discover a miracle—a cure, a treatment that could turn back even her cancer. But two weeks? No one was going to save her that fast. She might as well be dead already.

She tried to regain her equilibrium. What could she accomplish in two weeks? First she thought she might organize the boxes of photographs in the garage, but then she decided against it. If she set out a project for herself and completed it she would surely die. She decided to leave the photos alone, mildly concerned that Gary might throw them out someday, but far more frightened that God would think she had finished what she needed to do, and take her.

* * *

Suzy savored the last days, because for once Dee allowed her friends and family to wait on her. Suzy hovered near her bed, always ready to fulfill the slightest request, and watched as Dee floated in and out of consciousness. She was on stronger pain medication by then; there were fewer and fewer chances to talk with her.

When the condo was fairly empty one afternoon, Suzy sat on the edge of Dee's bed and took her hand.

"I love you," Suzy said, and bent down to kiss her friend on the forehead. She lay down and they rested together, quietly, watching the boats slide by in the bay outside the bedroom window.

In the haze Dee remembered three things. Once she woke up in bed alone and heard Gary crying downstairs. The next time she awoke she was still alone, and she heard him praying aloud. The third time she woke he was lying next to her on the bed, stroking her arm, not saying a word.

Three days after the funeral, about forty of Dee's family members and friends congregated at the harbor in San Pedro to board the *Spirit,* the boat that would take them out to sea so that Dee's ashes could be scattered on the ocean. Everyone received a small program bound in pink ribbon.

"Safe passage, Braveheart," read the inscription at the top of the first page, "during your transition from apprentice to full-fledged Angel."

"Dena Yvette Smith Wieman, 'Dee.' Enhanced our lives October 25, 1948, Evansville, Indiana. Ascended October 21, 1995, Long Beach, California. Cherished Mommy, Grammy, Wife, Daughter, Sister and Friend."

There was a copy of a poem Dee's uncle had read at the funeral, followed by two pages of photographs of her, from 1950 to the mid-1970s. On the last page was her 1985 wedding picture—a jubilant, beaming Dee, her shining blond hair crowned with a wreath of fresh flowers, wearing a low-cut white dress. The picture below it was from 1995, just weeks before she died—Dee with cropped hair and a more tentative grin, as though she had to be reminded of what to do in front of a camera.

Suzy could not go up to the top deck when it was time to scatter the ashes; she could not bear to see her friend's life reduced to a handful of nothing. She looked out to sea and saw a growing gray stain next to the boat, as the ashes fell into the water. The boat turned and circled once, twice, and headed back to shore.

36

DANCING WITH
THE DEVIL

THERE WAS A REVOLUTION, ALTHOUGH IT WAS NOT THE ONE LOVE HAD so eagerly anticipated. President Clinton's health care reform package, with its central dream of universal medical coverage, had gone down to ignominious defeat in September 1994, a victim of its own impractical idealism. It was like one of Love's own grand ideas—sweeping, born of the best intentions, but difficult to implement. His critics dismissed the defeated plan as "fantasy," and business stepped in where politics had failed.

Industry engineered the upheaval; insurance companies acted as though Clinton's defeat was the signal for them to take over. During 1995, the managed care revolt that had begun when Love was still in private practice had spread. There was no one left to pay the kinds of fees doctors were used to charging. The ranks of private indemnity patients dwindled because that type of insurance was prohibitively expensive, and patients found the gap between their new insurance reimbursements and their bills intolerable. By the time Love began her salary negotiations for fiscal 1997, in April 1996, business owned medicine.

She found herself confronting the same dilemma she had faced back in Boston, four years before: the only way to stay in business, even in a university setting, was to see more patients. The lower overhead and subsidized salary were no longer enough to protect her. It was as though insurers were now in a conspiracy with her employer to force her to trim the time she spent with each patient and give up her political work. The previous year UCLA had for the first time tied a portion of her salary to volume, but she had more than compensated for a slight dip in salary when she accepted an $850,000 offer from Times Books to write a book on hormones.

She knew what this year promised, though—an even heavier clinical workload and lower guaranteed reimbursements. She had to take time off to write the book, and that, combined with her political work, would make it virtually impossible to maintain her earnings as a surgeon. Love anticipated that she would make about one-third less than the $300,000 she had received when she first arrived. The move downstairs to the new Revlon/UCLA Center for Women's Health was scheduled for early 1997, meaning higher operating costs—and worse numbers, and undoubtedly more complaints from Denny Slamon.

She went through the motions of asking for more, and got the university to raise its guarantee slightly, but even as she did so she realized that money was not really the issue. After more than twenty years of seeing patients, Love was too tired, she said, "to keep churning them out." If she could not see patients on her terms, she would not see them at all.

Her situation was hardly unique. Doctors everywhere were being paid less for what they did or opting for early retirement. This was the revolution—not the glorious revolt that would allow her to spend more time with women, debate speculative ideas with her colleagues, provide quality care no matter which insurer was footing the bill. It was piecework in the name of affordable health care.

Love obstinately held out hope for the future of managed care; she believed in the concept of doctors' accountability that was supposed to stand at the center of it. But the first phase was not a viable system. It was an overreaction to what had come before—after too many years of padded fees and deified physicians, the pendulum had swung to the other extreme, bare-bones coverage and an assembly-line mentality. There were still huge profits to be made, but by insurance companies rather than by doctors.

She did not want to be part of it, not yet, and she had the luxury of being able to walk away.

This is unacceptable, she thought. It was time to move on.

Love decided to leave the university. In May 1996 she drafted two letters. The first went to Dave McFadden, the chairman of the Division of Surgery and her one-time colleague at the Breast Center; to E. Carmack Holmes, the chairman of the Department of Surgery and McFadden's boss; and to the dean of the School of Medicine. The second letter was for Denny Slamon and the people at Revlon, who expected Love to be the director of their breast program.

Love's relationship with Slamon had deteriorated during the last half of 1995, as they reached a stand-off on the structure and operation of the new center. He was in charge of the money for it, but she always did better as her own boss. There was no longer any common ground. Slamon, exasperated, had given up trying to keep her in line—and Love stopped telling him what she was doing. They had not spoken for months when he first heard that her salary negotiations were in trouble. He decided to stay out of it. Susan was going to do what Susan was going to do.

He did not reply to her letter. No one responded save McFadden, who sent her an e-mail saying, "Sorry."

That spring, just as Love and the university began their talks, the Defense Department awarded her dogged efforts at grantsmanship with a $700,000 grant to pursue her duct endoscope research. If she left UCLA she would have to turn down the grant—but once Love embraced a new idea she found it hard to negotiate with the past. She announced to her intimates at the Center that she was prepared to sacrifice that money to buy her freedom.

It was a big gesture, but it made no sense. The money was important to her, and to the university, so Love accepted an offer to become an adjunct professor, which enabled her to keep the grant. It was a slim thread. She had no clinical practice, and no ties to the Breast Center; just the occasional lecture to medical students. She would work from home. Her last day at UCLA would be May 15, 1996.

*   *   *

The real question was how to tell the patients. She sent out a letter informing them of her decision and encouraging them to continue to take advantage of the Breast Center's expanding list of services. She had the facilitators call a handful of women—the ones who had broken past the usual doctor-patient boundaries, Dottie Mosk, Laura Wilcox, Jerilyn Goodman, Shirley Barber, Ann Donaldson, Barbara Rubin—to ask them to make one last appointment. Laura declined; she preferred to move forward. The others came in, as did many patients who were told that there were no more appointments available. They showed up anyway and sat in the General Surgery waiting room without an appointment, determined to see Love one last time before she left. Her last days were a glimpse, in miniature, of the future she had rejected: patients in, patients out, and hardly enough time to catch her breath in between.

Shirley Barber's daughter, Kim, anxiously inquired about what her mother was to do if someday she needed another surgery.

"She won't," replied Love. "But if she does, just drop by the house. I'll set up in the garage."

Once again she had walked away, and her critics were quick to condemn what they perceived as irresponsible behavior. Love was used to it. Many doctors in Boston had scorned her—and when news of her decision to leave UCLA became public, some of her colleagues there turned on her as well, insisting that they were relieved to see her go. She had expected as much. Her opinions on current treatment and the right way to practice medicine—and her disdain for academic camaraderie—had alienated a lot of doctors who had prospered under the old, private practice model.

Love was not about to mourn what she had left behind. The opportunity here was to make the brave transition. She began to talk, not to other doctors, but to people who understood business.

An economist she knew told her that the reason for the managed care revolution was simple. Medicine, she said, was a cartel. There was no way to foment change from inside the cartel, because its doctor members were stakeholders in the old system. Businessmen took over medicine because doctors could not make the necessary reforms. They had priced themselves out of the market, and it took outsiders to bring them under control.

"The business people," as she called anyone involved in the insurance industry, were in fact great potential allies. They believed, as she always had, in what she called "evidence-based medicine"—they wanted to pay for proven treatments and not for anecdotal experimentation. They had the nerve to talk about cost-benefit ratios, which their critics condemned as medical rationing. Love preferred to think that they were trying to distinguish between what worked and what did not—an honorable goal, even if they had overdone it in their first few months of power.

One way to keep health care costs down was to keep people from developing illnesses that required dramatic, expensive treatments. What looked like less care could turn out to be better care, if insurers ended up paying for preventive regimens. The only prevention against breast cancer to have surfaced in the last year was regular exercise, three to four hours each week, but the dearth of possibilities did not diminish Love's enthusiasm. If there was financial support for prevention, then research might turn in that direction—just as it had turned to breast cancer when the Defense Department started spending money.

Love wanted to create a nonprofit think tank for women's health issues, as well as a for-profit consulting firm to work with managed care providers on service packages for breast patients. The insurance companies may have wrested control from the medical community, but Love had something they needed—a plan for standardized care. Her attempt to define a set of basic practice guidelines had finally borne fruit; "The Revlon/UCLA Breast Center Practice Guidelines for the Treatment of Breast Cancer," had been published in January 1996 in *Science* magazine's publication, the *Cancer Journal*.

She wanted to clone the programs she had created at UCLA and teach managed care providers to supply quality at a reasonable cost. It was time, as far as she was concerned, for doctors to stop complaining about their diminished status. She was ready to embrace the enemy.

"I think the first wave of managed care was ratcheting down the cost," she said. "Making it as cheap as you could. But what's going to happen is, pretty soon, we're going to be down where you can't make it any cheaper. And then people are going to differentiate by quality. That's where I hope to be able to come in and say, 'Okay, this is how you make your HMO health plan services of a higher quality than the next one.' "

She had already heard about a study showing that many people were willing to pay a $250 monthly charge for the privilege of choosing their doctors; more than that and they balked. If she could figure out how to help provide comprehensive breast services in that price range she would have a new, even larger constituency.

She was just where she wanted to be—on the edge, on the front line of a new movement. She thought about pursuing a master's degree in public health, but decided instead to go after a master's in business administration, beginning in the fall of 1996. The long and finally fruitless series of meetings she had had with UCLA's Managed Care Contracts department had failed to yield a relationship with a managed care provider, and in great part Love blamed herself. She had not bothered to learn the native dialect. She had been that thing she so disdained, the arrogant surgeon.

This time around she would behave differently. If the only way to prevail was to learn to "speak business," as she put it, that was what she would do. Once she had a seat at the table, she could be the one to teach them medicine.

The science remained maddeningly out of reach. If the September 1994 discovery of BRCA-1 heralded the beginning of a new era in breast cancer research, the following year put science on notice. There would be no quick solutions, not with breast cancer. Doctors and patients alike wanted desperately to believe in gene therapy as the answer to their prayers, but BRCA-1 did not cooperate.

The gene was in no hurry to give up its secrets. Natalie Angier reported in *The New York Times* that the gene proved "to be as frustrating and recalcitrant as the disease," in the months following its discovery. One Utah researcher was finishing a report that listed a total of eighty possible mutations to BRCA-1, and estimates of the final count ran into the hundreds.

Worse, scientists were having trouble detecting mutations in some women whom they suspected of having a damaged gene. And they could not find a mutation in tumor samples from women with sporadic breast cancer—though they had hoped to find a link that might shed light on the majority of patients, who had no known risk factors. Women who had hoped for information, if not answers, were going to have to wait a good while longer.

The first break came almost a year after the initial discovery. In September 1995 the National Institutes of Health linked a BRCA-1 defect to a high risk of breast and ovarian cancer among Jewish women of European ancestry. National Center for Genome Research director Dr. Francis Collins said that the finding—which could account for as much as sixteen percent of breast cancers in women under fifty in that ethnic group—represented a "sea change in how people think about genetics and public health." Jewish women could be screened for the genetic alteration, just as they were screened for Tay-Sachs disease, a hereditary disease that drastically increased the chances of severe birth defects.

But Mary-Claire King saw the danger in widespread testing. She, like Love, supported genetic testing only within a research setting. Science did a woman no favor by telling her she had the gene, only to abandon her to conflicting medical advice and the possibility of job and insurance discrimination.

"There was bound to be a stage when we could identify people at risk (for breast cancer) and not be able to do anything about it," King told a reporter. "We are there now. We're stuck."

It was, at this point, a purely philosophical debate. The term "screening test" implied a simple blood test that yielded a definitive yes or no. The truth was far more complex. Myriad Genetics wanted to develop a comprehensive test, one that screened for all known mutations—and once its revised patent application was approved, it would be the only company legally authorized to provide a test.

In the meantime, though, other labs were scrambling to put together tests that screened for some of the existing mutations. OncorMed Inc. had started testing patients and their family members, as part of a research program, in the summer of 1995. They and other labs could do business until Myriad got the patent, at which point they would have to enter into a licensing agreement with Skolnick's company—a license he was not inclined to issue, at least not to a commercial company that represented direct competition. He planned to allow researchers to use Myriad's test without paying a licensing fee, but anyone else who sold a test without permission would be violating his patent. He was prepared to get an injunction to stop the other labs, if need be, and if they ignored him to pursue legal action to collect damages.

But he saw what was coming, in the months it would take to devise Myriad's test and win patent approval: tests of varying scope and accuracy, sold to women who were anxious to know something and unaware of the tests' limitations. A high-risk woman could pass one of the early tests and still carry a mutation. There was going to be a lot of aggressive salesmanship before a comprehensive test was available.

He was emphatically optimistic about what that test would mean. Skolnick wanted to test women and then offer them options: close monitoring for young high-risk patients, more aggressive biopsies—or possibly prophylactic mastectomy, "if she has had multiple breast cancer deaths in the family, has a stable, secure marital situation, or for whatever reason wishes to reduce her risk of dying as much as possible, and has no negative feelings" about the procedure. He hoped that would be an infrequent choice, though, and looked instead to "the advances that one can anticipate in the near future which may reduce risk, such as preventive therapeutic options."

He held out hope for tamoxifen as a preventive. He also thought that women with a mutated gene might consider the prophylactic removal of their ovaries, "a much different type of operation, surgically and cosmetically. It does have the severe effect of creating an artificial menopause," but it eradicated the threat of ovarian cancer risk and lowered breast cancer risk.

Skolnick likened attitudes about the procedure—with the attendant issue of whether to put a patient on hormone replacement therapy—to the early debate over lumpectomy. No one had suggested not operating while doctors studied the relative merits of lumpectomy and mastectomy. The only way to determine how well oophorectomy worked was to research it. Skolnick wanted high-risk women to be tested for BRCA-1 so they could make an informed decision about their risk—and he wanted future generations to have data.

"Wouldn't it be better to find out who should have it and who should not?" he said. "Let's do what we can do, and let's make sure that no women who test positive and are willing to participate in future research aren't utilized to the maximum," he said. Anything less seemed ridiculous to him. "That's like saying, 'Because breast cancer's not curable we shouldn't operate,' which is utterly stupid."

Skolnick insisted that people said there was no cure for breast cancer "because they can't think of what else to say. It's such total nonsense." To him, there was possibility everywhere. On one point he agreed with the activists and Mary-Claire King: "The need for further study," he said, "is immense."

He saw Myriad's test as a doorway to the future, a means for recruiting a new population of research subjects. Skolnick wanted to offer it to any interested high-risk woman. "In the spirit of freedom of choice, which this country's based on," he said, "women should be allowed to follow their own dictates."

On that issue the advocates took a more conservative stance. Susan Love advised women to have the test only if they already had been diagnosed—and not to let their daughters be tested, "or they'll never get medical insurance."

In November 1995 researchers at the University of Texas at San Antonio made a stunning announcement that guaranteed even more intense interest in screening for BRCA-1. In an article published in *Science* magazine, they showed that the gene did in fact have a relationship to sporadic breast cancer. Whatever researchers could learn about the gene, and about possible interventions to block its abnormal behavior, would hold far greater significance than originally thought. Women with no family history might eventually choose to be tested, to see if they carried a mutated copy of BRCA-1.

The elusive gene suddenly seemed full of potential. Taming it was a feasible challenge, compared to the endless effort involved in finding it. *The New York Times* ran a long article, "Surprising Role Found for Breast Cancer Gene," in March 1996, about the part BRCA-1 played in sporadic breast cancer, and ways in which it might yield to manipulation. Mary-Claire King, who had move the University of Washington in Seattle, and a group of researchers at Vanderbilt University published two reports on BRCA-1. The gene seemed to invite medical intervention: instead of being sequestered deep in the nucleus of the cell, it sat on the outer edge and secreted its protein into the fluid between cells. Under normal conditions the protein regulated cell growth; gone awry, it allowed malignant growth to begin.

It looked easy to get at, and quite possibly would respond to treatments that did not damage the rest of the body. There was hopeful talk of a "magic bullet." Researchers in one study gave injections to ten mice who had received grafts of human breast cancer cells. Five received a virus with a healthy copy of BRCA-1, and five received a defective version of the gene. After just over a week the mice with the mutant gene were dead of cancer, but the ones with working BRCA-1 lived as long as forty-one days. If there was a way to replace a damaged BRCA-1 in a human being, it might be possible to stop a breast cancer from developing.

Still, it was a long way from mice in the laboratory to an intervention for humans. "Provocative as the rodent results are," wrote the *Times*'s Natalie Angier, "viral delivery vectors are not likely to be terribly useful for human patients. Instead, researchers hope that their latest explorations of the protein's function will yield standard chemically based drugs to be taken orally or intravenously."

Despite the news of its accessible position, Susan Love feared that BRCA-1 was going to be as difficult to manipulate as any of the other mutated genes scientists were working on. It could be years before that painful window between understanding and action was closed.

But after twenty years' effort, Mary-Claire King allowed herself a small hope. She wondered if she might have arrived at the halfway point—if twenty years from now there might be an effective treatment for breast cancer. Not a cure or a preventive, but at least a treatment that worked.

"I'm getting more optimistic," she said, "as time goes on."

Early in 1996, OncorMed began offering its BRCA-1 test through doctors, medical centers, and clinics, the first time a screen-

de available outside a research setting. Despite
social ramifications of general testing, there was
the product—and some women complained that
est to researchers was just another example of pater-
inking. Women could make up their own minds, and they
wa ed a test. OncorMed would screen breast and ovarian cancer
patients, and their family members, at a cost of $150 to $1,650,
depending on the amount of screening that had to be done.

At the same time, Skolnick's group published a paper explaining that their early notions about a screening test had been wrong.
At first Skolnick had imagined that there would be a few common
mutations, and that creating a "mutation profile" to serve as the
foundation of a test would be a relatively simple matter. About
twenty research institutions had complied with his request for DNA
samples, in return for free screening once Myriad had a test—but as
Skolnick's team began to evaluate the samples, they found more
and more mutations. Devising a comprehensive test was going to be
far more complicated than they had thought. Skolnick revised his
estimate, and started telling people that he hoped to have a test
ready by the end of 1996.

Still, he reminded the participating researchers that they had got
a good deal, "millions of dollars worth of testing" for free. It was
worth the wait.

Fifteen months after the National Cancer Institute issued its
revised guidelines on mammography for women under fifty, a team
of Swedish researchers released the study Larry Bassett had heard
about, a meta-analysis of several smaller studies of mammography
for women between the ages of forty and fifty. Their March 1996
analysis looked at 150,000 women in that age group who had participated in randomized trials, and provided follow-up data twelve
years out, extending beyond the original studies.

It refuted the NCI's conclusion. Mammography did, in fact,
save young lives. According to the Swedish study, there was a
twenty-four percent reduction in mortality among women under
fifty who had annual mammograms. When the Swedes included
data from the controversial Canadian study that had shown no
improvement in mortality and first sparked the controversy, the

figure was still impressively high—a seventeen percent reduction in mortality.

Dr. Richard Klausner, who succeeded Dr. Samuel Broder as director of the National Cancer Institute in August 1995, felt that the Swedish study required the NCI to reconsider its recommendation. He announced that the NCI would reevaluate its data on mammography in the fall of 1996.

Dr. Barry Kramer, associate director for the Institute's early detection and community oncology program, told the *Boston Globe*, "We do plan to get all the world's investigators together again, to go over the most recent results."

Dr. Daniel Kopans, director of breast imaging at Massachusetts General Hospital, who had argued vehemently against the NCI's changed policy, now wondered what the cost of the past two years of confusion would be. Kopans estimated that nearly twenty percent of breast cancer cases involved women in their forties—about thirty-six thousand annually, he told the *Globe,* some of whom might have decided not to have a mammogram because of the NCI's position. "I have no idea exactly how many lives could have been saved by not confusing women in their 40s about the value of mammograms," said Kopans. "I would expect in the thousands."

Saving lives. Dr. I. Craig Henderson, the oncologist who in 1982 had hired Susan Love to see breast cancer patients at Boston's Dana Farber Hospital, thought that it was perhaps arrogant for the medical community to think it could eradicate breast cancer. A more appropriate goal was to keep the women who got it from dying of the disease. A woman's one-in-eight lifetime risk was not the important number. What mattered was that 1 in 28 American women died of breast cancer. That was the number doctors and researchers needed to improve.

Henderson stood aligned with Glaspy and Slamon at the far end of the treatment continuum, working to enhance the effectiveness of chemotherapy. He would have been happy if someone at the other end of the line came up with a preventive, but he was a realist. The likelier victory was better treatment. He worked doggedly to perfect Bernie Fisher's paradigm, and find a more effective way to combat systemic disease. He had become sorely tired of watching women with metastatic disease die.

John Glaspy was ever eager for a new idea, and toward the end of 1995 he had turned from his usual interest in chemotherapeutic drugs to what was for him an unlikely field—nutrition. Dave Heber and Susan Love had been unable to find funding for their study of soy, low-fat diet, and exercise, but Heber told anyone who would listen how intrigued he was by the idea. He kept the grant proposal on his shelf, unwilling to let go of the notion, proud of the science at its foundation.

It dovetailed nicely with Glaspy's curiosity about changing the levels of various polyunsaturated fatty acids in a woman's body, as well as his frustration with the tools he usually used. He embarked on a study of his most desperate and eager patients, women with metastatic disease who had undergone a transplant. They were so motivated to keep fighting; they were willing to endure a diet high in soy and fish oil, and very good about compliance.

By the fall of 1996 he had exciting results, although it would be years before he knew if they translated into an effective clinical regimen. Diet could change the makeup of breast tissue, which in turn might be enough to discourage a recurrence. Love had talked about figuring out ways to change the biological environment, and so disarm a cancer. Glaspy was having luck with the first half of that equation; in time, he would find out if he had in fact picked a promising path.

Whatever the outcome, Heber was ebullient. A real researcher working on a nutritional study. An oncologist using something other than drugs. He dove into his application for a third renewal of his NIH grant, and made plans for the opening of a $500,000, privately endowed center devoted to the study of nutrition. Heber's research had been a stepchild for a long time, but he believed it was about to take its rightful place at the center of breast cancer research.

Dr. Bernard Fisher sat out the future, a proud but sorrowful man who alternated between outrage at what had happened and a more somber fear of the consequences of his actions. Two and a half years after the *Chicago Tribune*'s disclosures about falsified NSABP data, the tamoxifen prevention trial was again under way, and the furor over the lumpectomy data had subsided. Bernie Fisher was still in exile, and he chafed at his new existence.

"When all this stops," he said, referring to his work in clinical trials, "then there's no point in continuing. That, I think, is one of the great tragedies that happened to me in my life. Not so much what happened to *me,* but what *happened.* There were many things in the pot, to get it boiling, and that was stopped. The flame went out under the pot. For me, personally, that has prevented me from progressing on to another dimension. So now what I'm trying to do is get the pot lighted."

His days were taken up with his two lawsuits, with depositions and legal documents and the costly, time-consuming process of obtaining what he defined as justice. For thirty-five years he had gotten up in the morning for "the excitement and thrill of making some kind of progress." Now he woke up wondering if he would ever get back to his life's work. But there could be no compromise: He insisted that justice come to him. He spoke bleakly of McCarthyism, of attacks on academic freedom and first amendment rights. He yearned for a return to the old order, even as science turned in a new direction.

Mark Skolnick learned humility, as months passed without a test. He referred to the "black eye" Myriad had, for making promises it could not keep. He began to forge tentative alliances with one-time adversaries.

He made an overture to Fran Visco, having realized that they had certain goals in common. They still disagreed on the proper setting for testing—Visco wanted to limit it to research, while Skolnick intended to take it into the marketplace—but they shared a frustration with governmental bureaucracy, and a desire to speed up work on new clinical therapies. Skolnick met with Visco over the summer of 1996 and came away wishing he had released the gene sequence as soon as the press got hold of the news about BRCA-1. He should not have alienated her by hanging on to it. There was enough divisiveness in the fight against breast cancer without looking for more.

He was not as successful with Mary-Claire King. She was not among the researchers who had contributed twelve hundred DNA samples to help Myriad develop a mutation profile; she was doing her own testing on the families who had participated in her research, and had had no contact with Myriad since the discovery of BRCA-1 had been announced.

King kept her distance, for she saw no reason to have any dealings with her ex-collaborator. Her position was simple: The gene sequence was now public; she insisted that she had no use for Skolnick's test. "All experienced laboratories, public or commercial, use the same range of methods to detect mutations in BRCA-1," she said. "I would not need to ask any other lab to carry out the work."

Skolnick disagreed. He believed that Myriad's test would be "superior to any other, research or commercial, in a number of aspects," and he could imagine a time when King might want access to it. He was still waiting for his patent approval, but had already decided not to impose any licensing requirements on King. He intended to extend the researcher's free use, even if she wanted to charge for screening in a clinical setting. The most he would do, once he had the patent, would be to ask her to limit the amount of paid testing she conducted.

He might have the right to demand more, but there was no point. How stupid would it be, he thought, to make trouble for Mary-Claire King?

Denny Slamon's research on metastatic patients got a boost in the spring of 1996. On April 22, 1996, UCLA issued a press release that caused a deluge of media attention: "New Antibody May Control Breast Cancer in Some Cases, Trials Show at UCLA's Jonsson Comprehensive Cancer Center." The cautious wording—the *may,* the *in some cases*—became a casualty of the media's enthusiasm. News programs introduced the segment with talk of a cure.

The previous summer Slamon had begun enrolling subjects for his Phase 3 clinical trial, which involved ninety sites in the United States, almost twenty in Europe, six in Canada, and three in Australia. The principal trial was for women who had never been treated for their metastatic breast cancer; half of them received chemotherapy plus a placebo, and the other half, chemotherapy plus the HER-

2/neu antibody. Six patients were enrolled at UCLA. One woman's tumor disappeared completely, three patients had their tumors shrink, one stayed the same, and only one saw her cancer progress.

"Our early findings are very promising, with some outstanding results," said Slamon. "But I want to emphasize that we don't yet have enough information for statistically meaningful evaluations. We certainly have come to no final conclusions." He knew he needed bigger numbers, and he knew about all the other promising treatments that had run dry after about four years. At the moment he had measurable clinical response in a handful of very grateful women—which might, in turn, help him achieve full enrollment of 450 patients for the study. Ten years after the discovery of the HER-2/neu alteration, he was a happy man.

It had been a satisfying year on several counts. In the fall of 1995, when his daughter started high school, Slamon had for the first time allowed himself a slight respite from his normal sixteen-hour days. He realized that if he did not find some time to spend with her she would be in college, out of his house, grown, before he had a chance to know her. So he decided to stay home in the mornings to have breakfast with his children, and reveled in the time they had to talk about school, and what had happened the day before. Sometimes he did not get to UCLA until nine, or even nine-thirty.

That was his only deviation from routine. Denny Slamon had banked his life on a single bit of research that might help a small group of breast cancer patients, and nothing mattered to him as much as that. When he heard about the trouble Love was having, it was like a noise heard at a great distance. Between their fractured relationship and this pivotal phase of his research, he had put her out of his mind. Slamon had been in thrall to Love's celebrity in the early days, without realizing it, eager to have someone of her stature run UCLA's program. Borrowed glory had mattered to him. Now all he cared about was that the Breast Center succeed, whether Love was there or not.

He had come to regard the Breast Center as a "failed experiment" under her administration, but failure meant something quite different to a medical researcher than it did to the rest of the population. He thought about his friend John Glaspy, the one person at

UCLA for whom Slamon expressed unabashed praise. Glaspy was simply "the smartest guy around," in Slamon's estimation, and more aware than most of the importance of failure. He worked the same long hours Slamon did, many of them devoted to the stem cell transplant, even though he did not expect it to become a standardized treatment. He was open to new ideas, but rigorous in his approach.

They both believed that there was always a contribution to be made, if a person was smart enough to recognize it.

Mary-Claire King had failed to locate BRCA-1, but her attempt was what had enabled Mark Skolnick to make the discovery. In Slamon's estimation Susan Love had failed to make the Breast Center a success—but she had left a legacy he could exploit, a framework for the comprehensive, innovative breast program he had envisioned when he first set out to find a director in 1991. It happened at the moment to lack leadership, but he could remedy that. For a second time Denny Slamon embarked on a search for someone to run the center—preferably a woman, preferably a breast surgeon.

He was finished being angry—relieved, in an odd way, that the sparring was over. He liked Susan in spite of himself; thought her valiant, if rash, and deeply committed, even if he took issue with the quality of that commitment. They were just different. Slamon's life was about the incremental adjustment; Love's, about the paradigm shift. Let her joust with the future. He had work to do.

EPILOGUE

W HEN SHIRLEY WOKE UP NOW IN THE MIDDLE OF THE NIGHT IT was not because of her breast pain. That had quietly disappeared. She woke up because she was used to having her sleep interrupted. Tracy had not responded to the chemotherapy, and the surgery that was supposed to save his life was instead a procedure to enable him to continue eating, so he would not starve to death before his body gave out. So Shirley napped on hospital couches; she collapsed in her own bed for a few hours and then drove back to see her husband. When he came home, vigilance kept her half-awake. He was officially a terminal patient.

A few weeks after the surgery, in April 1995, Shirley called Susan Love to report on her progress and Tracy's condition. When she got to the part about the surgery they both began to cry. This was the worst part of a clinician's job, standing by while a decent guy with rotten luck got sicker and sicker. All the empathy in the world was not going to save Tracy Barber or cheer up his wife. The most generous wish Love could offer was for a hasty end.

"I hope it shows up in the liver," said Love. "It's quick."

It did not. Pain pills bought Tracy the summer he wanted— lazy days with his wife, driving over to a local art show, renting movies to watch on videotape. The family saw Paris and Venice and Rome. Tracy got Mitch installed in a freshman dormitory at Boston's Northeastern University in September 1995—and then, as though he had kept his disease in check while he finished what he wanted to do, he came home and started to decline. The doctors had been right. Ten months after his diagnosis, and he felt worse.

The sicker her husband became, the more ferociously Shirley looked after him. She was his guardian, as he had been hers, and she would not hear of anything else. He had to have surgery again, to remove tumors in his abdomen. More nights of sleeping alone in their big bed. That woke her up too.

This was a different kind of loneliness. She could not toss the covers onto her husband and hope to wake him up, at least long enough for a sympathetic hug. Even the widow down the street had remembered how to sleep, so there were no more shared images reflected on Shirley's window. If she wanted to watch TV now she would have to acknowledge her insomnia. Instead she just sat there in the dark.

It was practice for the future. This was how it was going to be. Tracy had faced it. He had taken her to a lawyer so early on that she had had a panic attack in the poor man's office, while the lawyer attempted to get straight exactly which one of his clients was dying. Tracy made up the inscription for his tombstone: I AM LOST. I HAVE GONE TO FIND MYSELF. IF I SHOULD RETURN BEFORE I GET BACK, PLEASE ASK ME TO WAIT.

He made Shirley promise to throw a wake before he died, so he could enjoy the festivities along with everyone else. He wondered where to find a bagpipe player to play "Amazing Grace" at his funeral.

Tracy took what he called a leave of absence from his laminating business and embarked on a new project. He did not want Shirley to have to make any important decisions in the first year following his death, so he inventoried the house to see what needed fixing. They bought new appliances. Tracy took Shirley to a nearby Ford dealership and bought her a brand-new silver Mustang. He was so methodical that sometimes it made her angry.

One morning she picked up the remote control that ran their

TV, compact disc player, and VCR, the one she never used because she did not know how, and brandished it at her husband.

"Before you croak," she said, "tape the instructions on it."

It was either that or endless tears. The kids broke her heart on a regular basis, every time they thought of some new thing that their father would miss. Mitch suddenly realized that Tracy would not meet the children he expected to have someday, and plunged into a funk. Kim focused all her grief on the question of who would walk her down the aisle the day she got married. Shirley suggested four possibilities—her brother, Mitch; her uncle; her mom; or nobody; she could walk herself down the aisle—but those were not the answers Kim wanted.

The future, that speculative space Shirley had worked so hard to control, seemed full of nothing but sadness, and at night, awake, alone, she had to struggle not to give in to it. No future pain: how easy that had been when all she was fighting was two dots on a piece of film.

She kept up the tough front. When Tracy told her, in March 1996, that it was time for what he called his "practice wake," she sent out the invitations and ordered the souvenir T-shirts, black ones with a sunset logo and the words, THE TRACY BARBER FAREWELL TOUR, 1995, 1996 . . . ? She went with Tracy to the cemetery and picked out a nice spot next to a lovely tree that someone else had just paid to plant. When he needed to rest she laid down with him, threw her arm around his waist, and muttered softly, "Mine."

Sorrow waited for night. She racked her brain for some defense, and then it came to her. When she could not sleep she would tell herself the story of Kim's wedding. Kim was only fifteen. It would be eight, ten years before she found the man she wanted to marry. Some of this sadness would have faded by then, and Shirley, full of pride, full of remembered love for Tracy, would do his job. She would be the one to walk their daughter down the aisle.

She did not tell Kim. This was Shirley's private talisman, and she clung to it whenever the grief threatened to engulf her. She knew she could do it. After all, she had DCIS, not invasive cancer. Dr. Love called it "cancer light." She had two years left on what she believed was tamoxifen, which she just knew was working. In the meantime, doctors had the gene, and the army had its research program, and there were all sorts of promising headlines. Shirley was going to stay healthy, and medical science had eight years to build her a safety net in case anything did go wrong.

Kim's wedding day. Surely there would be answers by then.

AFTERWORD
TO THE
PAPERBACK EDITION

OCTOBER 1997

I N RETROSPECT, THE VICTORIES OF THE EARLY 1990S HAD COME WITH
relative ease. Past neglect had provided anyone who cared
about breast cancer with a vast frontier just waiting to be
colonized. The fights were linear struggles for more money, more
information, more attention. And the pioneers, the ones determined
to expand activism from service and education to lobbying and
social change, were part of an allied crusade. There was no competition between breast cancer activists, nor from representatives of
other causes. Imagination and will had plenty of room to maneuver.

Breast cancer had been an easier cause for policymakers to embrace than its model, AIDS. However tight the federal budget might
be, these were the mothers and wives of America asking for help.
The first skirmishes were frustrating, but with hindsight it was clear
that the timing had been perfect. In terms of start-up money and
sympathy, the country was ready to yield.

By the end of the decade the fight had become far more popular—and far more complicated. Progress changed the nature of the
choices to be made; as the new movement became more sophisticated, it also became more vulnerable. Funding success fairly guaranteed that others would copy the breast cancer activists' moves,
and in fact the activists quickly found themselves in the odd posi-

tion of being regarded as the establishment, partisans of a well-fed issue that ought to share its riches with the less fortunate.

Politicians envied their colleagues in Congress who could claim credit for increasing the research budget, so new bits of legislation sprang up, often having far less to do with a considered, long-term agenda than with sound bites and media coverage. Private and corporate money tripped over itself in an attempt to contribute.

The new research was a crazy quilt of possibility, with hundreds of studies racing in all directions—and the ironic consequence was that many women felt more, not less, afraid. They imagined that such variety betrayed the scientific community's uncertainty; women's anxiety continued at an exaggerated level, far higher than the statistics warranted.

In fact, all the commotion was an indication only that more people had joined the fray. What Visco and Love had envisioned in 1992 had come to pass: Researchers who had not worked on breast cancer before now devoted their efforts to it and saw answers in unexpected directions. The field was suddenly very busy.

The search for a cure or preventive for breast cancer was not unlike the hunt for the gene for a heritable form of the disease. A few people worked in isolation until an initial victory—acquiring Defense Department funding or the narrowing of the gene search to a stretch of a single chromosome—made success seem within reach. Then there was a rush to participate in what looked to be an easier final sprint. New players, new motives, and a new, less manageable agenda.

There were roadblocks everywhere—not just enemies, but competitors. The National Breast Cancer Coalition had borrowed a page from the AIDS activists when it came to federal funding, but their success at the Department of Defense (DOD) had inspired a copycat who threatened to erode the research program they had worked so hard to establish and, each year since, to maintain.

Financier and prostate cancer survivor Michael Milken and the prostate cancer activists did the same thing the Coalition had done four years earlier, demanding an increase in an existing DOD prostate cancer research allocation—which, if granted, could mean a cut in the breast cancer budget. Fran Visco's dream of "more pie" was still just that. What money there was had to be shared by the loud, the wealthy, the quick. It helped to be able to cite a history of neglect—but the breast cancer advocates could no longer claim that position exclusively.

The media suggested that breast cancer could not claim that place at all. The *New York Times Magazine* announced the movement's new status on December 22, 1996, in an article about private and corporate largesse entitled, "How Breast Cancer Became This Year's Hot Charity." The attention frightened Visco, as had her initial victory at the Defense Department. Every acknowledgment carried with it an attendant threat: that the troops would decide their services were no longer needed. To Visco, the reverse was true. The struggle would begin in earnest once the noise subsided, as it inevitably would, as people lost patience or interest— once breast cancer was no longer "hot" but just another unresolved medical issue.

As she slogged through 1997, she was often overcome by dark feelings of frustration and irritability. Every politician seemed to have his or her pet breast cancer legislation. "Everyone in Congress wants to have their breast cancer bill," she observed ruefully. "It's very popular." There were more researchers, more activist groups springing up around the country. What was missing was the clear sense of a shared agenda, an informed definition of progress.

"The field is very, very crowded," she said, "and there are so many people who want to be connected to this. They're well meaning, but they aren't very well informed." She agonized over a whole new array of questions that had nothing to do with finding a preventive or a cure. The Coalition was invited to ally itself with various umbrella groups trying to raise money for cancer research, but Fran was not sure that the fundraising efforts of such groups were beneficial to breast cancer, however high-profile they might be. Did the presence of more disparate groups enhance or dilute the movement? Fighting breast cancer now required internal strategies as much as it did the more single-minded pursuit of change.

The science continued to balk and start, as recalcitrant as ever; the complexities of breast cancer defied any attempt to define clear priorities for the coming decade. BRCA-1 and BRCA-2, a second gene that when mutated increased the risk of developing breast cancer, never did what was expected of them. Initial reports had put the lifetime risk of breast cancer at about eighty-five percent for a woman who tested positive for BRCA-1, which made for a flurry of articles about genetic testing and prophylactic mastectomies; the UCLA Breast Center saw an influx of women who signed up for the high-risk clinic certain that they were knocking on death's door, only to be told that their histories were not as dire as they believed them to be.

In early April 1997 Dr. Craig Malbon, a researcher at the State University of New York at Stony Brook, his university, and a public relations firm, briefly promoted the attractive notion that there was an easier answer—that breast cancer cells often had elevated levels of an enzyme linked with cell growth. After studying the breast cells of eleven women who had breast cancer and nineteen who did not, the researcher concluded that mitogen-activated protein kinase, or MAP kinase, was five to twenty times more abundant in cancerous breast cells than in nonmalignant ones.

They considered the discovery nothing short of a breakthrough. If this was the switch that triggered the malignancy, then researchers could focus their collective efforts on the single question of how to turn it on and off.

But other researchers were less impressed: MAP kinase was associated with cell growth in general; they expected to find high levels of it in cancer cells. A week later the excitement had abruptly subsided. A simple answer was an appealing notion but not a likely one.

Hope was once again focused on BRCA-1 and BRCA-2. Researchers had already established a link between BRCA-1 and sporadic breast cancers, which accounted for as many as eighty-five percent of cases and could not be traced to a genetic or familial predisposition. Toward the end of 1996 researchers found that women who had mutated genes and developed breast cancer seemed to have a slower-growing form of the disease than other patients—the first somewhat positive attribute to be connected to the mutations. Once the researchers determined definitively how the genes worked, and how they might be repaired, they could look for new clinical answers both for patients and for women at high risk.

In the spring of 1997 researchers announced that both genes seemed to be part of the body's "copyediting" machinery, assigned to correct mistakes in the cells' genetic code. In particular, a healthy BRCA-2 worked to repair damage from ionizing radiation, like X rays. A woman with a damaged copy of the gene might be vulnerable to radiation from mammograms—although, ironically, a cancer caused by a mutated BRCA-2 might respond well to radiation therapy.

Then, in May 1997, came a daunting reappraisal: the gene might be not an isolated villain, but a coconspirator with other, unidentified troublemakers. Knowing the identity of the ringleader was not enough to predict a woman's fate. As the *Washington Post* reported, "Women who inherit faulty versions of the two genes, called BRCA-1 and BRCA-2, are less likely to get breast or ovarian cancer than previous studies had indicated, and the mutations are present in a smaller number of breast cancers than had been anticipated. . . ." A woman who carried a mutation but lacked a strong family history probably had a fifty percent chance of developing the disease by age seventy—four times higher than the population at large, but far less than the original estimate. Another study showed that mutated genes were present in only sixteen percent of women with a family history—not forty-five percent, as had been previously reported.

The genes seemed to cause less damage, and to be present in fewer cases, than had originally been thought. On a practical level, the already controversial genetic screening tests "may have less medical value than had been believed for most women," according to the *Post*.

"At this time," said Margaret Tucker, one of the researchers in the National Cancer Institute study who arrived at the revised figures, "we cannot predict an individual's risk based on genetic testing alone." There had to be other variables—in the environment, in a woman's lifestyle, in the workings of other genes—that made some women develop the disease and others not.

But the entrepreneurs, driven both by faith and by economic imperative, continued to profess their belief in genetic testing. In October 1996 Mark Skolnick's Myriad Genetics finally introduced its $2,400 screening test, to immediate challenge. A Stanford University bioethics panel recommended that most women avoid having the test. A negative result meant only that a woman had the same risk level as the rest of the population, not that she was free from all worry. A positive result did not necessarily mean she was destined to develop the disease. Since guidelines were not yet in place to protect a woman's privacy, she would have to worry about insurance and job discrimination.

Skolnick dismissed all of it as "utter nonsense." He held to his belief that there was a right-to-know issue involved—women ought to be able to find out their risk level if they wanted to, particularly with all the media attention being given to prophylactic mastectomy as a preventive. Suggesting that women avoid the test was, he said, "a great disservice. . . ."

Skolnick talked about empowerment. Dr. Francis Collins, head of the government's Human Genome Project, worried about the consequences of making tests available to doctors who did not fully comprehend them, in a vacuum, without sufficient counseling or support for the patient.

"We're going to have a lot of people potentially faced with information that is puzzling and frightening and no one to explain it to them," he told the *Los Angeles Times*.

Ten months after introducing the test in August 1997, Skolnick still did not have his patents for BRCA-1 or its mutations, although Myriad had filed several applications. Other companies continued to offer their own screening tests, and could continue to do so until a patent allowed Myriad to demand licensing arrangements. OncorMed, the company Skolnick had intended to bring to heel for offering a test, surprised many by filing for, and receiving, what that company called a "significant patent." OncorMed was coming at the problem from another direction, isolating a healthy portion of the gene as a standard for possible treatments. According to the *New York Times*, their patent covered "a full-length sequence of a variation of BRCA-1 somewhat different from the 'wild type' gene that Myriad identified." The sequence contained no mutations that would cause cancer, but it was found in half the population. Since therapeutic treatments "are expected to be based on healthy versions of the gene," said the *Times*, OncorMed now owned a hefty chunk of genetic real estate, as well as the medical treatments and diagnostic tests that arose from it.

Peter Meldrum, Myriad's president, told the *Times*, "We just don't comment on other companies' activities."

As Skolnick faced frustrating new obstacles, Dr. Bernard Fisher saw his tarnished reputation restored, along with that of the lumpectomy research he had overseen as director of the National Surgical Adjuvant Breast and Bowel Project (NSABP). Fisher's 1994 lawsuits against the University of Pittsburgh, the National Institutes of Health, the National Cancer Institute, and the Office of Research Integrity were scheduled to go to trial jointly on April 7, 1997, but in March of that year the federal Office of Research Integrity cleared the seventy-eight-year-old Fisher of all scientific misconduct charges.

Although one of Fisher's lawyers complained that the full ORI report included "page after page of kicking the guy," the gist of the media coverage was that Fisher was not culpable for the falsified data that had surfaced in NSABP clinical trials, nor was there any greater risk for women who had chosen lumpectomy and radiation instead of mastectomy. The ORI agreed with an earlier reanalysis published in the *New England Journal of Medicine;* even with the falsified data deleted, the study findings were the same.

The trial was postponed until August 27 and the two sides quietly began negotiations toward a settlement, which was announced the day after they were to have met in court. Fisher had asked for unspecified monetary damages from the university and for attorneys' fees from the government, and in the end received $2.75 million from a "settlement fund" administered by the University of Pittsburgh and other sources, as well as $300,000 from the National Cancer Institute.

"I was always hoping this day would come," Fisher told the *Washington Post.* "The last three years have been holy hell. They took away my position, my reputation, my work. I was smeared in electronic databases. This was a terrible thing where people ran amok and they didn't know what they were running amok about."

He also got the public acknowledgment he had been waiting for—although it took three and a half years, and received only cursory coverage in the national press, compared with the headlines devoted to the original accusations of fraud. The university statement confirmed that "at no time was Dr. Fisher found to have engaged in any scientific or ethical misconduct concerning any of his work." The National Cancer Institute released a statement calling Fisher "a dominant force in the study of breast cancer for the last forty years."

Real progress—what Dr. Susan Love called "evidence-based medicine," theories backed up by substantial clinical data—was limited to reassurances and refinements. While the big headlines went to stories about potential breakthroughs, clinical researchers continued to work on existing therapies. By August 1997 a new technique for lymph node evaluation was being used at several hospitals around the country. Dr. Armando Giuliano, Dr. Love's predecessor at UCLA before he decamped for St. John's Hospital, had developed a less invasive method of lymph node dissection, called "sentinel node dissection," in which a blue dye was injected at the site of a breast tumor and tracked until it infused a lymph node. That single node was removed. If it was positive for cancer, the surgeon had to do the standard, more extensive procedure, removing a cluster of nodes. But if the first node tested negative a woman was spared any more surgery. Two months earlier, Giuliano had reported one hundred percent accuracy with a research group of one hundred patients; the single node procedure accurately predicted what he found when he examined additional nodes.

For women with small tumors, suggestive of an early-stage breast cancer, it was a tremendous relief, sparing them the uncomfortable side effects of a traditional dissection, like swelling of the arm, which could make a lymph node dissection more of a chronic problem than the breast surgery that caused it.

For women with larger tumors, there was more work on neoadjuvant chemotherapy—doctors found that they were often successful in shrinking the tumor in advance of surgery or radiation.

The simple passage of time brought other answers, although not always the ones doctors expected. As lumpectomy survivors got older there was more data on their progress—including the surprising finding that accompanying radiation therapy seemed to alter the way a woman survived, but not her eventual fate. A woman who had a lumpectomy without radiation therapy might have more frequent local recurrences, but survival rates were almost equal for both groups.

A study published in the *Journal of the National Cancer Institute* showed that women who did not have radiation had recurrences three times as often as those who did receive such treatment, but mortality figures in both groups were similar: ninety-nine of the women who did not have radiation died of breast cancer, compared to eighty-seven women who did have radiation. The 837 subjects had been followed for a median of 7.6 years.

One of the study's authors confessed that the findings were "difficult to explain," but they raised the possibility of further refining the trio of therapies—surgery, radiation, and chemotherapy—that women continued to depend upon.

There were pockets of hope, the most accessible of which made it into the mainstream press: Denny Slamon's work with a HER-2/neu antibody for women with aggressive disease; at Memorial Sloan-Kettering, an experimental vaccine for women who survived on the far side of a stem cell transplant; Dave Heber's soy regimen; every bit of news on BRCA-1 and BRCA-2.

What got the most attention, though, were the seemingly endless reports about isolated risk factors, many of which were beyond women's control: being an Ashkenazi Jew meant increased risk, a finding that affected ninety percent of the Jewish population of the United States. Being tall or having strong bones, which would prevent fractures later in life, increased the risk of breast cancer. Smoking was bad. Drinking was bad. Drinking while taking Estrace, a particular kind of hormone replacement therapy, was worse, since the combination boosted the amount of circulating estrogen in the body, and could make it a more comfortable place for cancer to grow. For a brief moment it looked like abortion increased a woman's risk—until other researchers faulted the proponents of that position for letting their political beliefs cloud their scientific conclusions.

As for finding the cancer, the debate about mammography for women under fifty continued without resolution, despite ongoing efforts to force unwieldy statistics to yield a definitive answer. Early detection became a political issue early in 1997, after the National Cancer Institute assembled a new panel to consider the issue.

"I'm hoping it's going to be clear," NCI director Dr. Richard Klausner told the *Washington Post*. It was not. On January 23 the panel decided that existing data was not sufficiently compelling to recommend routine mammograms for women in their forties. Klausner announced that he would ask the NCI's advisory board to consider the issue again in February. That panel decided to educate women to help them make an informed choice, but again stopped short of endorsing the test for women under fifty.

At that point the politicians stepped in and changed the face of the debate. The Senate voted 98 to 0 to endorse mammography for women under fifty in what Fran Visco dismissed as a "patronizing" effort to provide a clear message—as though women were not capable of coping with ambiguity.

"We know so little about this disease," she said. "It's not going to help us to pretend we know more. They were putting pressure on leaders of the scientific community to support a measure that has no scientific basis."

It worked, nevertheless. In March of that year, using the same data that twice had failed to convince experts of the need for annual mammograms for younger women, the NCI reversed itself and recommended that women in their forties have mammograms every one or two years. At a news conference President Clinton expressed his satisfaction with the finding: "Now women in their forties will have clear guidance based on the best science, and action to match it."

If more data was the answer, more money was the means; not even the DOD and the high-profile charities could fuel the expanding fight. Those successes only made people yearn for more— and the most impatient ones pushed in whatever way they could. Lilly Tartikoff informed Denny Slamon that she wanted to up the ante, to raise money for him with a nationally televised appeal. The Revlon money had done what it was intended to do, allowing Slamon to pick up the pace of his HER-2/neu research. Imagine if she could tap other financial resources: he could go even faster, or branch out to look at other oncogenes.

He refused. Slamon felt it would be inappropriate to be named the sole beneficiary of a national campaign, when there were other researchers and medical centers around the country who were as hungry as he was.

But Tartikoff would not be denied, so the question became how best to funnel her energies. The National Women's Cancer Research Alliance was formally launched in October 1997—a group of seven medical centers that would receive monies raised by a one-hour program on Lifetime Television. In addition to Slamon, the other six beneficiaries named were geneticist Mary-Claire King, now at the University of Washington in Seattle; Dr. Martin Abeloff, Director of the Johns Hopkins Oncology Center, where work centered on nongenetic cell alterations that led to cancer; Dr. Albert LoBuglio, Director of the Comprehensive Cancer Center at the University of Alabama, Birmingham, a leader in translational research that moved laboratory findings into clinical settings; Dr. Harvey Golomb, Professor of Medicine at the University of Chicago Medical Center, where work on hormone withdrawal therapy led to the development of the drug tamoxifen; Dr. Karen Antman, Director of New York's Columbia Presbyterian Comprehensive Cancer Center, a leader in the use of stem cell transplants as well as studies of environmental links to cancer; and Dr. William Neaves, Dean of the Medical School at the University of Texas Southwestern Medical School, a "younger" institution that had already become prominent for work on ways to inhibit the growth signals of cancer cells. Funds would also be set aside for the National Breast Cancer Coalition.

Slamon explained that the candidates were "all picked because they have a very active presence in women's cancer, breast and ovarian, or in the case of Texas, a chance to exploit basic science and bring it to bear on those two cancers." The Coalition, which would receive an equal portion of the money, would be the "conduit for information," charged with disseminating news to the public on what the Alliance members were doing.

This would be money to make things happen. In suggesting the beneficiaries Slamon had used as a model not just his own research but the recent work Dr. John Glaspy had done in modifying the diets of women with advanced breast cancer. Glaspy's hunches about soy and fish oil as a means of altering the physiological makeup of a woman's body were descended from Dr. David Heber's nutritional work, but Glaspy had not found favor with government funding sources. Revlon had enabled him to get started. There were more deserving projects than Revlon could reasonably handle, so Slamon wanted to expand both the available sources of money for speculative research and the network of doctors who benefited from it.

"We want to replicate something similar to the Revlon program," explained Slamon of his and Tartikoff's goals for the Alliance. "People who we think have good ideas, or have access to good ideas, have money made available to them to use to make things happen quickly. It can be clinical research, but it does have to be research. It's not for buildings, not for endowments, not for clinical care."

For the patients, after a while, it was all a distant hum of numbers and percentages, errant background sounds in lives that seemed deceptively mundane. Some days the volume increased unexpectedly—the surprise headline, the news of a friend's diagnosis, a doctor's fingers lingering over something new in the breast, a doctor's eye taking just a moment more than usual to study a mammogram. Mostly it was vague, irritating white noise, and nothing more.

Barbara Rubin did everything she could think of to ignore it. She continued most of the regimen she had begun when her biopsy first came back positive: an annual retreat at a health institute near San Diego, a weekly massage, and an assortment of therapies and workshops designed to help her maintain an inner peace. She remained convinced that physical health would flow from there.

She congratulated herself when she learned that new research bore out her instinctive decision not to have radiation. Her chances of survival were as good as they would have been with it; better, as far as she was concerned, given her suspicion about radiation's ill effects. So Barbara allowed herself to focus on the less formidable choices of daily life. She tried letting her hair grow out to its natural color, took one look at the gray, and became a soft ash blond. Her young boyfriend had taken an apartment of his own, but they continued to see each other, and Barbara had other dates, as well. She was not ready to face the calendar when she looked in the mirror every morning.

She was doing fine. The only question, six years after her first face-lift and almost four years since her lumpectomy, was whether it was time for a second face-lift. Barbara had no problem asking for medical assistance in making her physical being better reflect her current emotional state. She had excised the unhappy past from her soul; no reason to leave traces of it on her face.

Ann Donaldson was even more eager to walk away from her past. The drama of her pregnancy and diagnosis had resolved itself in Lisa, a toddler who seemed to her parents the epitome of happiness. Work was a familiar distraction, a comforting routine. But Lisa's every gesture was a slap at the past: she was some sort of magic elf who with a word or smile could erase the lingering effects of her mother's treatment.

Ann faced a considerable list of problems—although, ironically, they were all consequences not of her disease but of the treatment she had received for it. Between the standard chemotherapy and the drugs she had been given as part of the stem cell transplant, Ann endured a chronic hoarseness, a jarring transition into an abrupt menopause, and a memory that sometimes failed her. She tolerated an extra fifteen pounds, despite the fact that it made her clothing uncomfortable. She was cancer-free and she and Rick had a healthy daughter.

They began to make big plans: a daunting work schedule and a new house at the rim of Santa Monica Canyon; better to be exhausted at the end of the day than to let a moment go to waste. One afternoon, in the summer of 1996, Ann piled Lisa, the housekeeper, and a friend's kid into her new Jeep, tossed her handbag into the car at her feet, and roared off for a quick expedition to the park. She was in such a hurry that she did not notice the handle of her purse wrapped around her ankle—and when she tried to get out of the car she fell.

In that single moment her carefully constructed universe fell apart. Despite a searing pain in her hip, Ann got back in the car, drove everyone back to her house, and ignored her housekeeper's entreaties about calling 911. No one was going to take her back inside a hospital, where demons surely lurked behind every door. It was only when she tried to get up to go to the bathroom, and nearly passed out, that she called her oncologist and asked him what to do.

Ann had broken her hip and had to have a partial hip replacement. The doctor who saw her insisted the accident was a fluke, that her bones "look perfectly healthy," but she had learned not to trust either her own body or the first answers she got from doctors. She kept asking until she wore away at the doctor's resolve and he agreed to run a bone scan.

It showed "severe osteoporosis." What she grimly referred to as her "instant menopause" had given her the brittle bones of an old woman. She took an odd satisfaction in having been proven right. This was not an isolated incident. As a result of all the chemotherapy, she would have to be vigilant for the rest of her life. She began taking Fosamax, a drug used to treat osteoporosis by increasing bone mass and improving stability.

Ann had managed since her diagnosis to compartmentalize every crisis—do what she had to, and then move on. She and Rick dutifully registered Lisa in a Montessori preschool as the little girl approached her third birthday—assuming that she would be properly toilet-trained in time for the first day of school. When she wasn't, Ann and Rick debated what to do. They could spend the last three weeks of summer on a campaign to train Lisa, or they could delay preschool for a year.

They decided to wait. It was a practical decision, but it had a peculiar resonance for a woman who had been rushed through the end of her pregnancy and into treatment. Three years out and cancer free, Ann savored the opportunity to slow down—and the promise of more free time with her daughter. This was how a normal woman, specifically a last-minute working mother, ought to live: obsessed with that little package of shimmering life, all darker thoughts shoved into a back corner somewhere. There had been a time when Ann's natural ambition might have prevailed, and she would have pushed her daughter into the future, but no more.

*   *   *

Laura Wilcox had no one to worry about but herself, which only seemed to make matters worse: she too often felt there was no one in the world to care about her. She continued to believe that the solution was a physical one, first; that outer beauty would draw people—would draw a man—to her, at which point they would recognize her inner beauty. Having promised herself perfection, she continued to pursue it. A woman who was born with uneven breasts might tolerate them, and a slight sag came with the passage of time, but nothing about what had happened to Laura was normal. She had at her disposal one of the finest plastic surgeons in the country. If she was going to suffer, she wanted the best results.

She continued to complain to Dr. Shaw that her reconstructed right breast did not match her left, and to ignore anyone who pointed out that most women's breasts were not identical. He finally decided that the solution was to put a saline implant back in the left breast. She wished he had listened sooner. She had been saying all along that the reconstructed breast was both larger and a more pleasing shape, but rather than be pleased at his acquiescence, she took it as an insult.

There was nothing more that could be done, though, so she went out and bought a selection of new bras for her new body, and tried to get on with her life.

"They are beautiful," she told herself. She was not going back again.

As though to help distract her, an actress looking for a juicy vehicle suddenly decided to fund a project Laura had been trying to develop for years. Laura spent five months on the East Coast in production on the small independent film, and along the way struck up a wary romance with a cameraman. He was, she told her friends, "the first guy I'm comfortable with, who's comfortable with my body," but it was not easy. She yielded and backed off; she went away with him for a romantic weekend and then fled to the familiar solitude of home.

Laura was beginning to feel as though stability was always just beyond her reach. She complained of dizziness, problems with her left eye, and nausea. In her rational moments she knew it was all stress-related—and compounded by the fact that she no longer did her yoga or exercises consistently—but fear spoke louder than reason.

In the spring of 1997 she began badgering her oncologist for an MRI, an imaging test that might reveal malignant hot spots elsewhere in her body. "I've never had an MRI," she said. "I want one. I want to know what's inside there." He told her she did not need one. She continued to fret about it, and by the fall had resolved to start asking for one again.

It was as though vigilance was the only antidote to disease. A relaxed body was a vulnerable one; Laura had to be doing something lest her body, untended, start to make mischief on its own.

"It's about how we all have to cope and learn to overcome hardships," she said, but she was still fearful, still looking for a way out.

Having defied the odds so far, Dottie Mosk decided to up the ante. She was three years out, with eighteen positive lymph nodes and not enough strength even to have considered a transplant, one of the exceptions that made the rules so wobbly. She wanted a new challenge.

Over the summer of 1997 Dottie and Joe had decided to sell the home they had lived in for thirty-seven years and purchase an elegant condominium on an exclusive stretch of Wilshire Boulevard known as the Corridor. Their grandson had decided not to spend a year with them after all—"too many rules," Dottie speculated with a chuckle—so it was time to make a change. For some couples in their sixties, this would have been a chance to downsize, to trade a family home for a smaller, more manageable couple's house. Dottie wanted more, a project that, like the rose garden, demanded her continued survival. Stasis was her enemy, both emotionally and physically; she had to keep moving forward.

The roses had been beautiful, no question about that, but after the initial thrill Dottie began to focus on the disadvantages of the project. She was tired of the upkeep and maintenance involved; drained by her managerial responsibilities. She began, she said, "mentally starting to distance myself from the garden. I can give it up now. We're going to have a new, exciting adventure in life, a new beginning. I'm looking forward to a new environment for myself."

Her health was a mix of rigorous effort and dogged optimism. She continued her daily exercises to combat the fibromyalgia, and had regained her ability to drive, to have lunch out or do a little shopping. She and Joe went out to dinner every Saturday night and to the movies every Sunday. As for the breast cancer, she went to see Dr. Ganz twice a year, but beyond that biannual visit with her oncologist there was nothing more she could do. She had no interest in the Breast Center now that Dr. Love was gone.

She and Dr. Ganz were frank with each other. Dottie confessed that sometimes, in the back of her brain, a thought formed: "When will it come back?" But she refused to dwell on it. Dr. Ganz told her that if it did come back, if the breast cancer traveled its usual route from breast to bone to brain, it would be hard to diagnose, because Dottie already had such painful problems with fibromyalgia and osteoporosis. Those could mask the presence of metastases.

That was reality. Dottie decided not to wallow in it. She made sure her days were so full that sorrow had little chance to gain a foothold. The move became a six-month campaign. There were decorators to consult, closets to build, and old flooring to rip up. As long as she was active, she was living.

"I'm like a robot," said Dottie, with a mixture of pride and chagrin. "I just go forward; I have no other choice in life. There's no point to sit and dwell on every ache and pain, since it's not going to go away. I don't feel sorry for myself. I keep going. There are plenty of other people worse off than me."

A year after Dee Wieman's death, her best friend Suzy Drawbaugh, at fifty, was diagnosed with breast cancer—extensive ductal carcinoma in situ, and a small amount of invasive cancer. "Early, early, early," was what the doctors told Suzy; since the DCIS in her case was limited to a discrete area, rather than spread throughout the breast, she was a perfect candidate for a lumpectomy. Surgeons had begun to alter their approach to precancer, since only thirty percent of it turned into invasive cancer.

There was no need to perform a mastectomy if the problem was confined to a specific region of the breast.

Two days before her scheduled surgery Suzy went in for a pre-operative appointment, but this time the doctor was not so sanguine about her condition.

He changed his mind: she ought to have a mastectomy.

She thought of all the time Dee had lost debating what to do. Suzy had a mastectomy and began to take tamoxifen. She decided not to have simultaneous reconstruction because the description of it frightened her. It was enough to find out at the last minute that she was going to lose a breast. She did not want to delay, or face a more difficult recovery.

Her husband and two grown daughters were textbook examples of the supportive family. They all helped with her postoperative care, emptying the surgical drains and making sure she was comfortable. Her older daughter dismissed her mother's anxiety with, "Mom, what's a breast?" and her husband was adamant that none of this changed the way he felt.

For a year Suzy floated on that cushion of constant affection. "I'm fine," she told everyone. Then one morning, almost a year after her diagnosis, she got up, looked at herself in the mirror, and announced to her husband that she had changed her mind.

"I'm not fine," she told him in a wavering voice. She did not expect him to be able to do anything about that; she had no idea what she would do about it. But she finally needed to acknowledge that her appearance dismayed her, that she felt unattractive. It was a relief, in a way, to say so. She decided to let herself be not fine for a while, and see where it led her.

A few weeks later, in September 1997, she and her husband invited Gary Wieman over for dinner. In the months following Dee's death Suzy had stayed away from Gary. She heard stories, from friends, about his self-induced rehabilitation. He had stopped drinking, he went to church regularly, he was helping others. A changed man. After twenty-six years she found it hard to believe.

But he was one of her oldest friends, and finally curiosity and habit prevailed. Gary accepted the invitation and brought a date. Suzy was stunned at how much the woman resembled Dee—blond hair, green eyes, a great sense of humor. She had to admit: this woman was fun to be around.

"All night," she said, "I was laughing and feeling sad at the same time."

As for Gary, Suzy found him "kind, introspective, interested in people, intimate. Gary is not the same person. It's genuine. I was so skeptical; I thought, 'This isn't going to last.' Too bad it didn't happen sooner."

Jerilyn Goodman was browsing at Al's News in Beverly Hills when her gaze fell on the September 15 issue of *New York* magazine. The headline screamed CANCER REDUX, above a photograph of Joyce Wadler, the forty-nine-year-old journalist who had written another two-part article, five years earlier, about her battle against breast cancer. That piece had led to a feisty memoir, *My Breast,* which put the disease on notice: "This is a modern story. Me and my cancer. I won."

She had been right—and wrong. In 1995 Wadler was diagnosed with ovarian cancer, and in the new article she dubbed herself the Mutant Jewish Writer, on the assumption that a damaged gene had propelled her down this particularly hellish path.

Jerilyn picked up the magazine and started to read, but she was overcome by anger and fear. She knew she was being "totally irrational," as she put it, but she was furious with Wadler for "publicizing her problems and opening the floodgates for the rest of us." Just when Jerilyn had got to the point where she didn't think about breast cancer all the time, here was someone who had thought she was victorious, telling the world that good news was not necessarily permanent.

With some effort, she managed to put the magazine back on the rack rather than finish reading it. She told herself, This is not good for you. When she got back home she called Ann Coscarelli and Carol Fred at the Rhonda Fleming Mann Center. She called friends around the country. She was, she admitted, "hysterical," and she needed people to talk her down.

"My anguish, my worry, is there, below the surface," she said. She no longer felt it every day; Susan Love had been right when she said that it would diminish with time. But it was hard when she was caught by surprise. Serenity was not her natural state but the product of conscious effort.

She had devised routines that made her feel better—conversations with her friends back in Madison, Wisconsin, or, if she needed an immediate distraction, two slices of thin-crust cheese pizza and a Coke, which was as comforting as food got. Aside from the occasional crisis like the Wadler article, Jerilyn was pretty comfortable with her body—and given her experience with doctors, she depended on her own instincts, rather than their exams, to tell her if something was wrong. She found she did not miss Susan Love all that much, now that she was past the initial crisis of her diagnosis.

Medicine now was more about dutiful maintenance. She went to Sherry Goldman for her breast exams, and had annual mammograms, but she fully expected that she would be the first to know if the cancer ever came back. Her run-ins with misinformed radiologists and doctors had permanently altered her point of view.

"I have more faith in myself than any of them," she said.

In June 1996 the Barber family rented a specially equipped van for their annual jaunt to Yosemite, one large enough to accommodate not only Tracy's wheelchair but his brother and sister-in-law, who were joining the Barbers for the first time to help with logistics. Tracy managed the preparations from his bed downstairs, and Shirley ran back and forth from there to the driveway well into the night. It was insane, which was part of the appeal. Tracy was on round-the-clock pain medication and they were packing for a camp-out.

Around four in the morning Shirley woke up to the reassuring sound of her husband's light, relaxed breathing. She allowed herself a happy moment. Shirley was hardly a fool; she knew Tracy was dying. But perhaps fate was going to hand them a favor, and postpone the inevitable long enough for one last family trip.

Mitch came into his parents' bedroom at around six to wake them. He sat looking at his father for a long time. Then he woke his mother to tell her that Tracy was dead.

Since then she had coped by increments. She took the summer off and then went back to work. She groused after her August 1996 appointment at the UCLA Breast Center, because she felt things had slipped since Susan Love's departure: there was such confusion about the regular refill on her tamoxifen prescription that she left instructions for the nurse to send her the pills on her own Federal Express account. On subsequent exams she questioned Sherry Goldman closely about every change in her schedule for mammograms or blood work. Was it because the study requirements changed over time—or because she could no longer depend on the Center to get things right?

She had lost the two people who had guided her through her own medical crises, the ones upon whom she depended. With Tracy and Susan Love gone, Shirley focused on every little problem and complained vigorously about it.

In February 1997 Goldman ordered a fine-needle aspiration because Shirley had continued to have sporadic discharge from the right breast, which felt unusually heavy. But Love had been right not to worry, it seemed—the results showed necrosis, dead cells related to the DCIS, and nothing more.

In September 1997 Goldman found something else she did not like, this time in the left breast, the one with the chronic infection that had first brought Shirley to Dr. Love. It was not a lump, "more an oblong mass," said Shirley. It moved around like a cyst—a good thing, since all of Shirley's previous lumps had moved around, and proved to be benign fibroadenomas.

But given Shirley's history, Goldman ordered an ultrasound and another fine-needle aspiration. She would have the results after the weekend.

Shirley had lived in that limbo too many times before to get upset, but while she waited she thought about what she would do if there was trouble. She knew she could not be objective about UCLA—she adored Love too much for that—but as her objections began to pile up she thought, for the first time, about going somewhere else.

"You take a spark plug out of a car," she said, "and even though there are other spark plugs, when the car starts, it misses."

Both tests came back negative, but Goldman refused to let it go at that. She had an instinctive concern; she wanted Shirley to come back in to talk to a surgeon.

At that Shirley checked out, at least temporarily. Her reasoning was this: Sherry Goldman wanted her to see a surgeon. Her surgeon was Dr. Susan Love. Dr. Love was no longer in practice. Therefore, Shirley could not see her surgeon. She knew she would break down eventually and consult with someone else, but she was not prepared to make the move right away. Sherry thought there was something wrong about the mass. Maybe there was, maybe there wasn't. Rushing would not change it.

Maybe. It was the tired side of hope, with one foot in shadow: maybe Shirley would give herself a month in London or Paris once Kim was in college, or maybe a biopsy would send her down another path. It was harder to hold course alone—but Tracy was gone, and Shirley had never been one to spend time looking over her shoulder. Years before, Susan Love had told her she would know she beat breast cancer when she died at ninety of a stroke. At first she had focused on the potential triumph. These days she thought about the daily life of it—a long time, between now and ninety, peppered by exams and mammograms and biopsies and false fears. It could be draining. She kept laying promises out in front of her—London, Paris, grandchildren, someday a small romance—like stones across a river. Maybe she would get across, although that was really beside the point. No matter how tired she got, she had to keep moving.

The new Revlon/UCLA Breast Center opened quietly late in the summer of 1997, with plans for a formal opening sometime in October, once the new director had arrived. Dr. Helena Chang was an immunologist and surgeon, the director of the breast center at Brown University, and one of three candidates considered by Dr. Denny Slamon and the search committee. To him she was the perfect candidate: "She's a scientist with funded grants, she's published, and she's an accomplished surgeon and clinician," he said. "Very energetic, very enthusiastic about the job, not afraid to roll up her sleeves. She doesn't have the attitude that she needs a lot of worker bees to do the job."

Love had offered to come meet with Chang, but by the end of September no one had taken her up on it. It was not clear whether anyone would. "Helena's very confident, as all the candidates are," said Slamon. "I think everyone recognizes Susan for what her strengths were and her weaknesses. They all respected her, but they weren't in awe of her."

Susan Love had managed, by coincidence more than by conscious effort, to remove herself even further from the center of the fray. It had been a year of new challenges for Love, whose book, *Dr. Susan Love's Hormone Book*, sparked loud controversy over estrogen replacement therapy. That had always been one of the things Love did best—forcing debate by confronting a general readership with a new perspective on an old problem.

But this time the opposition was better prepared than when she first took a public stance on "slash, burn, and poison." In the wake of publication, articles appeared around the country considering the underappreciated advantages of hormone therapy—and the *New Yorker*, in an article entitled, "How Wrong Is Susan Love?" strongly attacked her interpretation of existing data on the relative risks and benefits of hormones. Love defended her conclusions in a letter to the editor, but the article was one of many that spoke of the compelling advantages of hormone replacement therapy in fighting heart disease, osteoporosis, and possibly Alzheimer's disease. Her new position met with far more resistance than had her call for a greater national commitment to breast cancer research.

Still, the book became a bestseller; there was always an enthusiastic audience for Love's outspoken skepticism about the status quo. And if her other activities did not move along quite as quickly as she had initially hoped, she chose to consider that an advantage. Without being explicit about it, she clearly had taken what happened at UCLA to heart. She had not rushed ahead with her think tank, which she now described as being "a little bit on the back burner." Instead, she was thinking about alternative ways to organize it, to avoid the problems she had encountered in the past.

She invited groups of people to her home, once a month, to discuss how best to proceed, and along the way started to think about "the charismatic model, where you attract people who are drawn to you, which is how I've often done things in the past." Perhaps there was a better way, based on a foundation of more people working together. She was more inclined to share the responsibility this time out, and in no hurry to get under way. Love was in her second year of business school, still determined to educate herself in the ways of managed care. She had also inherited research from a Santa Barbara doctor, which she used to establish the Santa Barbara Breast Cancer Research Institute, "a community-based resource center," a manageable local project limited only by her imagination. As October and Breast Cancer Awareness Month approached she prepared to "go out on the stump again," as she always did, but it seemed more a habit than a calling. Love was trying out new endeavors—looking for a proper role for the next decade, one that differed from the part she had played at UCLA.

It was as though she had changed gears for the long haul. Individual enterprise had initiated the first phase of the fight against breast cancer, one based on grassroots activism, new money, and a seismic shift in the relationship between those who conducted research and those who stood to reap its benefits. The initial assault almost demanded personalities—people like Susan Love, who could wield a sound bite with the best of Capitol Hill, or Fran Visco, who transferred her skills as a corporate lawyer to a new field of negotiation. High-profile heroes were essential. Celebrity drew attention; noise brought a response.

They were the guardians of the larger agenda. They had to make sure that it stayed on course—that energies were devoted to fundamentals, and not to what Susan called "*60 Minutes* legislation, where some show does a story that makes something sound like a horrible problem, and the next thing you know the legislators are falling all over each other to fix it." She did not want to hear the outcry about same-day mastectomies or mammography for women under fifty. These were, she insisted, "distractions" from more important concerns like how and where money got spent, and who was involved in the decisions.

"We need an enormous push to look at new ways of approaching things," said Love. "The whole movement of having women with breast cancer involved in the decision-making, we've barely had success with that; the DOD and nowhere else. And there's work at the grassroots level. You think you've been there and done everything, but then you go to places where they're just beginning to wake up and get involved."

To Fran Visco, it required a "revolution," not just improvements within the NIH and Congress, but a whole new system of scientific research. "It may sound like a boring topic," she said, "but we would like to change the way scientists collaborate and share information. You can't put that on a placard or do a sound bite, but if it happened it would make a big difference. Much more revolutionary than getting more money for the National Cancer Institute."

The future required work on two levels at once—the push for philosophical change that Love and Visco talked about, and the sort of work they used to do, effecting change on a more immediate level. They had spent the first part of their lives as activists making something out of nothing. Now they needed to make it better—and permanent—and leave the administration of what they had built to those who followed.

For they understood just how long a struggle they faced. Annual skirmishes over the DOD money or new sources of private funding eclipsed the larger truth, which was that the fight was just barely getting under way.

"The further you go, the successes are less dramatic," said Love. "Also, the more you know about the science, the harder it is to stand out there and scream—because you realize things just aren't that simple, The same thing happened with AIDS: part of the reason we can't find the cure is because it's really not easy to do. That's a hard thing to face."

Ironically, the activists were catching up with a truth the medical community had known for decades. This was not an easy puzzle to solve. The threat lurked behind every ambiguous study or failed research effort—that breast cancer might remain just out of reach of even the best intentions.

Although Susan Love might never be invited to drop by and meet Helena Chang, they depended on each other. In the early days of the UCLA multidisciplinary clinic, Love had told the patients that one of the reasons she moved from private practice in Boston to UCLA was to expand her sphere of influence. She wanted to work in a university teaching setting so that she could educate young doctors in a different clinical model. If her approach worked only within the confines of a small private practice, she said, then it was a failure.

By the same reasoning, Dr. Chang had to succeed as Love's successor. She had to convince women that the approach was what mattered, not the public visibility of the doctor who administered it.

"She'll provide the bridge" to the new center, was the way Denny Slamon explained it. "It's not like Helena has a new charge. She has the same charge Susan always had."

Chang was now part of the continuum of change, along with Love, Visco, Slamon, and the patients who had made their way through UCLA's multidisciplinary program. The one thing that was certain was reciprocity: however she might choose to change the program, the program would undoubtedly change her. As Denny Slamon well knew, the fight against breast cancer was more than a medical battle, and it was impossible to step to the fore without learning about other aspects of the fight—the politics, the changing relationship between patients and their doctors, the endless scramble for money.

Chang herself sensed that the job would have an impact. She came to UCLA armed with more traditional notions than Susan Love had; Chang believed in mammography for women under fifty and was less worried than her predecessor about hormone replacement therapy. But she was about to encounter Susan Love's legacy—skepticism, challenge, a patient-oriented environment—and knew she would come out the other end a different person.

"I don't understand too much about politics," Chang told the *Los Angeles Times* when she arrived in town in late September, in an eerie echo of the way Susan Love had viewed the world a decade earlier. "But in the future I may get more involved."

ADDENDA

ACKNOWLEDGMENTS

Four years ago I approached Dr. Susan Love about doing a book. She cut me off ten minutes into what would have been a half-hour explanation and said it was fine with her. When did I want to start? She never asked for any editorial input or control; she had her work, I had mine, and for a while we did them in the same place.

There would be no book without her. I thank Susan for taking a chance and letting a stranger stand at her side. She was a patient guide and an excellent tutor.

Dr. Dennis Slamon, who acquired an onlooker by default, proved a willing teacher as well, and I am very grateful to him for finding time he did not have, to talk with me. Dr. John Glaspy and Dr. Michael Zinner also contributed generously to this book.

The women I wrote about, and their families, made a different kind of contribution, a far more intimate one, because they felt that it would do some good. I admire their honesty and courage, and thank all of them: Shirley, Tracy, Mitch, and Kim Barber; Ann and Rick Donaldson; Jerilyn Goodman; Dottie and Joe Mosk; Barbara Rubin; Dee and Gary Wieman, Suzy Drawbaugh, and Laura Wilcox.

I offer a special, added word of thanks to Tracy Barber, a man of great grace and humor, who taught me what this book was really about.

Fran Visco, president of the National Breast Cancer Coalition, took on my continuing education as a personal challenge. I appreciate her astute analysis of the political scene and her fine, footnoted sense of outrage. Colonel Irene Rich, of the army's breast cancer research program, was a happy revelation to me, and I thank her for keeping me apprised of all her efforts.

Other doctors, researchers, and staff at UCLA took the time to explain their particular field of interest, and allowed me to watch them at work. They provided a comprehensive sense of how UCLA's breast program worked: Drs. Larry Bassett, Linnea Chap, Ann Coscarelli, Patti Ganz, David Heber, David McFadden, Michael Racenstein, William Shaw, and David Wellisch; adminstrator Mary Bading; research nurses Linda Norton and Stephanie Chang; social worker Carol Fred; nurse-practitioner Sherry Goldman, and Breast Center staff Leslie Laudeman, Connie Long, Shannon Tucker, Christi Dearborn, and Lisa Gotori-Koga.

Clinicians at medical centers around the country helped to broaden the book's perspective. I thank Dr. Armando Giuliano for discussing his work and ideas with me. I also thank Drs. Larry Norton, Jeanne Petrek, David Spiegel, Peter Boasberg, I. Craig Henderson, Jay Harris, Daniel Kopans, and Marc Lippman for sharing their perspectives as well as information on their clinical work.

Researchers helped to translate often arcane scientific information into civilian language and concepts. I am very grateful to Dr. Harold Varmus, director of the National Institutes of Health, geneticists Dr. Mary-Claire King and Dr. Mark Skolnick, Dr. Bernard Fisher, Dr. Samuel Broder, Dr. Helene Smith, and Dr. Kay Dickersin for discussing the current state of breast cancer research—and for providing a valuable sense of history as well as an informed glimpse of what the future holds.

With President Clinton's stated commitment to fight breast cancer, the federal government became an active participant in the drama. Health and Human Services Secretary Donna Shalala, Dr. Susan Blumenthal, Ed Long, Sen. Patrick Leahy and Rep. Patricia Schroeder helped to articulate the government's changing role in the fight against breast cancer.

Amy Langer, executive director of the National Alliance of Breast Cancer Organizations, and Nancy Brinker, founder of the

Susan G. Komen Foundation, put the advocates' long fight for change into an historical framework. Lobbyist Joanne Howes, of Bass & Howes, gave me an insider's look at breast cancer funding battles.

I thank Adi Herman for explaining the philosophy behind his work, and Mark Gelhaus and Beth Winter for explaining how a medical center does business.

As the private sector became more involved in breast cancer research, the role of philanthropists and fund-raisers took on new importance. I am grateful to Lilly Tartikoff for explaining how an ex-ballerina, a scientist, and a cosmetics magnate came to do business together—and to Giorgio Armani and Ralph Lauren for discussing their relationship to the cause. Evelyn Lauder kindly took the time to explain how the Evelyn H. Lauder Breast Center at Memorial Sloan-Kettering came into existence.

Several people helped with the preparation of this book, and I appreciate their efforts. Dr. Lauren Pinter-Brown reviewed all the medical material. Jacquelyn Cenacveira was a tireless researcher and an invaluable asset, and Freddie Odlum and Sue Clamage provided tape transcriptions.

At Delacorte Press, Carole Baron's passion for the project exceeded the usual professional enthusiasm, and was greatly appreciated. Tracy Devine's insightful editing was disciplined and full of heart. We were surrounded by dedicated allies—Linda Steinman, Carisa Hays, Laura Rossi, Leslie Schnur, Susan Schwartz, Amanda Kimmel, Johanna Tani, Phil Rose, and Brenden Hitt.

My agent, Kathy Robbins, is a true believer, and I am always grateful for her fierce support and sound advice. My thanks to Bill Clegg, too, for his enthusiasm.

Susan Kamil and Peter Gethers encouraged me from the sidelines.

My friends listened to stories that were often hard to hear, and then the next time we were together they asked again how the book was going. Ginger Curwen, Marcie Rothman, Carolyn See, Harry Shearer, and Judith Owen have been right beside me all along. I am very lucky to have such friends.

I also want to thank those who provided various forms of sustenance along the way—good talk, good food, a quiet place to read, the occasional shoulder to lean on: Annette Duffy and David Odell, Jack Nessel, Vicky and Hummie Mann, Lori and Roy Rifkin, Joel Siegel, David Shaw and Lucy Stille, Patty Williams and Kenny Turan and Jo Ann Consolo. Piero and Stacy Selvaggio and Mark Peel and Nancy Silverton provided the best possible homes away from home.

Larry Dietz, my husband and in-house editor, has an enduringly good heart in the former role, and an elegant eye in the latter. I am the happy beneficiary of both. We have collaborated only once, with excellent results: I thank Sarah Dietz simply for being her luminous self. I love her more than words.

Karen Stabiner
Santa Monica, California
January 1997

VOCABULARY

adjuvant and neo-adjuvant chemotherapy: drugs used to fight cancer, traditionally administered after surgery, but in neo-adjuvant therapy, administered before surgery to shrink the tumor.

AMRMC: Army Medical Research and Materiel Command, which oversees the Defense Department's breast cancer research program.

axillary node dissection: removal of lymph nodes located in the armpit, to determine the likelihood of micrometastasis.

autologous stem cell transplant: a more sophisticated descendant of the bone marrow transplant. This procedure is used in combination with high-dose chemotherapy for women with advanced disease. After taking toxic doses of drugs, a woman receives a life-saving infusion of her own stem cells—young bone marrow cells, harvested from her bloodstream before treatment—which have been enhanced with a synthetic growth hormone. Still, the procedure has a five percent mortality rate.

biopsy: removal of tissue to check for malignancy.

BRCA-1: a gene for heritable breast cancer, located by Dr. Mark Skolnick's research team in September 1994. BRCA-1 has since been shown to play a role as well in sporadic breast cancer—disease in women who do not have a family history of breast cancer.

carcinoma: cancer found in epithelial tissue, which includes the skin, glands, and the lining of internal organs.

clinical trials: trials of new treatments or procedures, in a research setting, to determine toxicity levels, proper dosage, and efficacy compared to existing treatments.

Double-blind study: a clinical trial in which neither the patients nor the medical personnel know who is receiving an experimental treatment and who is receiving standard therapy or a placebo.

Randomized control study: a trial in which women are assigned at random—either to receive a new treatment or procedure, or to be given a placebo or standard treatment. The control group provides an essential basis for comparison for the treatment group's results.

cooperative oncology groups: four groups comprised of a network of doctors conducting clinical trials research, including the East Coast Oncology Group (ECOG), the Southwest Oncology Group (SWOG), Cancer and Leukemia Group B (CALGB), and the National Surgical Adjuvant Breast and Bowel Project (NSABP).

cyst: a fluid-filled sac.

DCIS: Ductal Carcinoma in Situ, a noninvasive cancer, limited to the breast's ductal system, sometimes referred to as "precancer." Improved detection technology has enabled doctors to detect microcalcifications—tiny dots on a mammogram—that sometimes signal the presence of DCIS. If a biopsy confirms it, the standard treatment is mastectomy—though only thirty percent of DCIS cases progress to invasive cancer.

dirty margins: malignant cells at the edge of a pathology slide from a surgical biopsy, which means that not all the cancerous tissue has been removed.

DNA: Deoxyribonucleic acid, the chemical that comprises an individual's genetic code. Two pairs of interlocked bases match up in specific patterns; in a damaged gene those pairs are altered, either by heredity or the environment.

DOD: Department of Defense, which undertook a $210 million breast cancer research program in fiscal 1993.

epithelial: a type of cell that lines the ducts of the breast.

estrogen receptor: a receptor on some cells to which an estrogen molecule can attach. Estrogen-receptor-positive tumors are often more responsive to hormone treatment than are receptor-negative cancers.

fibroadenoma: a hard, benign growth usually seen in young women.

fine-needle aspiration: removal of fluid or cells to determine whether a lump is benign or malignant, using a hypodermic needle.

gene: a unit of DNA, which carries the instructions to make a protein. Genetic material is contained in the nucleus of a cell. A damaged gene can send faulty instructions, which can result in malignant growth.

HHS: the Department of Health and Human Services, the federal agency that oversees the National Institutes of Health, the Women's Health Initiative, and the National Action Plan on Breast Cancer.

hyperplasia: literally, "too many cells." The two stages that precede DCIS are intraductal hyperplasia, where more than the normal number of cells are crowded into the breast duct, and intraductal hyperplasia with atypia, where some of those cells have an abnormal appearance.

intraductal papilloma: a benign tumor in the lining of the breast duct.

invasive carcinoma: also known as infiltrating carcinoma. Cancer that has the ability to spread.

IOM: Institute of Medicine, a division of the National Academy of Sciences, contracted by the Defense Department to develop a framework for that department's breast cancer research program.

lumpectomy: also called a wide excision. Breast-conserving surgery in which the doctor attempts to remove malignant tissue and a small rim of healthy tissue.

mastectomy: according to Dr. Love, "the ultimate wide excision." The current procedure involves removing all the breast tissue and a wedge of skin that includes the nipple, as well as some lymph nodes. The radical mastectomy, introduced in the United States in the 1890s by Dr. William Halsted, involved removing pectoral muscles and lymph nodes above the breast as well.

metastasis/micrometastasis: metastasis is the spread of cancer to a distant organ. Micrometastasis is the as-yet-undetectable spread of tumor cells.

microcalcifications: dots of calcium that can show up on a mammogram; benign eighty percent of the time, but, if small and clustered together, a possible indication of DCIS.

NABCO: National Association of Breast Cancer Organizations, a service and education umbrella organization for over 250 advocacy groups nationwide. Founded in 1986.

National Action Plan on Breast Cancer: President Clinton's attempt, under HHS Secretary Donna Shalala's supervision, to define a national strategy against breast cancer.

NBCC: National Breast Cancer Coalition, a grass-roots lobbying and advocacy group founded in 1991 by Dr. Susan Love and Susan Hester, with breast cancer survivor Fran Visco as its first president.

NCI: National Cancer Institute, the largest division of the National Institutes of Health, created by a special act of Congress in 1937 and funded separately under a bypass budget.

NIH: National Institutes of Health, the federal government's center for medical research, founded in 1887 and located in Bethesda, Maryland.

oncogenes: tumor genes that can, if damaged, encourage uncontrolled malignant cell growth.

ORI: the federal government's Office of Research Integrity, called the Office of Scientific Integrity until a 1993 restructuring. Responsible for investigations into allegations of falsified data in the NSABP lumpectomy and tamoxifen clinical trials.

recurrence: the reappearance of a cancer. Local recurrence can occur at the site of a lumpectomy, and is not considered a metastasis. More serious recurrences can show up in lymph nodes, the mastectomy scar or chest wall, in the second breast, or in distant organs.

simultaneous reconstruction: in autologous simultaneous reconstruction, the plastic surgeon builds a breast for a mastectomy patient out of her own tissue, at the same time as her mastectomy. Two procedures are most common: the tunnel tram-flap, in which a segment from the abdomen is tunneled up to the chest, its blood supply intact; and the free-flap, in which the tissue and skin are severed and attached to a new vein and artery pulled down from the armpit.

staging: there are four stages of cancer, listed in order of increasing severity. Stage 1 cancer, the least threatening, means the disease has been caught at an early stage—no positive lymph nodes and a tumor less than two centimeters in diameter. Patients in this group usually do not have chemotherapy, since seven will survive without it, two will die in spite of it, and only one will survive because of it.

Stage 2 can mean several things—a small tumor with positive but mobile axillary lymph nodes; a tumor up to five centimeters with positive mobile nodes or negative nodes; or a tumor over five centimeters with negative nodes.

Stage 3 is a large tumor, over five centimeters, with positive nodes; or a small tumor with fixed nodes.

Stage 4 means that a woman's cancer has obviously spread to distant organs.

stereotactic core biopsy: use of a high-speed needle, guided by computer, to remove tissue samples; an alternative to some surgical biopsies.

tamoxifen: an estrogen blocker used to prevent recurrence—and in a clinical trial, to prevent breast cancer in high-risk patients.

taxol: a drug first derived from the Pacific yew tree, now produced synthetically. A common treatment for women with advanced disease and for those who have failed to respond to high-dose chemotherapy.

Women's Health Initiative: a fifteen-year, $625 million National Institutes of Health study of breast cancer, osteoporosis, and heart disease, incorporating both randomized clinical and observational trials.

PATIENT HISTORIES

NAME PERSONAL HISTORY	**Shirley Barber** Forty-three years old Married to Tracy Barber since 1974 Two children: Mitch (17) and Kimberly (13) Occupation: Flight attendant, United Airlines
SYMPTOMS & DIAGNOSIS	Persistent infection in a sebaceous gland in left nipple. Mammography showed no abnormalities on the left, but a cluster of microcalcifications on the right. Benign condition called intraductal papilloma diagnosed after surgical biopsy on right breast; Dr. Love also operated on infected gland in left breast. Symptoms of the infection returned. Residual calcifications shown by follow-up mammogram. After 2nd operation on both breasts, biopsy showed ductal carcinoma in situ (DCIS) in right breast. "Dirty margins" on pathology slides indicated cancerous cells still present.
MEDICAL RECOMMENDATIONS	Several options following the surgical excision: a mastectomy, another wide excision, no further treatment, or a national clinical trial of tamoxifen and radiation. Chose the clinical trial, a five-year, double-blind study in which neither patients nor medical personnel know who is receiving tamoxifen and who is receiving a placebo.

Ann Donaldson
Forty-six years old
Married
Pregnant with first child
Occupation: Owner of a small public
relations firm

First felt a lump in May 1993;
mammogram showed nothing. Lump
seemed to disappear. Became pregnant
in November 1993, after years of
infertility treatments including
surgeries and fertility drugs. Felt lump
again in early April 1994.

Infiltrating lobular cancer, a tumor
over 2 cm in diameter, and dirty
margins revealed by surgical biopsy.
Lymphatic invasion suggested by
pathology slides.

At 27th week of pregnancy, several
options: immediate lumpectomy (with
risk of premature labor), followed by
chemotherapy and radiation; no
treatment until child is born naturally;
or one cycle of chemotherapy
immediately, induced labor at 30 to 31
weeks, and completion of treatments
after the birth.

Chose the 3rd option which was
recommended by multi team.

Jerilyn Goodman
Forty-three years old
Single
Occupation: Freelance television
producer
Family history of breast cancer (aunt
and grandmother)

Complained of a mass in left breast in
1988, which was dismissed by her
doctor; radiologist saw nothing
suspicious on mammogram.

In fall 1993 mass biopsied at
suggestion of new internist. Atypical
cells revealed by needle aspiration;
surgical biopsy scheduled. Stage 1
small invasive cancer and extensive
DCIS subsequently diagnosed.

Mastectomy and axillary node
dissection recommended and
performed; no chemotherapy, since
nodes were negative. Declined
reconstructive surgery.

Embarked on a regimen of ancillary
therapies: weekly acupuncture, visits to
a healer, a support group for women
with early-stage cancer, and a low-fat
diet.

NAME	**Dottie Mosk**
PERSONAL HISTORY	Sixty-four years old
	Married to Joe since 1948
	Mother of two
	Grandmother of two

SYMPTOMS & DIAGNOSIS	Bothered by a lump in armpit, which was dismissed as a swollen hair follicle after clean mammogram. Needle aspiration performed by another doctor on the lump yielded malignant cells.
	Diagnosed with an "occult primary"—no palpable lump in her breast, no detectable mass, but the cancer had already spread to a lymph node.

MEDICAL RECOMMENDATIONS	Mastectomy and axillary node dissection performed by Dr. Love; 35 lymph nodes removed from under arm, eighteen positive indicating Stage 3 breast cancer. Because of debilitating rheumatologic condition, not strong enough to be considered as candidate for autologous stem-cell transplant. Underwent standard chemotherapy and radiation treatments.

Barbara Rubin
Fifty-three years old
Divorced twice
Three children
One grandchild
Occupation: private psychotherapist

Felt a lump in her breast. Benign finding with two needle aspirations. Radiologist insisted on third biopsy, which revealed a small invasive ductal cancer, barely over 1 cm in diameter.

Declined recommended lumpectomy. Embarked on two-month program of visualization and meditation to shrink the tumor herself. Tumor appeared smaller on first visit to Dr. Love, who then performed a lumpectomy. Standard radiation therapy recommended, with an axillary node dissection.

Declined further treatment despite greater risk of recurrence. Developed own regimen—diet including soy, wheat grass juice, organic produce, and weekly sessions with body-work masseuse.

Dee Wieman
Forty-five years old
Married to Gary Wieman since 1985
An adult daughter from Dee's first marriage and one grandchild

Complained in spring 1993 about a hard lump in right breast, which was diagnosed as a fibroadenoma, a benign lump more common in younger women. In November 1993 noticed a change in the color of right nipple. Bilateral mammogram showed no abnormalities on the right, but irregularity on the left. Biopsy revealed a small amount of invasive ductal breast cancer.

Invasive cancer and extensive DCIS on the left confirmed by additional biopsies. Invasive lobular cancer on the right, DCIS, and 26 out of 28 positive lymph nodes also discovered.

Mastectomy and chemotherapy, followed by high-dose chemotherapy with autologous stem-cell transplant, recommended by one surgeon. Neo-adjuvant chemotherapy (drugs preceding surgery), followed by a lumpectomy, a mastectomy if there were dirty margins, and the transplant offered by Dr. Love

Resisted the idea of mastectomy for months; continued to visit specialists at several Los Angeles area hospitals, seeking a consensus.

NAME	**Laura Wilcox**
PERSONAL HISTORY	Thirty-eight years old
	Single
	Occupation: Development executive for Hollywood production company. First diagnosed with invasive cancer and single positive lymph node, 1988. Had a lumpectomy, radiation, and chemotherapy
SYMPTOMS & DIAGNOSIS	Discovered new lump in October 1993; surgical biopsy in December showed malignancy.
	New malignancy considered by Dr. Love a "leftover" cancer from first lumpectomy, and less of a threat than a new primary cancer or a recurrence right after the initial surgery would have been. However, pathology report also showed extensive DCIS.
MEDICAL RECOMMENDATIONS	Mastectomy to eliminate DCIS recommended by UCLA multidisciplinary team. Mastectomy performed with simultaneous reconstruction using Laura's own tissue.
	Embarked on a discipline of vitamins, meditation, and exercise. Also took shark cartilage pills, believed by some to be an effective cancer fighter.

NOTES ON SOURCES

This is a work of nonfiction. The book is based on research conducted between December 1993 and November 1996—primarily personal interviews and my observational notes. During 1994 I was at UCLA on a regular basis, chronicling daily events there: patient appointments and procedures, staff and administrative meetings, and the encounters between people that appear in these pages. I accompanied patients to medical appointments outside UCLA, to alternative treatments, to support groups, and I traveled with their doctors to research conferences. I continued to follow their stories throughout 1995 and 1996.

In addition, I relied on medical journals—the *Journal of the American Medical Association*, the *Journal of the National Cancer Institute*, the *New England Journal of Medicine*, *Science* magazine—as well as weekly news magazines and major daily newspapers, including *The New York Times, The Wall Street Journal*, the *Chicago Tribune, The Washington Post*, the *Los Angeles Times*, the *Seattle Post-Intelligencer*, and others.

Government reports contained information about budgetary allocations, statistics on incidence and mortality, demographics, and the history of the disease. They also provided a history of this country's research effort against breast cancer. I used as references many recent books about breast cancer and about cancer in general, including individual patient memoirs and books on science and policy. Those books are listed in the "Selected Bibliography" that follows these notes.

I had access to the patients' complete medical records. Material that pertained to their diagnoses and treatments was reviewed both with their doctors and with two oncologists who were not involved in their treatment. Those two doctors also reviewed all the medical information in this text.

The following section is intended more as a resource guide than a traditional list of citations. Information on a given topic often came from a number of sources—a patient interview, a medical journal, a newspaper article, a doctor's comments—and stories overlap within chapters. In the interest of clarity, I have listed references alphabetically, on a chapter-by-chapter basis.

Prologue

Personal interviews: Kimberly, Mitch, Shirley, and Tracy Barber.

Chapter 1

Personal interviews: Dr. Susan Love, Health and Human Services Secretary Donna Shalala, Fran Visco.

Anderson, Christopher. "Healy Slams Clinton's NIH Budget." *Science*. May 21, 1993.

Brody, Jane. "Personal Health." [Article on health risks.] *The New York Times*. February 24, 1993.

"Call to Action." National Breast Cancer Coalition Quarterly Newsletter. Volume 1, Nos. 1 and 2. Winter/Spring 1994.

Clymer, Adam. "Tests Added for Women in Health Plan." *The New York Times*. October 7, 1993.

C-SPAN videotape. October 18, 1993.

Eley, Dr. J. William, et al. "Racial Differences in Survival From Breast Cancer." *Journal of the American Medical Association*. September 28, 1994.

Ferraro, Susan. "The Anguished Politics of Breast Cancer." *The New York Times Magazine*. August 15, 1993.

Johnson, Judith A. "Breast Cancer." Congressional Research Service Report for Congress, pp. 4–6, 28–37. March 15, 1994.

Klemesrud, Judy. "A Woman's Fight Against Breast Cancer." *The New York Times*. August 5, 1985.

Kolata, Gina. "Weighing Spending on Breast Cancer." *The New York Times*. October 20, 1993.

———. "Deadliness of Breast Cancer in Blacks Defies Easy Answer." *The New York Times*. August 3, 1994.

Levine, Judith. "Donna Goes to Washington: Secretary of Health and Human Services Donna Shalala." *Harper's Bazaar*. July 1994.

National Breast Cancer Coalition 1994 Annual Report.

Rosenthal, Elisabeth. "Does Fragmented Medicine Harm the Health of Women?" *The New York Times*. January 13, 1993.

U.S. Centers for Disease Control, Surveillance Report, 1982–1994.

"Vital Statistics of the United States." U.S. National Center for Health Statistics. 1991.

Chapter 2

Personal interviews: Dr. Ann Coscarelli, Sherry Goldman, Leslie Laudeman, Dr. Susan Love, Dr. David McFadden, Dr. Dennis Slamon, Dr. Michael Zinner.

Observational notes.

"Let the (Quality-Based) Competition Begin!" *Rand Research Review*. Vol. XVII, Number 3. Winter 1993–94.

Loomis, Carol. "The Real Action in Health Care." *Fortune.* July 11, 1994.

Meier, Barry. "Health Plans Promise Choice But Decisions May Be Hard." *The New York Times.* March 31, 1994.

O'Neill, Molly. "Dr. Susan M. Love: A Surgeon's War on Breast Cancer." *The New York Times.* June 29, 1994.

Chapter 3

Personal interviews: Dr. John Glaspy, Linda Norton, Laura Wilcox.

Observational notes.

O'Shaughnessy, Joyce A. and Cowan, Kenneth H. "Dose-intensive therapy for breast cancer. (Grand Rounds at the Clinical Center of the National Institutes of Health)." *Journal of the American Medical Association.* November 3, 1993.

Chapter 4

Personal interviews: Dr. Jay Harris, Dr. I. Craig Henderson, Dr. Susan Love, Dr. David McFadden, Dr. Michael Zinner.

Colker, David. "Telling It Like It Is." *Los Angeles Times.* November 16, 1992.

Gleick, Elizabeth. "Susan Love: A Surgeon Crusades Against Breast Cancer." *People.* July 25, 1994.

O'Neill, Molly. "Dr. Susan M. Love: A Surgeon's War on Breast Cancer." *The New York Times.* June 29, 1994.

Chapter 5

Personal interviews: Nancy Brinker, Dr. Samuel Broder, Dr. Bernard Fisher, Joanne Howes, Amy Langer, Sen. Patrick Leahy, Ed Long, Dr. Susan Love, Col. Irene Rich, Rep. Patricia Schroeder, Donna Shalala, Fran Visco.

Correspondence: Fran Visco to Richard Darman, Director, Office of Management and Budget. September 29, 1992.

Correspondence: Fran Visco to Ed Long. October 16, 1992.

"Army Cancer Chief Gives NIH a Cold Shoulder." *Science.* December 4, 1992.

Boodman, Sandra. "The Rise of 'In-Your-Face' Activism." *The Washington Post.* April 19, 1994.

"Breast Cancer Research Funds." Senate Congressional Record. September 30, 1992.

Fisher, Bernard. "Personal Contributions to Progress in Breast Cancer Research and Treatment." *Seminars in Oncology.* Vol. 23, No. 4, August 1996.

Kolata, Gina. "Why Do So Many Women Have Breasts Removed Needlessly?" *The New York Times.* May 5, 1993.

Marshall, Eliot. "An Expert Panel Advises, and the Army Consents." *Science.* May 21, 1993.

Norman, Jane. "Move to Quash Breast Cancer Research Funds." *The Des Moines Register.* October 1, 1992.

Oparil, Suzanne, et al. "Strategies for Managing the Breast Cancer Research Program: A Report to the U.S. Army Medical Research and Development Command." National Academy of Sciences' Institute of Medicine Committee report. National Academy Press. 1993.

"Research Hearings of the Breast Cancer Coalition: Hearings Summary and Conclusions of the Breast Cancer Coalition Research Task Force." March 1992.

Saxon, Wolfgang. "Dr. George Crile, Jr., 84, Foe of Unneeded Surgery, Dies." *The New York Times*. September 12, 1992.

———. "Oliver Cope, 91, a Top Surgeon Who Was a Harvard Professor." *The New York Times*. May 3, 1994.

Slatella, Michelle. "The Lagging War on Breast Cancer." *Newsday*. October 3, 1993.

"U.S. Army Broad Agency Announcement for Breast Cancer." United States Army Medical Research and Development Command. September 15, 1993.

Zuckerman, Mortimer. "Battling Breast Cancer" Editorial in *U.S. News & World Report*. November 23, 1992.

Chapter 6

Personal Interviews: Shirley Barber, Tracy Barber, Jerilyn Goodman, Dr. David Heber, Dr. Mary-Claire King, Evelyn Lauder, Ralph Lauren, Dr. Dennis Slamon.

Observational notes.

"America's Worst Toxic Polluters; Eight Companies with Poor Environmental Records." *Business and Society Review*. January 1993.

Angier, Natalie. "Quest for Genes and Lost Children." *The New York Times*. April 27, 1993.

Brody, Jane. "Breast Cancer Weapons: Fruit, Vegetables and, Maybe, Olive Oil." *The New York Times*. January 18, 1995.

Bukro, Casey. "Edison Is Criticized on Environment." *Chicago Tribune*. December 6, 1993.

Castleman, Michael. "Why?" *Mother Jones*. May–June 1994.

"Is *In Situ* Breast Cancer Always a Precursor of Invasive Disease?" The State of Breast Cancer 1994: An Interactive Symposium. Presentation and panel discussion. University of California San Francisco School of Medicine. September 26, 1994.

Johnson, Judith A. "Breast Cancer." Congressional Research Service Report for Congress, March 15, 1994. pp. 4–6, 28–37.

"Judge Dismisses Suit Against Chemical Companies on DDT Cleanup." From the Associated Press. *The New York Times*. March 24, 1995.

Krieger, Nancy, et al. "Breast Cancer and Serum Organochlorines: A Prospective Study Among White, Black and Asian Women." *Journal of the National Cancer Institute*. April 20, 1994.

Page, Dr. David, and Dr. Roy Jensen. "Ductal Carcinoma In Situ of the Breast: Understanding the Misunderstood Stepchild." *Journal of the American Medical Association*. March 27, 1996.

Paulsen, Monte. "The Cancer Business." *Mother Jones*. May–June 1994.

———. "BCAM Scam." Editorial in *The Nation*. November 15, 1994.

Wittman, Juliet. "I'm Alive and Angry." *Mother Jones*. May–June 1994.

Chapter 7

Personal interviews: Jerilyn Goodman, Dr. Jeanne Petrek, Laura Wilcox.
Observational notes.
Petrak, Dr. Jeanne. "Pregnancy Safety after Breast Cancer." *Cancer Supplement.* Vol. 74, No. 1. July 1, 1994.
————. "Breast Cancer During Pregnancy." *Cancer Supplement.* Vol. 74, No. 1. July 1, 1994.

Chapter 8

Personal interviews: Dr. Armando Giuliano, Sherry Goldman, Dr. Dennis Slamon, Lilly Tartikoff, Dr. Michael Zinner.
Observational notes.
Love, Dr. Susan, and Dr. Sanford Barsky. "Breast Duct Endoscopy as a Means of Obtaining and Studying Precancerous Ductal Epithelial Cells." Grant proposal.
Muchnic, Suzanne. "A Chance to See Barbra's Other Hits." *Los Angeles Times.* February 16, 1994.

Chapter 9

Personal interviews: Dr. Peter Boasberg, Dr. Armando Guiliano, Dr. John Glaspy, Dr. Susan Love, Dottie and Joe Mosk, Dr. William Shaw, Dee and Gary Wieman, Laura Wilcox.
Observational notes.
Caprino, Mariann. "Managed Care Industry Caught Between High Costs, Patient Welfare." From the Associated Press. *Los Angeles Times.* February 20, 1994.
Eckholm, Erik. "$89 Million Awarded Family Who Sued H.M.O." *The New York Times.* December 30, 1993.
Gorman, Tom. "Jury Adds $77 Million Against HMO That Denied Coverage." *Los Angeles Times.* December 29, 1993.
Kolata, Gina. "Study of Insurance Sees Decisions as 'Arbitrary.' " *The New York Times.* February 17, 1994.
Lee, Don. "Health Net Ordered to Pay $12.1 Million." *Los Angeles Times.* December 28, 1993.
Peters, Dr. William, and Dr. Mark Rogers. "Variation in Approval by Insurance Companies of Coverage for Autologous Bone Marrow Transplantation for Breast Cancer." *New England Journal of Medicine.* February 17, 1994.
Weinstock, Cheryl. "Lawyers Debate the Insurability of Bone Marrow Transplants." *The New York Times.* March 20, 1994.

Chapter 10

Personal interviews: Shirley Barber, Dr. Patricia Ganz, Sherry Goldman, Jerilyn Goodman, Dr. Mary-Claire King, Dottie Mosk, Dr. Larry Norton, Dr. David Wellisch.
Observational notes.

Bondy, Melissa, et al. "Validation of a Breast Cancer Risk Assessment Model in Women with a Positive Family History." *Journal of the National Cancer Institute.* April 20, 1994.

"Identification of Individuals at High Risk." The State of Breast Cancer 1994: An Interactive Symposium. Presentation and panel discussion. University of California San Francisco School of Medicine. September 25, 1994.

Kolata, Gina. "New Data on Risks Prompts Debate on Using Drug to Prevent Breast Cancer." *The New York Times.* March 16, 1996.

Roan, Shari, and Sheryl Stolberg. "Risk Estimate Raised for Those in Breast Cancer Study." *Los Angeles Times.* February 18, 1994.

Slattery, Martha, and Richard Kerber. "A Comprehensive Evaluation of Family History and Breast Cancer Risk." *Journal of the American Medical Association.* October 6, 1993.

Spiegelman, Donna, et al. "Validation of the Gail et al. Model for Predicting Individual Breast Cancer Risk." *Journal of the National Cancer Institute.* April 20, 1994.

Chapter 11

Personal interviews: Dr. David Heber, Dr. Susan Love, Donna Shalala, Dr. Dennis Slamon, Dr. Mark Skolnick, Dr. Harold Varmus (10/4/94, 3/30/95), Fran Visco, Laura Wilcox.

Angier, Natalie. "Harold E. Varmus: Out of the Lab and Into the Bureaucracy." *The New York Times.* November 23, 1993.

Kirschstein, Ruth. "Largest U.S. Clinical Trial Ever Gets Under Way." *Journal of the American Medical Association.* October 6, 1993.

Laurence, Leslie. "Women's Health Initiative Starts with Thousands of Eager Volunteers." *Chicago Tribune.* April 18, 1993.

Leary, Warren. "Study of Women's Health Criticized by Review Panel." *The New York Times.* November 2, 1993.

Marshall, Eliot. "Varmus: The View from Bethesda." *Science.* November 26, 1993.

———, and Jon Cohen. "Varmus Tapped to Head NIH." *Science.* August 13, 1993.

Marwick, Charles. "Coordinated Effort to Fight Breast Cancer Begins." *Journal of the American Medical Association.* January 19, 1994.

Marx, Jean L. "Cancer Gene Research Wins Medicine Nobel." *Science.* October 20, 1989.

McBride, Gail. "Women's Study in U.S. Criticised by Expert Committee." *British Medical Journal.* November 20, 1993.

Painter, Kim. "Slow-Starting Women's Health Study Aims High." *USA Today.* October 31, 1995.

Schwartz, John. "Federal Women's Health Study Faulted." *The Washington Post.* November 2, 1993.

Shalala, Donna. Speech at the International Human Genome Conference. October 4, 1994.

Shepard, Robert. "2nd Opinions: Critics, Legislators Debate Women's Health Initiative." *Chicago Tribune.* January 30, 1994.

Varmus, Dr. Harold. Keynote Address, the Secretary's Conference to Establish a National Action Plan on Breast Cancer. December 14, 1993.

Weiss, Rick, and John Schwartz. "Nobel Winner Harold Varmus Takes Charge at NIH." *The Washington Post.* November 23, 1993.

Chapter 12

Personal interviews: Suzy Drawbaugh, Dr. Bernard Fisher, Jerilyn Goodman, Dr. Susan Love, Barbara Rubin, Fran Visco, Dee and Gary Wieman, Laura Wilcox.

Observational notes.

Altman, Dr. Lawrence. "Federal Officials to Review Documents in Breast Cancer Study with Falsified Data." *The New York Times.* March 27, 1994.

Baue, Dr. Arthur. "Breast-Conservation Operations for Treatment of Cancer of the Breast." *Journal of the American Medical Association.* April 20, 1994.

Crewdson, John. "Fraud in Breast Cancer Study; Doctor Lied on Data for Decade." *Chicago Tribune.* March 13, 1994.

Farnsworth, Clyde. "Doctor Says He Falsified Cancer Data to Help Patients." *The New York Times.* April 1, 1994.

Hooper, Judith. "Unconventional Cancer Treatments." *Omni.* February 1993.

Jones, Charisse. "Flawed Cancer Study Haunts Many Women." *The New York Times.* March 16, 1994.

Kolata, Gina. "Breast Cancer Advice Unchanged Despite Flawed Data in Key Study." *The New York Times.* March 15, 1994.

Mitric, Joan McQueeney. "Sharks Swim into Cancer Picture." *The Plain Dealer* (Cleveland). April 27, 1993.

"National Breast Cancer Coalition Statement in Response to NSABP Data Falsification." April 6, 1994.

Plotkin, Dr. David. "Good News and Bad News About Breast Cancer." *The Atlantic Monthly.* June 1996.

Sawyer, Kathy. "Cancer Researchers' Credibility Ailing." *The Washington Post.* April 13, 1994.

Schwartz, John. "Experts Try to Allay Cancer Fraud Fears." *The Washington Post.* March 15, 1994.

Chapter 13

Personal interviews: Dr. Lawrence Bassett, Dr. Daniel Kopans, Dr. Susan Love, Col. Irene Rich, Fran Visco.

Observational notes.

Brody, Jane, and Gina Kolata. "Breast Cancer Screening Under 50: Experts Disagree if Benefit Exists." *The New York Times.* December 14, 1993.

Harris, Dr. Russell. "Breast Cancer Among Women in Their Forties: Toward a Reasonable Research Agenda." *Journal of the National Cancer Institute.* March 16, 1994.

"How Much 'Early Diagnosis' Can Women Tolerate and Society Afford?" Breast Cancer Symposium. Presentation and panel discussion. University of California San Francisco School of Medicine. September 26, 1994.

Johnson, Judith A. "Breast Cancer." Congressional Research Service Report for Congress, pp. 4–6, 28–37. March 15, 1994.

Kerlikowske, Karla, et al. "Positive Predictive Value of Screening Mammography by Age and Family History of Breast Cancer." *Journal of the American Medical Association.* November. 24, 1993.

Kinsley, Michael. "TRB From Washington: Screen Test." *The New Republic.* April 11, 1994.

Kolata, Gina. "Avoiding Mammogram Guidelines." *The New York Times.* December 5, 1993.

———. "Mammogram Debate Moving from Test's Merits to Its Cost." *The New York Times.* December 27, 1993.

———. "Studies Say Mammograms Fail to Help Many Women." *The New York Times.* February 26, 1993.

Love, Dr. Susan. "The Untold Truth Behind the Mammogram Dispute." *Los Angeles Times.* March 13, 1994.

Plotkin, Dr. David. "Good News and Bad News About Breast Cancer." *The Atlantic Monthly.* June 1996.

Purnick, Joyce. "Editorial Notebook: The Mammogram Controversy." *The New York Times.* January 16, 1994.

Rovner, Sandy. "Standards Set for Mammograms." *The Washington Post.* November 15, 1994.

Russell, Christine. "The Debate Over Mammography." *The Washington Post.* April 19, 1994.

Tanouye, Elyse. "Mammograms: Should She or Shouldn't She?" *The Wall Street Journal.* February 22, 1994.

Chapter 14

Personal interviews: Dr. Peter Boasberg, Dr. Bernard Fisher, Dr. David Heber, Dee Wieman, Beth Winter (UCLA Dept. of Managed Care Contracts).

Observational notes.

Fisher, Dr. Bernard. "The Evolution of Paradigms for the Management of Breast Cancer: A Personal Perspective." *Cancer Research* 52, 2371–2383. May 1, 1992.

———. "Personal Contributions to Progress in Breast Cancer Research and Treatment." *Seminars in Oncology.* Vol. 23, No. 4. August 1996.

Kolata, Gina. "Tests to Assess Risks for Cancer Raising Questions." *The New York Times.* March 27, 1995.

Weiss, Rick. "Tests' Availability Tangles Ethical and Genetic Codes." *The Washington Post.* May 26, 1996.

Chapter 15

Personal interviews: Mary Bading, Shirley and Tracy Barber, Dr. Bernard Fisher, Cindy Gensler, Jerilyn Goodman, Leslie Laudeman, Dr. Susan Love, Dottie Mosk, Barbara Rubin, Dee Wieman, Laura Wilcox, Dr. Michael Zinner.

Observational notes.

Kantrowitz, Barbara, and Nina Archer Biddle. "The Tempest in a D-Cup." *Newsweek*. March 28, 1994.

Levine, Joshua. "Bra Wars." *Forbes*. April 25, 1994.

Prager, Emily. "Underwire Wars." *The New York Times*. January 16, 1994.

Chapter 16

Personal interviews: Mary Bading, Dr. Bernard Fisher, Dr. John Glaspy, Dr. Susan Love, Dottie Mosk, Linda Norton, Dr. Dennis Slamon, Dee Wieman, Fran Visco, Dr. Michael Zinner.

Observational notes.

"Breast Cancer Advocate Involvement in Research Process." National Breast Cancer Coalition. April 6, 1994.

Fessenden, Ford. "A Study Under Fire." *Newsday*. April 14, 1994.

Fisher, Dr. Bernard, et al. "A Randomized Clinical Trial Evaluating Tamoxifen in the Treatment of Patients With Node-negative Breast Cancer Who Have Estrogen-receptor-positive Tumors." *New England Journal of Medicine*. February 23, 1989.

———. "Endometrial Cancer in Tamoxifen-Treated Breast Cancer Patients: Findings from the National Surgical Adjuvant Breast and Bowel Project B-14." *Journal of the National Cancer Institute*. April 6, 1994.

Friedman, Dr. Michael, et al. "Tamoxifen: Trials, Tribulations, and Trade-offs." *Journal of the National Cancer Institute*. April 6, 1994.

Kolata, Gina. "Patients' Lawyers Lead Insurers to Pay for Unproven Treatments." *The New York Times*. March 28, 1994.

Leovy, Jill. "Biotech's Victory Is on Hold." *Los Angeles Times*. July 12, 1994.

———. "Amgen's Latest Home Run in a Winning Streak?" *Los Angeles Times*. July 18, 1994.

Reynolds, Tom. "Breast Cancer Prognostic Factors—The Search Goes On." *Journal of the National Cancer Institute*. April 6, 1994.

Silvestrini, Rosella, et al. "The Bcl-2 Protein: A Prognostic Indicator Strongly Related to p53 Protein in Lymph Node–Negative Breast Cancer Patients." *Journal of the National Cancer Institute*. April 6, 1994.

Trump, Dr. Donald L. Letter to participants in NSABP Breast Cancer Prevention Trial. April 16, 1996.

Chapter 17

Personal interviews: Dr. Peter Boasberg, Dr. Bernard Fisher, Dr. John Glaspy, Dr. Susan Love, Dr. David McFadden, Dr. Dennis Slamon, Fran Visco, Dee Wieman, Dr. Michael Zinner.

Observational notes.

Altman, Dr. Lawrence. "Scientist Ousted from Cancer Study Declines to Testify to House Panel." *The New York Times*. April 12, 1996.

———. "Health Officials Apologize for Problems with Falsified Data in Cancer Study." *The New York Times*. April 14, 1994.

———. "Probe into Flawed Cancer Study Prompts Federal Reforms." *The New York Times*. April 26, 1994.

Bivens, Dr. Lyle W. Statement Before the Congressional Subcommittee on Oversight and Investigations Hearing, Committee on Energy and Commerce, U.S. House of Representatives. April 13, 1996.

Dingell, Rep. John. Opening Statement Before Congressional Subcommittee on Oversight and Investigations Hearing. April 13, 1994.

Herman, Robin. "Research Fraud Breaks Chain of Trust." *The Washington Post.* April 19, 1994.

Plourde, Dr. Paul. Conversation with Dr. Fisher (NSABP) and Dr. Ford (NCI). Internal memorandum. Zeneca Pharmaceuticals Group. July 7, 1993.

Ross, Michael. "Lapses Admitted in Cancer Data Scandal." *Los Angeles Times.* April 14, 1994.

Seligmann, Jean. "How Safe Is Lumpectomy?" *Newsweek.* March 28, 1994.

Chapter 18

Personal interviews: Dr. Patricia Ganz, Dr. John Glaspy, Amy Langer, Dr. Susan Love.

Observational notes.

Chapter 19

Personal interviews: Dr. William Shaw, Laura Wilcox.

Blakeslee, Sandra. "Implant Maker Had Conflicting Findings on Silicone's Effects." *The New York Times.* May 9, 1994.

Kolata, Gina. "Implants: Courts Dispose While Science Unfolds." *The New York Times.* June 19, 1994.

———. "A Case of Justice, or a Total Travesty?" *The New York Times.* June 13, 1995.

McCarthy, E. Jane, et al. "A Descriptive Analysis of Physical Complaints from Women with Silicone Breast Implants." *Journal of Women's Health.* Vol. 2, No. 2, 1993.

Shaw, Dr. William. "Bilateral Free-Flap Breast Reconstruction." *Clinics in Plastic Surgery.* Vol. 21, No. 2. April 1994.

Wade, Nicholas. "Method and Madness; Trials and Errors." *The New York Times.* July 24, 1994.

Weinstein, Henry. "When Law, Tragedy Intersect." *Los Angeles Times.* March 26, 1994.

Weiser, Benjamin. "Feud in Breast Implant Case Stirs Debate on Tactics." *The Washington Post.* May 11, 1994.

Chapter 20

Personal interviews: Shirley and Tracy Barber, Jerilyn Goodman, Adi Herman, Dottie Mosk, Barbara Rubin, Dee Wieman.

Observational notes.

Baum, Dr. Michael. "Breast Cancer 2000 BC to 2000 AD—Time for a Paradigm Shift?" *Acta Oncologica.* Vol. 32, No. 1, 1993.

Saltus, Richard. "Taxol: New Drug Playing Wider Role." *The Boston Globe.* July 17, 1995.

Verrengia, Joseph. "Taxol Gets Yellow Light." *Rocky Mountain News.* December 18, 1994.

Chapter 21

Personal interviews: Shirley Barber, Dr. Ann Coscarelli, Carol Fred, Cindy Gensler, Jerilyn Goodman, Dr. Susan Love, Dr. David Spiegel, Laura Wilcox.

Altman, Dr. Lawrence. "Flawed Breast Cancer Study Faces Cutoff of Financing." *The New York Times.* May 4, 1994.

Classen, Catherine, et al. "Brief Supportive-Expressive Group Therapy for Women with Primary Breast Cancer: A Treatment Manual." Psychosocial Treatment Laboratory, Stanford University School of Medicine. 1993.

Contavespi, Vicki. "Faith Healing." *Forbes.* July 4, 1994.

Erickson, Jane. "Fisher Given New Role in Cancer Project." *Science.* March 24, 1995.

Evans, Sandra. "Counseling: A Crucial Aspect of Care." *The Washington Post.* April 19, 1994.

Ganz, Dr. Patricia, et al. "Breast Cancer Survivors: Psychosocial Concerns and Quality of Life." *Breast Cancer Research and Treatment.* Vol. 38, pp. 183–199. 1996.

"Psychosocial Aspects and Patient Advocacy." The State of Breast Cancer 1994: An Interactive Symposium. Presentation and panel discussion. University of California San Francisco School of Medicine. September 27, 1994.

Schmuckler, Eric. "Oh, What a Beautiful Morning; Fox Children's Network Forges Ahead of Competition." *Mediaweek.* April 18, 1994.

Spiegel, Dr. David. "Compassion Is the Best Medicine." *The New York Times.* June 12, 1994.

Chapter 22

Personal interviews: Ann Donaldson, Dr. Susan Love, Dr. Jeanne Petrek, Dr. Dennis Slamon, Lilly Tartikoff, Dr. Michael Zinner.

Correspondence: Dr. Lillian Yin, Food and Drug Administration Office of Device Evaluation, to Dr. Susan Love. April 1994.

Chapter 23

Personal interviews: Dr. Susan Love, Dee Wieman, Beth Winter.

Altman, Dr. Lawrence. "Cancer Study Overseers Are Assailed at Hearing." *The New York Times.* May 12, 1994.

———. "Doctors Gets an Ovation and a Rebuke." *The New York Times.* May 19, 1994.

Angell, Dr. Marcia, and Dr. Jerome Kassirer. "Setting the Record Straight in the Breast-cancer Trials." Editorial in the *New England Journal of Medicine.* May 19, 1994.

Broder, Dr. Samuel. "Statement Before Congressional Subcommittee on Oversight and Investigations." June 15, 1994.

Brody, Jane. "New Clues in Balancing the Risks of Hormones After Menopause." *The New York Times.* June 15, 1995.

Davidson, Nancy. "Hormone-Replacement Therapy—Breast Versus Heart Versus Bone." Editorial in the *New England Journal of Medicine.* June 15, 1995.

Detre, Dr. Thomas. "Statement Before Congressional Subcommittee on Oversight and Investigations." June 15, 1994.

Dingell, Rep. John. "Opening Statement." Congressional Subcommittee on Oversight and Investigations. June 15, 1994.

Fisher, Dr. Bernard. "Statement Before Congressional Subcommittee on Oversight and Investigations." June 15, 1994.

Grady, Dr. Deborah, et al. "Guidelines for Counseling Postmenopausal Women about Preventive Hormone Therapy." *Annals of Internal Medicine.* Vol. 117, No. 12. December 15, 1992.

Herberman, Dr. Ronald. "Statement Before Congressional Subcommittee on Oversight and Investigations." June 15, 1994.

O'Connor, J. Dennis. "Statement Before Congressional Subcommittee on Oversight and Investigations." June 15, 1994.

Patterson, Dr. John. "Statement Before Congressional Subcommittee on Oversight and Investigations." June 15, 1994.

Sawyer, Kathy. "Breast Cancer Drug Testing Will Continue; Potential of Tamoxifen Is Said to Outweigh Risks." *The Washington Post.* May 12, 1994.

———. "Panel to Review Cancer Researcher's Work." *The Washington Post.* May 30, 1994.

Steinberg, Dr. Karen, et al. "A Meta-analysis of the Effect of Estrogen Replacement Therapy on the Risk of Breast Cancer." *Journal of the American Medical Association.* April 17, 1991.

Chapter 24

Personal interviews: Ann Donaldson, Dr. Susan Love, Dr. Dennis Slamon. Observational notes.

Chapter 25

Personal interviews: Suzy Drawbaugh, Dr. Armando Giuliano, Sherry Goldman, Leslie Laudeman, Dr. Susan Love, Dr. Dennis Slamon, Maynard Smith, Cynthia Jones, Dee and Gary Wieman.
Letter: Dee Wieman to Dr. Susan Love.

Chapter 26

Personal interviews: Shirley Barber, Ann Donaldson, Mark Gelhaus (Manager, Physician Relations, Department of Marketing and Planning), Jerilyn Goodman, Dr. Armando Giuliano, Dee and Gary Wieman, Laura Wilcox, Beth Winter.

Brody, Jane. "Smokers Have Higher Breast Cancer Death Risk." *The New York Times.* May 25, 1994.

"Cancer Drug Can Cause Problems in Womb, Study Says." From Reuters Wire Service. *Los Angeles Times.* May 27, 1994.

McFadden, Robert. "Death of a First Lady: Jacqueline Kennedy Onassis Dies of Cancer at 64." *The New York Times.* May 20, 1994.

Chapter 27

Personal interviews: Mary Bading, Dr. David Heber, Leslie Laudeman, Dr. Susan Love, Dr. David McFadden, Dottie Mosk, Dr. Dennis Slamon.

Observational notes.

Cooke, Robert. "Blocking Menstruation to Block Breast Cancer." *Newsday.* January 1, 1991.

Loscocco, Laurie. "Hormone, Drug Regimen Studied as Way to Curb Female Cancers." *The Columbus Dispatch.* April 5, 1992.

Saltus, Richard. "Hint to Cut Breast Cancer: Late Puberty, Early Menopause." *The Boston Globe.* May 17, 1996.

Tanne, Janice Hopkins. "Everything You Need to Know About Breast Cancer . . . But Were Afraid to Ask." *New York.* October 11, 1993.

Chapter 28

Personal interviews: Dr. Bernard Fisher, Sherry Goldman, Dr. John Glaspy, Dr. Susan Love, Dr. Dennis Slamon, Dee and Gary Wieman, Dr. Michael Zinner.

Observational notes.

Roselli Del Turco, Dr. Marco, et al. "Intensive Diagnostic Follow-up After Treatment of Primary Breast Cancer." *Journal of the American Medical Association.* May 25, 1994.

Broder, Dr. Samuel. "Statement on Oversight of Clinical Research at the National Surgical Adjuvant Breast and Bowel Project, Before the Subcommittee on Oversight and Investigations, House Committee on Energy and Commerce." June 15, 1994.

Detre, Dr. Thomas. "Statement Before the Committee on Energy and Commerce, Subcommittee on Oversight and Investigations, United States House of Representatives." June 15, 1994.

Dingell, Rep. John. "Opening Statement." United States House of Representatives Subcommittee on Oversight and Investigations hearing. June 15, 1994.

Eliot, Marshall. "Tamoxifen: Hanging in the Balance." *Science.* June 10, 1994.

Fisher, Dr. Bernard. "Statement Before the Committee on Energy and Commerce, Subcommittee on Oversight and Investigations, United States House of Representatives." June 15, 1994.

Herberman, Dr. Ronald. "Statement Before the Committee on Energy and Commerce, Subcommittee on Oversight and Investigations, United States House of Representatives." June 15, 1994.

"Impact of Follow-up Testing on Survival and Health-Related Quality of Life in Breast Cancer Patients." The GIVIO Investigators. *Journal of the American Medical Association.* May 25, 1994.

O'Connor, J. Dennis. "Statement Before the Committee on Energy and Commerce, Subcommittee on Oversight and Investigations, United States House of Representatives." June 15, 1994.

Patterson, Dr. John. "Zeneca Pharmaceuticals Group Statement to the Subcommittee on Oversight and Investigations, Energy and Commerce Committee, U.S. House of Representatives, Re: Federally Funded Breast Cancer Research Projects." June 15, 1994.

Chapter 29

Personal interviews: Shirley and Tracy Barber, Dr. John Glaspy, Jerilyn Goodman, Dr. David Heber, Dr. Susan Love, Dr. William Shaw, Jan Thielbar, Dee Wieman, Laura Wilcox.

Allison, Kathleen, and Michele Wolf. "Eat to Beat Cancer." *American Health*. October 1993.

Guinee, Dr. Vincent, et al. "Effect of Pregnancy on Prognosis for Young Women with Breast Cancer." *The Lancet*. June 25, 1994.

Maugh, Thomas. "Pregnancy and Breast Cancer Pose Lethal Risk." *Los Angeles Times*. June 24, 1994.

Meera, Jain, et al. "Premorbid Diet and the Prognosis of Women with Breast Cancer." *Journal of the National Cancer Institute*. September 21, 1994.

Chapter 30

Personal interviews: Dr. Susan Love, Dr. William Shaw, Dr. Michael Walker, Laura Wilcox.

Observational notes.

Chapter 31

Personal interviews: Shirley Barber, Dr. Susan Blumenthal, Dr. Peter Boasberg, Dr. David McFadden, Suzy Drawbaugh, Dr. Bernard Fisher, Dr. Mary-Claire King, Linda Norton, Dr. Mark Skolnick, Dr. Dennis Slamon, Maynard Smith, Dr. Harold Varmus, Fran Visco, Dee and Gary Wieman, Dr. Michael Zinner.

Observational notes.

"Pitt Cancer Researcher Sues Over Removal from Project." News Services. *The Washington Post*. July 9, 1994.

Angier, Natalie. "Vexing Pursuit of Breast Cancer Gene." *The New York Times*. July 12, 1994.

"Inventory of Breast Cancer Activities." Office on Women's Health, U.S. Department of Health and Human Services [Draft]. July 19, 1994.

Snyder, Christel. "Money, Clout Needed to Fight Breast Cancer." *The Santa Barbara News-Press*. May 29, 1994.

Chapter 32

Personal interviews: Giorgio Armani, Dr. Jay Harris, Dr. Mary-Claire King, Ralph Lauren, Ed Long, Dr. Susan Love, Col. Irene Rich, Dr. Mark Skolnick, Dr.

Dennis Slamon, Dr. Helene Smith, Lilly Tartikoff, Dr. Harold Varmus, Fran Visco.

"Activists Respond to Investigators' Failure to Disclose Location of Breast Cancer Gene." The National Breast Cancer Coalition. September 18, 1994.

Angier, Natalie. "Scientists Identify a Mutant Gene Tied to Hereditary Breast Cancer." The New York Times. September 15, 1994.

———. "Fierce Competition Marked Fervid Race for Cancer Gene." The New York Times. September 20, 1994.

Brownlee, Shannon, and Traci Watson. "Hunting a Killer Gene." U.S. News & World Report. September 26, 1994.

"Dispute Arises Over Patent for a Gene." From the Associated Press. The New York Times. October 30, 1994.

"Fashion Targets Breast Cancer." The New York Times. October 9, 1994.

Kaiser, Jocelyn. "Army Doles Out Its First $210 Million." Science. October 14, 1994.

Maugh II, Thomas. "Discovery of Breast Cancer Gene Called Major Advance." Los Angeles Times. September 15, 1994.

"Presymptomatic Genetic Testing for Heritable Breast Cancer Risk." The National Breast Cancer Coalition. September 18, 1994.

Shapiro, Laura, and Karen Springen. "Zeroing in on Breast Cancer." Newsweek. September 26, 1994.

Waldholz, Michael. "Scientists Say They've Found Gene That Causes Breast Cancer." The Wall Street Journal. September 14, 1994.

———. "Finding Breast-Cancer Gene Is Battle, Not War, Won." The Wall Street Journal. September 15, 1994.

———. "Feud Brewing Over Breast-Cancer Gene Patent." The Wall Street Journal. October 17, 1994.

Weiss, Rick. "Breast Cancer Gene's Impact Limited." The Washington Post. September 20, 1994.

Chapter 33

Personal interviews: Kim, Mitch, Shirley and Tracy Barber, Dr. Peter Boasberg, Ann and Rick Donaldson, Jerilyn Goodman, Dr. Susan Love, Dottie Mosk, Barbara Rubin, Dr. William Shaw, Dee Wieman, Laura Wilcox.
Observational notes.

Chapter 34

Personal interviews: Giorgio Armani, Ed Long, Dr. Susan Love, Dr. Mary-Claire King, Dr. Larry Norton, Dr. Jeanne Petrek, Col. Irene Rich, Donna Shalala, Dr. Dennis Slamon, Lilly Tartikoff, Dr. Harold Varmus, Fran Visco.
Observational notes.

Angier, Natalie. "Put on Your Best Chest—It's Time to Preen." The New York Times. April 2, 1995.

Brown, David. "Pentagon May Hold Up AIDS Study Funds; Breast Cancer Research Also in Danger; Both Are Regarded as Not Essential to Military." The Washington Post. February 10, 1995.

"Defense Secretary Rebuked Over Research Money." From the Associated Press. *The New York Times.* February 12, 1995.

"Gene Patent Dispute Is Settled." From the Associated Press. *The New York Times.* February 16, 1995.

Higgins, Bill. "Fire and Ice Ball Draws the 'A' List and Nets $2.4 Million for Cancer Research." *Los Angeles Times.* December 8, 1993.

Kattlove, H., et al. "Benefits and Costs of Screening and Treatment for Early Breast Cancer: Development of a Basic Benefit Package." *Journal of the American Medical Association.* January 11, 1995.

Olmos, David. "Blue Shield to Cover Experimental Breast Cancer Treatment." *Los Angeles Times.* January 19, 1995.

Priest, Dana. " 'Non-Defense' Projects Targeted." *The Washington Post.* February 10, 1995.

"Revlon Foundation Gives $7.5 Million to Women's Health Programs At UCLA." Press release. December 6, 1994.

Stein, Jeannine. "A Warm Turnout for Fire and Ice Ball." *Los Angeles Times.* December 6, 1991.

———. "New Orleans Connection for the Fire & Ice Ball." *Los Angeles Times.* December 4, 1992.

———. "Proof that Dreams Do Come True." *Los Angeles Times.* December 9, 1994.

Weiss, Rick. "NIH Cancer Chief Vents Frustration; Departing Broder Defends Government as Vital to Science." *The Washington Post.* December 24, 1994.

Chapter 35

Personal interviews: Dr. Peter Boasberg, Suzy Drawbaugh, Dee and Gary Wieman.

Chapter 36

Personal interviews: Shirley Barber, Ann Donaldon, Dr. Bernard Fisher, Dr. John Glaspy, Jerilyn Goodman, Dr. David Heber, Dr. I. Craig Henderson, Dr. Susan Love, Dottie Mosk, Barbara Rubin, Dr. Mark Skolnick, Dr. Dennis Slamon, Fran Visco, Laura Wilcox.

Letter: Dr. Susan Love to colleagues. May 7, 1996.

Angier, Natalie. "Breast Cancer Gene Isn't Making Screening Easy." *The New York Times.* November 30, 1994.

———. "Scientists Find Surprising Role for Gene in Breast Cancer Cases." *The New York Times.* March 5, 1996.

Church, George. "Teaching Hospitals in Crisis." *Time.* July 17, 1995.

Clymer, Adam. "National Health Program, President's Greatest Goal, Declared Dead in Congress." *The New York Times.* September 27, 1994.

———, et al. "The Health Care Debate: What Went Wrong? How the Health Care Campaign Collapsed." *The New York Times.* August 29, 1994.

Cooke, Robert, and Ridgely Ochs. "New Breast Cancer Test Ready." *Newsday.* January 12, 1996.

FitzGerald, Michael, et al. "Germ-Line BRCA1 Mutations in Jewish and Non-

Jewish Women with Early-Onset Breast Cancer." *New England Journal of Medicine.* January 18, 1996.

Hotz, Robert Lee. "Gene Defect May Provide Cancer Test." *Los Angeles Times.* September 29, 1995.

Kolata, Gina. "Breast Cancer Gene in 1% of U.S. Jews." *The New York Times.* September 29, 1995.

———. "Research Links One Gene to Most Breast Cancers." *The New York Times.* November 3, 1995.

Kong, Dolores. "Mammogram Guidelines Are Called Into Question." *The Boston Globe.* May 7, 1996.

———. "Mammogram Wars: The Debate Begins Again." *The Boston Globe.* May 27, 1996.

Langston, Dr. Amelia, et al. "BRCA1 Mutations in a Population-Based Sample of Young women with Breast Cancer." *New England Journal of Medicine.* January 18, 1996.

Lindfors, Dr. Karen, and Dr. John Rosenquist. "The Cost-effectiveness of Mammographic Screening Strategies." *Journal of the American Medical Association.* September 20, 1995.

Loomis, Carol. "The Real Action in Health Care." *Fortune.* July 11, 1994.

Love, Dr. Susan, et al. "The Revlon/UCLA Breast Cancer Center Practice Guidelines for the Treatment of Breast Cancer." *Cancer Journal.* January 1996.

Morgan, Dan. "From Some in Health Fields, No News Is Bad News; Lack of Legislative Safeguards, Subsidies Could Mean a Rougher Transition to 'Managed Care.'" *The Washington Post.* August 31, 1994.

Rosenblatt, Robert. "The Changing Health Care Industry." *Los Angeles Times.* February 21, 1995.

Tumulty, Karen, and Edwin Chen. "Mitchell Declares Health Reform Dead for Session." *Los Angeles Times.* September 27, 1994.

"Will We Be Able to Prevent Breast Cancer 10 Years from Now?" The State of Breast Cancer 1994: An Interactive Symposium. Presentation and panel discussion. University of California San Francisco School of Medicine. September 25, 1994.

Epilogue

Personal interviews: Kim, Mitch, Shirley, and Tracy Barber.

Following is a list of both personal and telephone interviews, with the date each interview was conducted. These are in addition to ongoing conversations with sources as part of the observational research for this book.

Giorgio Armani 12/9/94
Mary Bading 7/5/96
Kimberly Barber 3/20/94, 12/29/94
Mitch Barber 3/20/94, 12/29/94
Shirley Barber 2/28/94, 4/25/94, 5/20/94, 6/21/94, 7/19/94,
12/29/94, 3/17/95, 4/26/95, 6/16/95, 8/22/95, 10/31/95, 1/4/96,
4/13/96, 7/1/96, 7/5/96

Tracy Barber 3/20/94, 12/29/94, 4/13/96
Dr. Lawrence Bassett 6/2/94
Dr. Susan Blumenthal 2/23/95
Dr. Peter Boasberg 5/9/96
Nancy Brinker 2/16/94
Dr. Samuel Broder 2/15/94
Dr. Ann Coscarelli 10/21/94
Ann Donaldson 7/5/94, 10/15/94, 11/10/94, 4/9/96
Dr. Kay Dickersin 6/11/95
Suzy Drawbaugh 10/23/95, 11/1/95, 9/16/96
Dr Bernard Fisher 9/19/96
Dr. Patricia Ganz 5/25/94, 6/17/94
Mark Gelhaus 5/3/94, 9/27/94
Cindy Gensler 12/14/94, 12/28/94, 6/21/95, 8/21/95
Dr. Armando Giuliano 7/1/96
Dr. John Glaspy 3/24/94, 6/28/94, 9/6/96
Jerilyn Goodman 3/1/94, 3/21/94, 3/31/94, 4/8/94, 4/28/94,
5/5/94, 5/12/94, 6/8/94, 7/21/94, 8/11/94, 8/25/94, 9/27/94,
10/17/94, 10/28/94, 11/1/94, 11/17/94, 1/1/95, 2/9/95, 4/22/96
Dr. Jay Harris 9/26/94
Dr. David Heber 9/12/96
Dr. I. Craig Henderson 9/25/94
Adi Herman 9/22/94
Joanne Howes 3/31/95
Dr. Mary-Claire King 6/10/95
Dr. Daniel Kopans 9/26/94
Amy Langer 8/18/94
Leslie Laudeman 3/25/94
Evelyn Lauder 4/4/95
Ralph Lauren 4/4/95
Sen. Patrick Leahy 10/4/94
Dr. Marc Lippman 4/11/95
Ed Long 10/4/94
Dr. Susan Love 1/2/94, 3/7/94, 6/30/94, 5/13/96, 9/25/96, 11/4/96
Dr. David McFadden 7/28/94
Dottie Mosk 4/12/94, 4/27/94, 4/29/94, 5/5/94, 5/11/94, 5/18/94, 6/3/94,
6/30/94, 7/13/94, 8/11/94, 9/20/94, 11/2/94, 11/9/94,
11/12/94, 12/30/94, 5/18/95, 10/6/95, 8/13/96
Dr. Larry Norton 4/5/95
Linda Norton 7/1/94, 7/8/94
Dr. Jeanne Petrek 8/17/94
Col. Irene Rich 10/6/94, 2/22/95, 3/29/95
Barbara Rubin 2/25/94, 3/22/94, 4/4/94, 5/5/94, 5/26/94, 7/13/94, 9/9/94,
11/4/94, 5/19/95, 10/29/96
Rep. Patricia Schroeder 10/3/94
Donna Shalala 10/5/94, 3/30/95
Dr. William Shaw 7/14/94, 7/15/94
Dr. Mark Skolnick 9/30/96

Dr. Dennis Slamon 3/8/94, 4/19/94, 6/2/94, 6/30/94, 11/29/94,
3/22/95, 5/29/96, 10/21/96
Dr. Helene Smith 9/27/94
Maynard Smith 10/20/96
Dr. David Spiegel 9/27/94
Lilly Tartikoff 12/12/94
Dr. Harold Varmus 10/4/94, 11/7/94, 3/30/95
Fran Visco 7/9/94, 9/21/94, 9/29/94, 3/29/95, 6/9/95, 10/15/95,
5/14/96, 10/17/96
Dee Wieman 3/2/94, 3/17/94, 3/30/94, 4/6/94, 4/20/94, 4/22/94, 5/11/94,
5/13/94, 5/20/94, 5/23/94, 5/27/94, 6/13/94, 6/22/94, 7/22/94, 8/15/94, 11/2/94,
11/16/94, 1/9/95, 1/25/95, 2/10/95, 3/6/95, 3/20/95, 6/21/95
Gary Wieman 5/31/94, 9/26/95, 9/11/96, 10/21/96
Laura Wilcox 3/3/94, 3/18/94, 4/14/94, 4/16/94, 4/29/94, 5/9/94, 5/23/94,
6/23/94, 6/28/94, 7/8/94, 8/31/94, 9/12/94, 10/27/94,
11/8/94, 11/17/94, 2/8/95, 5/11/96
Beth Winter 4/13/94
Dr. Michael Zinner 4/12/94, 6/15/94, 6/17/96

SELECTED BIBLIOGRAPHY

Altman, Roberta. *Waking Up/Fighting Back: The Politics of Breast Cancer.* Boston: Little, Brown and Company, 1996.

Benjamin, Harold. *From Victim to Victor: The Wellness Community Guide to Fighting for Recovery for Cancer Patients and Their Families.* Los Angeles: Jeremy P. Tarcher, Inc., 1987.

Davies, Kevin and Michael White. *Breakthrough: The Race to Find the Breast Cancer Gene.* New York: John Wiley & Sons, Inc., 1995.

Feldman, Gayle. *You Don't Have to Be Your Mother.* New York: W. W. Norton & Company, 1994.

Hayes, Dr. Daniel, editor. *Atlas of Breast Cancer.* United Kingdom: Mosby Europe Limited, 1993.

Kaye, Ronnie. *Spinning Straw into Gold.* New York: Simon and Schuster, 1991.

Love, Dr. Susan, with Karen Lindsey. *Dr. Susan Love's Breast Book.* Reading, Mass: Addison-Wesley, 1990.

Nuland, Dr. Sherwin. *How We Die.* New York: Alfred A. Knopf, Inc., 1993.

Siegel, Dr. Bernard S. *Love, Medicine & Miracles.* New York: Harper & Row, 1986.

Sontag, Susan. *Illness as Metaphor.* New York: Farrar, Straus and Giroux, 1978.

Spiegel, Dr. David *Living Beyond Limits.* New York: Times Books, 1993.

Wadler, Joyce. *My Breast.* Reading, Mass: Addison-Wesley, 1992.

Wolf, Naomi. *The Beauty Myth.* New York: Doubleday, 1991.

INDEX